Anesthesia in Emergency Medicine

Anesthesia in Emergency Medicine

Anesthesia in Emergency Medicine

Edited by
Glenn S. Vanstrum, M.D.
*Clinical Instructor in Anesthesiology, University of
California, San Diego, School of Medicine; Staff
Anesthesiologist, Sharp Memorial Hospital, San Diego*

Foreword by
Peter Safar, M.D.
*F. S. Cheever Distinguished Service Professor of
Resuscitation Medicine and Anesthesiology, and Director
of the International Resuscitation Research Center,
University of Pittsburgh, Pittsburgh*

Little, Brown and Company
Boston/Toronto/London

Contents

Contributing Authors

Kris Bjornson, M.D.
Staff Anesthesiologist, Sharp Memorial Hospital, San Diego

H. Shannon Carson III, M.D.
Associate Clinical Professor of Anesthesiology, University of California, San Diego, School of Medicine; Senior Staff, Department of Anesthesiology, Children's Hospital and Health Center, San Diego

Thomas G. Karagianes, M.D.
Assistant Clinical Professor, Departments of Anesthesiology and Surgery, University of California, San Diego, School of Medicine; Associate Director, Surgical Intensive Care Units, University of California, San Diego Medical Center, San Diego

Marie Csete Prager, M.D.
Assistant Professor of Anesthesiology, University of California, San Francisco, School of Medicine; Attending Physician, Department of Anesthesiology, Moffitt-Long Hospital, San Francisco

Christopher A. Mills, M.D.
Staff Anesthesiologist, Sharp Memorial Hospital, San Diego

Benjamin Shwachman, M.D., J.D.
Chief, Department of Anesthesiology, Intercommunity Hospital Medical Center, Covina, California

Alan R. Snyder, M.D.
Clinical Associate, Department of Anesthesiology, Maricopa Medical Center, University of Arizona, Phoenix; Staff Anesthesiologist, Good Samaritan Regional Medical Center, Phoenix

Richard J. Unger, M.D.
Assistant Clinical Professor of Anesthesiology, University of California, San Diego, School of Medicine, San Diego

Glenn S. Vanstrum, M.D.
Clinical Instructor in Anesthesiology, University of California, San Diego, School of Medicine; Staff Anesthesiologist, Sharp Memorial Hospital, San Diego

Foreword

Advances in medicine depend on both the focused knowledge of specialists and the integrating concepts of generalists. In Glenn Vanstrum's book, *Anesthesia in Emergency Medicine,* he has successfully integrated the actual and potential contributions of specialists and generalists of two medical disciplines—from airway control to disaster medicine. This is a laudable accomplishment.

Physicians and nurses whose principal territory of operation is the operating room, and those who are based in the emergency department, have much to learn from each other for their daily practices. Anesthesiologists have much more to offer than teaching tracheal intubation, and emergency physicians have much more to offer than prehospital resuscitation. Inseparable from these two specialties is a third one—the multidisciplinary subspecialty (or regeneralized "superspecialty") of Critical (Intensive) Care Medicine (CCM). A fourth related field is "traumatology," that is, severe polytrauma-focused practice and research by interested anesthesiologists, surgeons, emergency physicians, intensivists, and others. Traumatology, of course, must be more than emergency orthopedics. Trauma surgery combined with CCM has recently received a subspecialty board status within the American Board of Surgery. Advanced trauma care needs a team leader, usually a general surgeon committed to traumatology. Modern care for victims of severe trauma, however, requires more than surgical expertise in the operating room. It should be managed with a team to include emergency physicians (particularly to stabilize the trauma victim in nontrauma centers), anesthesiologists, general surgeons, and intensivists. The team also includes nonphysician helpers. The unmet needs of the patient of major polytrauma and civilian emergency care are considerable.

Integrating the knowledge, skills, experience, and judgment of various disciplines and applying them in concerted efforts toward common goals become particularly important in acute situations. Collaboration between anesthesiology and emergency medicine benefits the emergency patient who has severe pain, and the critically ill or injured patient in need of resuscitation and life support.

In the United States, many patients seen by physicians in hospitals' emergency departments have non-life-threatening conditions. Once these conditions are recognized, care is usually passed on to specialists. Anesthesiologists have little role in this process. Other patients need relief of pain. Although acute pain control is a very important aspect of emergency medicine, the anesthesiologist may best contribute as teacher and adviser. He or she should guide, not resist, safe analgesia administered by nonanesthesia personnel. Major advances in acute pain management have recently been made and may well prove applicable in the emergency room setting. A smaller proportion of patients (about 5 percent of emergency room admissions in the United States and up to 20 percent abroad) require resuscitation and life support for the reversal of acute life-threatening medical and surgical emergencies, with or without the need for resuscitative anesthesia and surgery. The care of these patients presents the principal challenge for interdisciplinary collaboration.

Until World War II, much anesthesia and emergency care worldwide was practiced by physicians unskilled in these fields. Since the 1940s, in the United States, anesthesiology [1], resuscitation medicine [2], critical care medicine [3–6], emergency medical services (EMS) [7], emergency medicine [8], and disaster medicine [9–11] have evolved in this chronologic sequence. All were developed in response to recognized needs and perceived opportunities. They form the "emergency and critical care medicine (ECCM) continuum" [12] that has as a common scientific base, "reanimatology" [13, 14]—the science of resuscitation and life support. Cardiopulmonary-cerebral resuscitation (CPCR), the sequence of basic, advanced, and prolonged life support (BLS, ALS, PLS), has been developed since the 1950s through the collaboration of members of various base disciplines. The goal of CPCR is to reverse terminal states and clinical death to survival with human mentation. This requires more than "blowing and pushing." CPCR has its historic roots in a peculiar mix of observations and contributions by laboratory researchers, field researchers, technologists, and medical practitioners [15]. CPCR determines the quality of the EMS life support chain, which is only as effective as its weakest link. These links, from the scene, via transportation and the emergency department, to the operating room and ICU, are tied together by planning, education, organization, communication, and continuing evaluation. The latter is necessary to identify weaknesses in the chain. The multiple providers in each link of the life-saving chain should be integrated into an ECCM system [16].

Anesthesiology became a medical specialty in the 1930s in the United States and Britain, and in the 1950s in other countries. Critical care medicine was initiated in the 1960s [3–6] and since then has achieved multidisciplinary subspecialty status in the United States and abroad. Emergency medicine, however, is a rather recent phenomenon, peculiar to the United States: Before the 1960s (and still in other countries) emergency room needs were largely met by general practitioners and primary physicians of medicine, pediatrics, and surgery when life support was not required; and by anesthesiologists alone or participating in teams with other specialists when the patient needed resuscitation and life support.

Anesthesiology and emergency medicine have much in common. Both are concerned with the episodic management of acute problems. Both are hospital based. Both anesthesiologists and emergency physicians are "unsung heroes." Both must be skilled in "titrated" patient care, or moment-to-moment adjustment of physical and pharmacologic treatments according to changes in monitored variables. This titrated care, which is so important for patients with acutely life-threatening illness or injury, differs greatly from the care by "rounding" (or office visit) and prescription that is the pattern of general medical practice for chronic and subacute conditions.

Anesthesiology practice, being a mix of pain relief and multiple organ systems life support, calls for titrated care in almost every case in the operating room. The operating room setting is ideal for learning titrated life support. Thus, anesthesiologists in the 1950s pioneered the development of intensive care units (ICUs) and copioneered the development of CPCR. Unfortunately, most anesthesiologists have withdrawn from these settings, but some are reconsidering this [17]. Experienced anesthesiologists, who have become sophisticated life supporters for the most critically ill patients in the operating room, have much to offer outside the operating room. Their expertise should be applied to the care of patients in the emergency department and even the prehospital arena.

Intensive care practice by definition should be concerned only with patients in need of intensive monitoring or life support. While at the beginning of CCM most intensivists came from anesthesiology, most now come from internal medicine (or pediatrics) or one of its subspecialties. Many intensivists have become isolated in ICUs, and thereby have lost skills in emergency resuscitation. Intensivists, irrespective of their base specialty, should be trained in titrated life support in the operating room setting, through a sufficiently long, well-organized rotation supervised by anesthesiologists. They should also gain experience in the emergency department and in the prehospital setting.

The initiators of the Society of Critical Care Medicine (SCCM) [4–6] envisioned a multidisciplinary subspecialty of ECCM, consisting of internists, pediatricians, anesthesiologists, and surgeons who have specialty interest and expertise in life support. In teams, they would be responsible for the quality of care of critical cases throughout the EMS system [7]. In the early 1970s, they attempted to create a Federation between the SCCM and the then newly founded American College of Emergency Physicians (ACEP). The Federation concept failed, but friendly collaboration continues. Historically, anesthesiologists provoked pulmonologists, and cardiothoracic surgeons provoked cardiologists, into becoming reanimatologists. The most challenging CCM patients are those with multiple organ failure. Recovery of the central nervous system is the overriding goal. It is inappropriate to consider a medical subspecialist without additional ECCM (reanimatology) experience an "intensivist." With added experience, knowledge, commitment, competence, and availability, any medical or surgical specialist may become an intensivist. The fragmentation of critical care medicine into subspecialty boards controlled by different base specialties is unfortunate. A common ECCM (reanimatology) board for physicians of various base specialties, as suggested by the founding members of SCCM, might have avoided the present fragmentation.

Emergency medicine practice involves primarily noncritical cases. Although only a minority of the patients seen first by emergency physicians are in need of short-term titrated resuscitative care, the importance of that care is great. After emergency resuscitation, the emergency physician usually must turn long-term life support over to intensivists or trauma surgeons.

In the 1960s, most of the initiators of emergency medicine and the ACEP were formerly general practitioners who responded to apparent societal needs and practice opportunities. Patients with urgent problems did not find 24-hour coverage by primary physicians and flooded community hospitals' emergency rooms, where adequate physician coverage was not provided by general medicine and surgery. The emergency medicine initiators, through their wisdom and leadership over the past 20 years, developed emergency medicine into a recognized base discipline, with attractive residency programs, a specialty board, and increasing academic recognition. This new base specialty is also becoming established in university medical centers of the United States. Therefore, in the future, emergency physicians will increasingly come from emergency medicine residencies. These provide some experience in operating room anesthesia, as well as intensive care. Some programs also provide education in reanimatology for appropriately guided experiences in laboratory and pathophysiologic patient research. Emergency medicine specialists must also be allowed to train and to become certified in CCM, just as anesthesiologists, internists, pediatricians, and surgeons.

Despite the unfortunate fragmentation of medicine into technology-focused subspecialties, and of ECCM into economy-based territories, I look toward the future with optimism. Anesthesiologists, emergency physicians, intensivists, and trauma surgeons should learn via some practical guided experience in each others' territories. By learning together they would be better motivated to implement future breakthroughs in reanimatology.

The clinical interaction of team members from various specialties depends much on personalities. When collaboration between surgeons and anesthesiologists in the operating room is smooth, it can be a model for any multidisciplinary collaboration outside the operating room as well. The resuscitation environment requires either a strong predetermined team leader or automatic synchronization of team efforts for the benefit of the patient. The latter requires team members who are used to working with each other. An analogy for the automatic synchronization of efforts is the chamber music group composed of friends, the ideal team, which serves the "opus" (the patient) without the need of a conductor. This is difficult in teaching hospitals with rotating house staff, but more likely to occur in community hospitals with stable staff.

The negative effects of fragmentation of the ECCM system have become obvious to those who have tried to evaluate the course of critically ill or injured patients from the accident scene to discharge from the ICU. Examples of functional integration of care through all links of the lifesaving chain are the ECCM Systems of Hannover, West Germany (only for trauma), and of Brugge, Belgium (for all critical emergencies). Surgeons and anesthesiologists in the former and anesthesiologists-intensivists in the latter coordinate life support from the scene through the ICU, and draw in other specialists as needed. In the United States, the formation of the National Association for Emergency Medical Services Physicians (NAEMSP) is a step in the right direction. The NAEMSP will succeed if it opens its doors to interested physicians of any base discipline.

Medical leadership of community-wide EMS systems—including treatment at the scene and during transportation—is essential. This requires, however, more than just an M.D. degree. Medical care on the streets by physicians is an art that is learned only by first-hand experience [18]. The base specialties of these future (prehospital) EMS leaders are less important than their competence, leadership ability, interest, and availability. Their competence must include clinical skills in resuscitation medicine. Leadership, prioritizing, and quality control of EMS systems should be delegated not to administrators, but to people with first hand experience in resuscitating patients. Most EMS physician leaders will be based in the emergency departments of major trauma hospitals. These leaders must defend the principle that the performance of advanced and prolonged life support is integral to the practice of medicine, which, even if carried out by paramedics, must be under the predirected or moment-to-moment, radio-controlled guidance of experienced ECCM physicians. Also, the future introduction of novel resuscitation methods into the prehospital arena, and the conduct of prehospital research, will require reanimatologists (physician specialists) to work personally as members or leaders of ambulance (mobile ICU) teams, to deliver and study these new treatments outside the hospital. The Center for Emergency Medicine of Pittsburgh (Western Pennsylvania) is an example of such an effort.

For the future, it is less important to ponder why the fragmentation of acute medicine has occurred, and more important to decide whether it is bad, and if so, what to do about it. There is a need for regeneralizing of medicine (including surgery) and of resuscitation medicine in particular—for integrating the many needed specialties into more concerted efforts. No one can be a specialist in all the fields from which a patient with multiple organ failure can benefit. We should counteract the present fragmentation of the ECCM system through intellectual and functional links between ECCM-oriented specialists of various disciplines. Anesthesiology, emergency medicine, multidisciplinary CCM, and traumatology all belong to general surgery and medicine, from which they have emerged. Meeting identified patient needs and responding to new lifesaving opportunities must have priority over territorial disputes.

Research relevant for ECCM (reanimatology) has traditionally been without specialty boundaries. Both focused and integrating research programs are needed. Research in ECCM should be carried out at multiple levels:

molecule, cell, organ, organism, and community. Reanimatology can become a force to help integrate the fragmented disciplines of acute medicine into the ECCM system that the founders envisioned 30 years ago [3–6].

Finally, anesthesiology and emergency medicine can jointly help to develop disaster medicine, one of the special interests of Dr. Vanstrum. "Disaster reanimatology" [9–11], a new field of inquiry, concerns itself with individual victims of mass disasters, such as major earthquakes or conventional wars, who might be saved by immediate initiation of the lifesaving chain. Life-supporting first aid can be started by bystanders within minutes and should be continued by advanced life-support emergency medical teams. So far, disaster medicine has been advanced by public health experts who have focused on prevention and on supporting uninjured survivors; by epidemiologists who learn from past events; and by administrators who focus on planning and preparation of resources. A clinical resuscitation- and traumatology-oriented approach to disaster medicine is badly needed. Programs of National Red Cross Societies are in need of medical leadership. In 1981 we brought leaders of military medicine, disaster medicine, and peace medicine (International Physicians for the Prevention of Nuclear War) into dialogue [9] to carry out rational planning for mass disasters. A few anesthesiologists have become interested in trauma care and disaster medicine, even in peace time [9–11, 17]. Anesthesiologists and emergency physicians can work jointly, better than separately, toward adding resuscitation components to National Disaster Medical Systems worldwide. To determine specifics will require research into the early life-saving potentials in mass disasters, and the logistics that would be required to meet such challenges [11]. Disaster reanimatology would improve everyday EMS by enforcing universal training of the public in life-supporting first aid, ways to bring advanced life-support teams rapidly to the scene, and regionalization of major trauma hospitals.

Medicine in general and anesthesiology and ECCM in particular are creations of humanism. Their common goal is to help an increasing proportion of human beings live full lives with healthy minds in healthy bodies. At present, probably one-fourth of all deaths worldwide occur before old age, from potentially reversible emergency conditions, without an incurable lethal illness or injury and without severe irreversible brain damage. Man's potential biologic life span is more than 100 years. The promise of reanimatology is the gift of added meaningful years. The implementation of reanimatology needs scientists and physicians of many disciplines. Those who are logical promoters of ECCM, because of their special expertise, interest, and availability, should jointly pursue this common goal.

Peter Safar, M.D.

References

1. Dripps, R. D., Eckenhoff, J. E., and Vandam, L. R. *Introduction to Anesthesia.* Philadelphia: Saunders, 1988.
2. Safar, P., and Bircher, N. G. Cardiopulmonary Cerebral Resuscitation. An Introduction to Resuscitation Medicine. World Federation of Societies of Anaesthesiologists (3rd ed.). London: Saunders, 1988.
3. Safar, P. The Anesthesiologist as "Intensivist." In J. E. Eckenhoff (ed.). *Science and Practice in Anesthesia.* Philadelphia: Lippincott, 1965.
4. Weil, M. H. The society of critical care medicine, its history and its destiny. *Crit. Care Med.* 1:1, 1973.
5. Safar, P. Critical care medicine—quo vadis? *Crit. Care Med.* 2:1, 1974.
6. Shoemaker, W. C. Interdisciplinary medicine: Accommodation or integration? *Crit. Care Med.* 3:1, 1975.
7. American Society of Anesthesiologists, Committee on Acute Medicine (Safar, P., Chairman). Community-wide emergency medical services. *J.A.M.A.* 204:595, 1968.
8. Schwartz, G., Safar, P., Stone, J., et al. (eds.). *Principles and Practice of Emergency Medicine.* Philadelphia: Saunders, 1986.
9. Safar, P. (ed.) Disaster Resuscitology. Proceedings of the Second World Congress on Emergency and Disaster Medicine (Club of Mainz), Pittsburgh, 1981. *Prehospital. Disaster Med.* 1:1, 1985; 1(Suppl I), 1985.
10. Baskett, P., and Wellder, R. (eds.). *Medicine for Disasters.* London: Butterworth, 1988.
11. Safar, P., Klain, M., Ricci, E., et al. Disaster reanimatology for National Disaster Medical Systems (NDMS) planning and response. Interview studies of earthquakes. *Pre-hosp. Disaster Med.* August 1989.
12. Safar, P. The Critical Care Medicine Continuum from Scene to Outcome. In J. E. Parrillo and S. M. Ayres (eds.). *Major Issues in Critical Care Medicine.* Baltimore: Williams & Wilkins, 1984.
13. Negovsky, V. A. *Essays on Reanimatology.* Moscow: Mir Publishers, 1986.
14. Safar, P. Reanimatology—the science of resuscitation. *Crit. Care Med.* 10:134, 1982.
15. Safar, P. History of Cardiopulmonary-cerebral Resuscitation. In W. Kaye and N. Bircher (eds.). *Cardiopulmonary Resuscitation.* New York: Churchill Livingstone, 1989 (in press).
16. Safar, P., Grenvik, A., Abramson, N. S., and Bircher, N. (eds.). Reversibility of clinical death: Symposium on resuscitation research. *Crit. Care Med.* 16:919, 1988.
17. Grande, C. M., Stene, J. K., and Barton, C. R. The trauma anesthesiologist. *Maryland Med. J.* 37:531, 1988.
18. Caroline, N. L. Medical care in the streets. *J.A.M.A.* 237:43, 1977.

Preface

This book has evolved to its present form after much helpful criticism from a wide range of practitioners of both emergency medicine and anesthesiology. It has developed into an interface between two exciting and closely related specialties that combines these two bodies of knowledge. One plus one synergistically makes three. As we initially explored this interface, the common ground shared by the two disciplines became more and more apparent, from preoperative preparation, to airway management, to the striking similarities of their political problems. Each specialty has developed a different and valuable perspective on these common points of issue, and it is our challenge to unveil these perspectives for the benefit of the clinician.

There is much for anesthesiologists to learn from emergency physicians, and the need for knowledge transfer in the opposite direction is just as apparent. For example, trauma patients may present to the operating room volume replenished, but with hypothermic solutions. Patients with elevated intracranial pressure may be intubated in the emergency department without pharmacologic attempt to ameliorate the resulting pressure increase. Muscle relaxants may or may not be optimally utilized. On the other hand, many anesthesiologists are unfamiliar with important advances in the pharmacology and treatment of cardiac arrest. Others may benefit from emergency physicians' expertise in many aspects of trauma management. Finally, there are areas in which the specialties need to combine forces, as in the use of inhalational agents for status asthmaticus and status epilepticus, or in disaster planning and management.

Our goal in exploring the interdigitation between these two specialties is to create a clinically oriented, highly readable volume to aid the emergency medicine practitioner and the anesthesiologist. Although our target audience are the physician bodies of these specialties, there is much of value herein for trauma surgeons, critical care physicians, advanced nursing and paramedic personnel, and medical personnel-in-training. A vigorous attempt has been made to provide current and classic references and complete tables when appropriate. Each chapter will no doubt contain some information which is review material for one or the other specialist. We have endeavored, however, to supplement and keep fresh such material with discussion of current controversies and interesting clinical examples. Each chapter will also contain information that might at first seem extraneous to a rigid specialty definition. We have adopted the philosophy that the clinical problem takes precedence over specialty considerations, and that knowledge of what has been done to a patient in the past or will happen in the future is always invaluable. Thus, even if an emergency physician will not place the pulmonary artery catheter, he or she should be familiar with its use and indications. Even if an anesthesiologist does not work in a trauma center, he or she can still benefit from familiarity with the use of autotransfusion techniques. We have, however, limited the material covered to information that should be of practical value and interest to both emergency physicians and anesthesiologists. In the interest of keeping the volume readable, we have endeavored to examine specific areas in detail, rather than presenting the kind of encyclopedic overview that is already available in excellent standard specialty textbooks such as Rosen's *Emergency Medicine* [1] or Miller's *Anesthesia* [2].

The reader will concede, we hope, that medicine today is practiced in a wide range of settings, from urban to rural, and from teaching center–based to private practice. Certain treatment options viable for a busy inner city teaching hospital with full specialist back-up are not realistic in a rural emergency department with a two-hour transport time to a major center. A rural practitioner, however, must be cognizant of such options in order to aid in transport decision making. Performance of certain surgical procedures by nonsurgeons might seem heroic and out of place in an academic, urban emergency department that has residents of all specialties in-house, but such procedures are sometimes justified in a remote setting. For this reason we have included brief descriptions of anesthetic and surgical management of several life-threatening situations, such as emergent cesarian section during the cardiac arrest setting, or emergency thoracotomy for penetrating trauma.

While this book could conceivably offend those who engage in "turf warfare," we hope the reader will understand that we find it important for both specialties to recognize the potential succor one's colleague in a related specialty might render. Most "turf" arguments stem from a fear of erosion of a given specialty's sphere of influence and loss of resulting monetary reward and job security. While both specialties are hospital based and do face an uncertain future, they have much to gain by combining forces. Our goal is to help forge a bond between these two sophisticated and intelligent groups of physicians, not to promote one specialty over the other.

The final chapter, on disaster management, was written not only to educate, but to stimulate. No man is an island, and no specialty or pair of related specialties is separated from the rest of the world. Thus, in this chapter we have endeavored to examine the anesthesiology-emergency medicine interface and the macroenvironment. We feel no current work on modern medicine is complete without discussing this area, however briefly, and we trust the reader will find the change of direction provided by this section to be of value.

As a concluding note, we have consistently favored the flexible over the algorithm approach to clinical problems. Any situation often has several treatment options, each with risks and benefits. One must always steer one's course between the Scylla and Charybdis of over- and undertreatment, and rigid adherence to formula can lead to a clinical shipwreck. While some would argue with this, we feel there has been sufficient emphasis on recent algorithm-based physician protocols (i.e., ACLS and ATLS). This work attempts to provide a contrasting, nondogmatic philosophy as a balance to this trend.

We have had many pleasurable and enlightening hours researching and writing this book, and we hope and trust the reader will find the reading equally as enjoyable. We encourage any comments, criticisms, or suggestions from interested readers. These will be utilized in future editions, and may be directed to the following address: *Anesthesia in Emergency Medicine,* Glenn S. Vanstrum, M.D. (Editor), Anesthesia Service Medical Group, P.O. Box 82807, San Diego, CA 92138-9004.

G.S.V.

REFERENCES

1. Rosen, P. (ed.). *Emergency Medicine* (2nd ed.). St. Louis: Mosby, 1988.
2. Miller, R. D. (ed.). *Anesthesia* (2nd ed.). New York: Churchill Livingstone, 1986.

Acknowledgments

We would like to extend special thanks to the staff of the Sharp Memorial Hospital Library and to the office staff of the Anesthesia Service Medical Group, San Diego. Their help and encouragement in producing this volume was invaluable.

A special note of thanks also needs to be extended to the spouses, significant others, and dear ones who supported the contributors to this volume.

Finally, we would like to dedicate this book to those who still take the time to turn off the television, open up a book, and read and think about things. This book, then, is dedicated to you, the reader.

NOTICE

Medicine is an art as well as a science, and it is ever-changing. Ongoing research and clinical experience constantly alter drug therapy and treatment. The editor, contributors, and publisher of this work have made every effort to ensure that the drug dosage schedules herein are accurate and in accordance with accepted standards and practices of the medical community at the time of publication. The medications described do not necessarily have specific approval by the Food and Drug Administration for use in the diseases and dosages for which they are recommended. Readers are advised, however, to check the package insert of each drug they plan to administer to be certain that changes have not been made in the recommended dose or in the contraindications for administration. This recommendation is particularly important in regard to new or infrequently used drugs.

Anesthesia in Emergency Medicine

1. Introduction

Glenn S. Vanstrum

In exploring the intersection of the two specialties of anesthesiology and emergency medicine, certain similarities and dissimilarities stand out. Both specialties utilize invasive procedures and require a commitment of care for the seriously ill. Both specialties require knowledge and experience in dealing with cardiopulmonary arrest, trauma care, and disaster management. Physicians in each specialty have intermittent patient contact, although this is less true for anesthesiologists. In terms of hospital politics and power, this lack of primary care contact puts both specialties at a disadvantage. Finally, the specialties are alike in that physicians in both were once solely hospital based but are now starting to become independent, owing to outpatient ambulatory centers and outpatient surgery centers.

What are the dissimilarities? The obvious one is the location of practice, with the emergency physician spending time in the emergency department (ED) and the anesthesiologist in the operating suite (OR). Less obvious is the fact that, with the exception of obstetric anesthetic practice, anesthesiology puts the physician in a one-on-one relationship with a single patient. This is not the case for a busy emergency physician, who must often deal with five to ten serious problems simultaneously. This puts incredible stress on the shoulders of these clinicians. Unfortunately, emergency physicians are held by our legal system to a standard of one-on-one care. Thus, one cannot offer that the ED was extremely busy at the time as a legally valid excuse for some egregious error.

A further burden placed on the emergency physician is that he or she is responsible, in a sense, for delivering a specialist's level of care in a multiplicity of areas, even if only for that first hour in the ED. Gone are the days of the dermatologist moonlighting in the "accident room." Since the advent of emergency medicine as a specialty, an ongoing philosophic problem has been the definition of limits on the body of knowledge prerequisite for an ED specialist. Aspects of surgery, internal medicine, obstetrics, anesthesiology, psychiatry, and pediatrics are incorporated into the field, and judging from this author's personal experience in emergency medicine board examinations, these subjects are covered in depth. Emergency medicine is a generalist specialty, although the temporal problems of emergent patients limit the body of knowledge to prehospital care and somewhere around the first hour of in-hospital care. Nevertheless, performance of care during that time period is now held to a specialist level.

Anesthesiology is not without its stresses, even given the predominant one-on-one care pattern. These physicians are often required to take a patient who is awake and very much alive to a deep anesthetic plane not so far from death, where surgeons perform a variety of physiologic insults and body cavity violations. Things can and do go awry, and, given that most operations are indeed performed on patients with something very wrong to start with, unplanned results do occur. When disasters happen, although rare, they often involve major disability, such as paralysis, or death. The ever present element of causation involved in these unexpected results adds a great amount of stress to the anesthesiologist's existence.

What exactly is anesthesia? This state may be defined as the combination of the following five conditions: analgesia or insensibility to pain; amnesia or the inability to remember; hypnosis or the loss of consciousness; physiologic homeostasis or the preservation of intact cardiopulmonary, renal, hepatic, cerebral, and other organ system function; and, finally, muscle relaxation or the provision of optimal surgical conditions. Anesthesiology is the science and art of the provision of anesthesia through varying combinations of these five ingredients. Although it is usually considered in reference to surgical and obstetric operations or diagnostic procedures of one sort or another, the involvement of anesthesiology in such areas as pain management shows that this is not always the case.

That there are many aspects of anesthesia intimately involved in the practice of emergency medicine will become obvious as one reads this volume. Because the emergency physician is held to a standard of practice at or near the specialist level, the importance of the anesthesiologist's perspective on the practice of emergency medicine should also be clear. But just as important, although perhaps less obvious, is the generalist nature of anesthesia— the fact that anesthesia is required for all types and ages of patients and for surgery on nearly all organ systems and the importance of the perspective of the emergency physician to the anesthesiologist. Thus, as for emergency medicine, it is difficult and perhaps improper to draw strict boundaries limiting the body of knowledge that defines the specialty of anesthesiology.

Although there are dissimilarities between the specialties, underlying the major differences is a common undercurrent that develops from delivering care to extremely ill patients in today's stressful socioeconomic and medical-legal climate. To get a better feel for some of these similarities and differences, we conducted a research poll among two equal groups of anesthesiologists and emergency physicians. Four hundred physicians were selected at random from nationwide specialty listings provided by the American Society of Anesthesiologists and the American College of Emergency Physicians. Seventy-five of two hundred ED physicians responded, for a return of 38 percent, and 70 of 200 anesthesiologists responded, for a return of 35 percent.

The demographic results of this poll are presented in Figures 1-1 through 1-5. The majority of these physicians work in hospitals that have 101 to 300 beds and are nonteaching hospitals, i.e., do not have house staff. Sixty-nine percent of the anesthesiologists who responded worked in urban centers, compared to 43 percent of emergency physicians, and 60 percent of the anesthesiologists work in cardiac surgical centers, compared to 28 percent of ED physicians. This preponderance of anesthesiologists in high level care facilities is also reflected by the greater number who work in designated trauma centers. Such a difference may reflect the use of nurse anesthetists in primary and secondary care hospitals, or it may simply reflect the fact

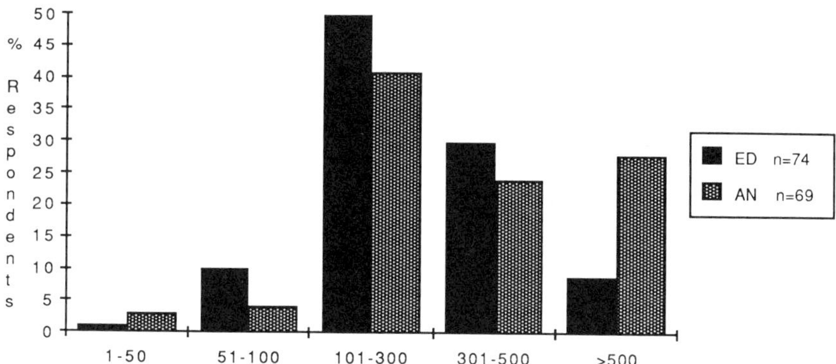

Fig. 1-1. Number of beds in hospital.

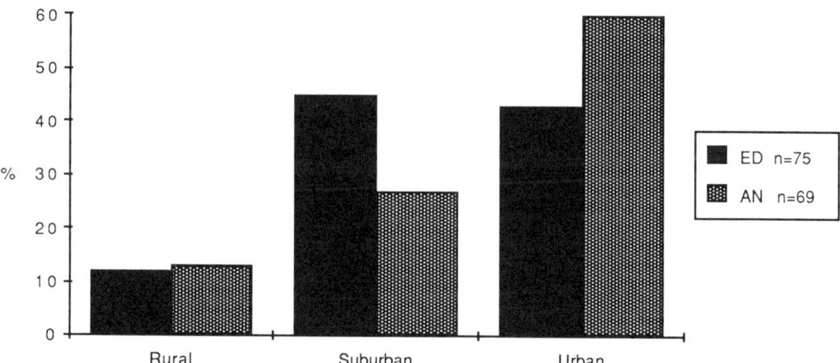

Fig. 1-2. Location of hospital.

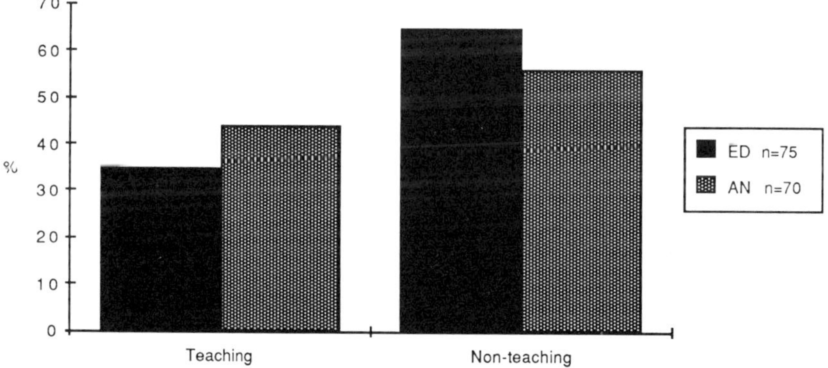

Fig. 1-3. Academic affiliation of hospital.

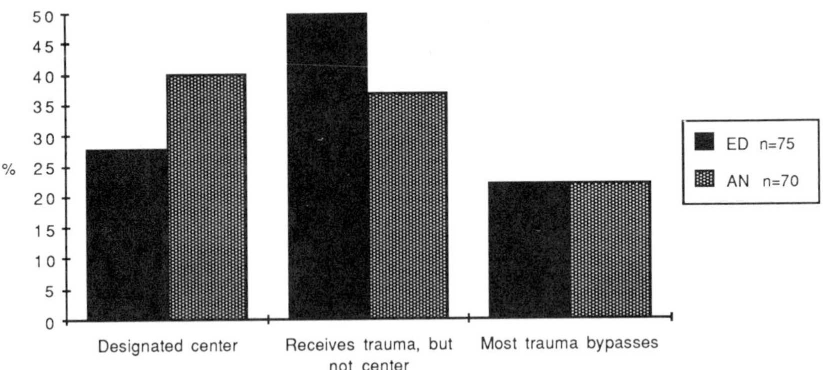

Fig. 1-4. Status of trauma center.

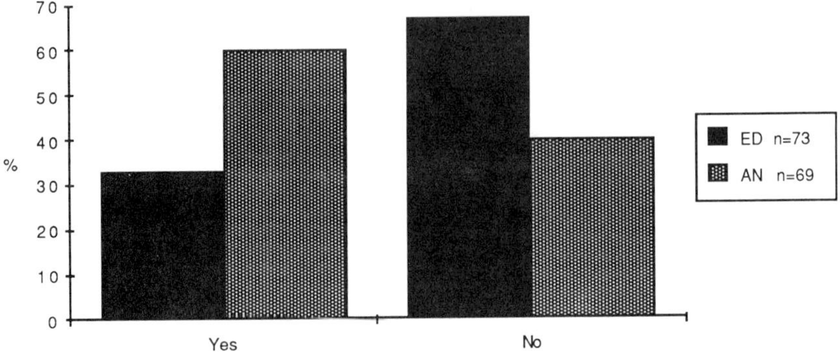

Fig. 1-5. Cardiac surgery performed at hospital.

that more surgery, and hence, more need for anesthesiologists, takes place in tertiary and quaternary care centers.

Such a finding reflects the importance of a good understanding of preoperative care in emergency physicians because many provide such care for patients who are transported to larger or more specialized facilities. Fifty-nine of the seventy-five ED physicians work in hospitals that do transport patients to higher levels of care, as opposed to 38 of the 70 anesthesiologists. Interestingly, the helicopter is used for this purpose by 37 percent of the emergency physicians and 34 percent of the anesthesiologists who transport patients (see Fig. 1-8).

The issue of response to cardiac arrest, or "Code Blue," was considered in this questionnaire (Figs. 1-6, 1-7). As a necessary part of defining the young specialty of emergency medicine, it has become accepted, not unreasonably, among the mostly academic emergency medicine hierarchy that it is improper for the emergency physician to abandon his or her patients in the ED to "run upstairs" to handle a cardiac arrest. Unfortunately, unless

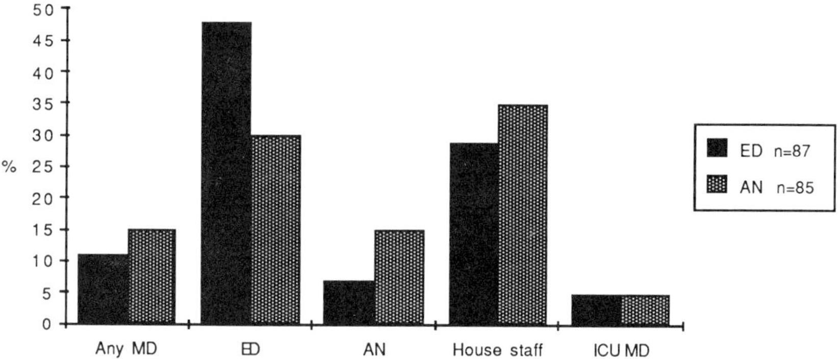

Fig. 1-6. Designated Code Blue responder.

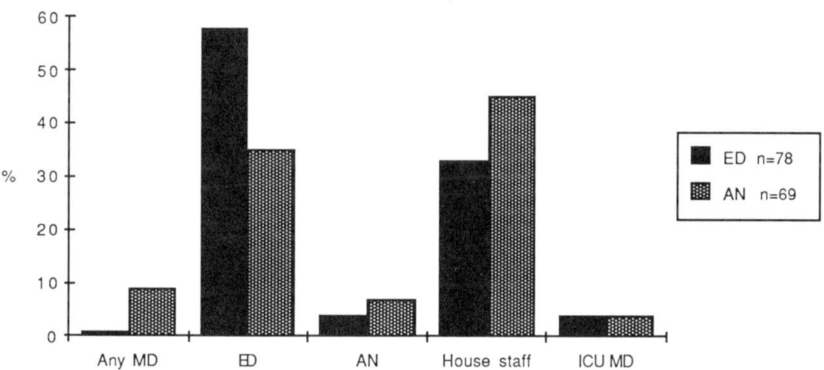

Fig. 1-7. Actual Code Blue responder.

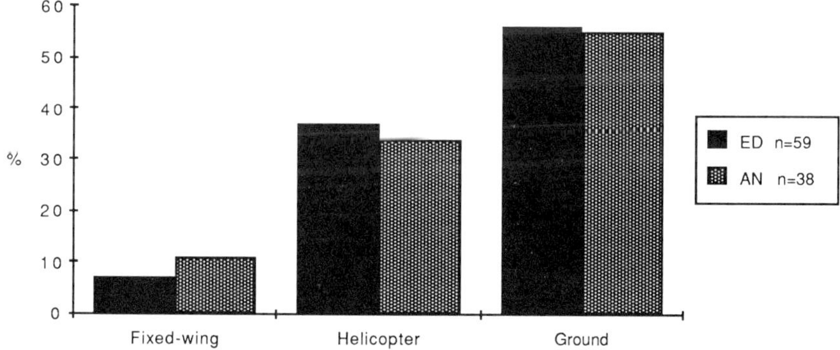

Fig. 1-8. Transport mode to larger center.

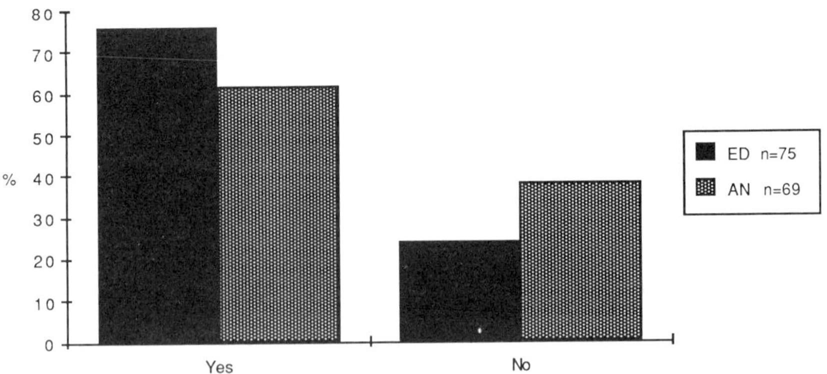

Fig. 1-9. Physicians involved in disaster medicine.

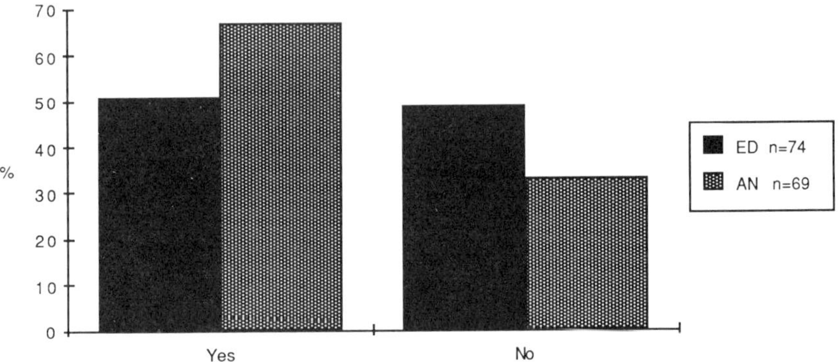

Fig. 1-10. Pain unit or referral source available.

house staff or an intensive care unit (ICU) physician is available, it seems clear from this poll that a majority of ED physicians (58 percent) still must respond to in-house arrest situations. Whether this does endanger the patient population in the ED remains to be demonstrated. Until major changes are made in many hospitals, however, it is clear that ED physicians do have to manage many cardiac arrests on the ward or in the ICU. Thus there is some rationale for these physicians to have an understanding of some of the peculiarities associated with in-house disasters, not the least of which are postsurgical problems.

It was heartening to see that a majority of both groups of physicians polled are involved in disaster medicine (Fig. 1-9). A significant minority remain uninvolved, however, and this may be considered by some to be cause for concern.

Nonavailability of pain units and referral resources is shown by the sizable minority in both specialties who lack either facility (Fig. 1-10). Similar room

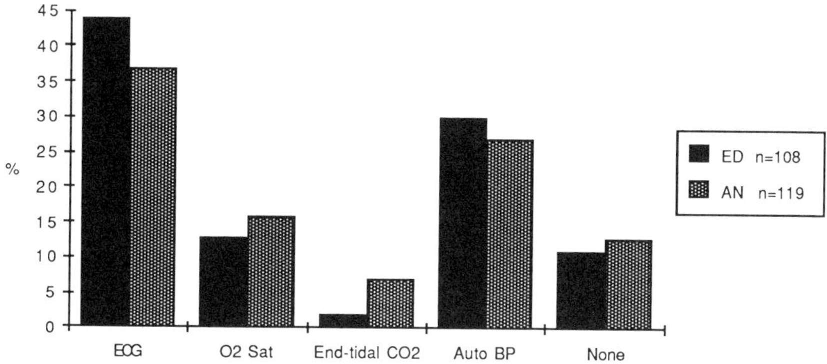

Fig. 1-11. Availability of CT monitoring. ECG = electrocardiography; O_2 sat = O_2 saturation; End-tidal CO_2 = end-tidal CO_2 measurement; Auto BP = automatic blood pressure.

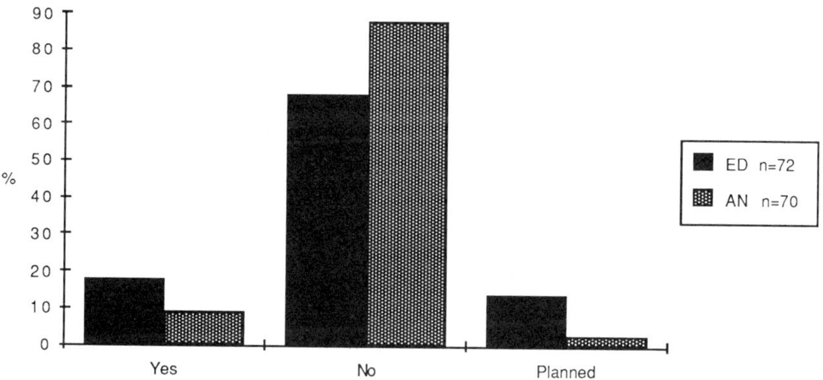

Fig. 1-12. Nitrous oxide used in emergency department.

for improvement is apparent in the response to monitoring availability of the computed tomography (CT) scan room (Fig. 1-11). If hundreds of thousands of dollars can be spent on each such device, several thousand dollars might well be spent to ensure homeostasis of critically ill patients by effective monitoring of those who require scanning.

Some 32 percent of emergency physicians polled either use or plan to use nitrous oxide in some capacity in their departments (Fig. 1-12). Hence, we have included a brief section in Chapter 5 on some of the more cogent volatile anesthetic principles.

It is interesting to note that 55 percent of the paramedics supervised by emergency physicians use endotracheal intubation for airway management. This reflects the force of the trend begun only recently to train these deliv-

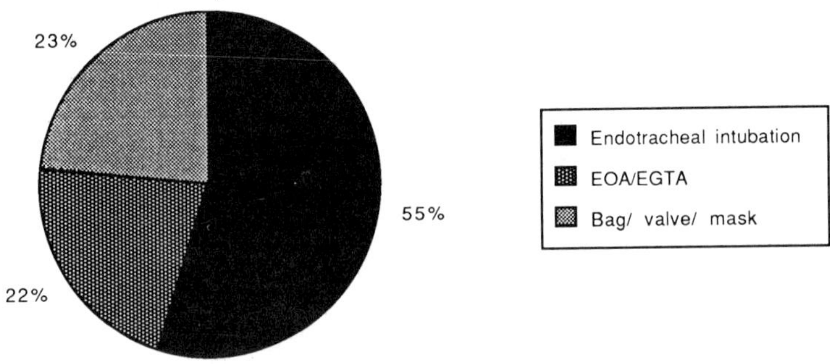

Fig. 1-13. Prehospital care of airway. EOA = esophageal obturator airway; EGTA = esophageal gastric tube airway.

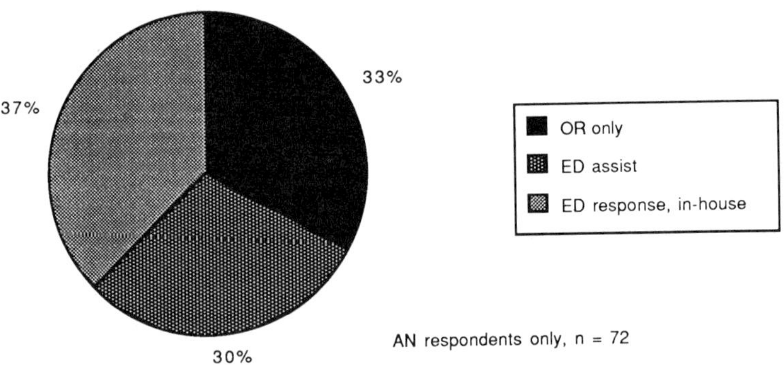

Fig. 1-14. Involvement of anesthesiologists in trauma resuscitation efforts.

erers of prehospital care in this modality (Fig. 1-13). Prehospital care is of special importance to both emergency physicians, who train and often assume responsibility for paramedic personnel, and anesthesiologists, who offer specialized airway training to prehospital personnel and ultimately receive patients in the operating suite whose condition depends on adequate field care.

Sixty-seven percent of the anesthesiologists assist in trauma resuscitation efforts in the ED, on either an on-call or in-house basis (Fig. 1-14). The close association of emergency medicine with this field reinforces the need for cross-over of information between the two fields.

We have endeavored to tailor the ensuing chapters to the audience delineated by this questionnaire. Considerable effort has been made to produce a book that will be of interest to both specialties because there is a need for both groups to learn from each other. In many countries in Europe, interestingly, the two specialties exist within a single encompassing field known as "reanimatology." This precedence should be kept in mind as we study this exciting intersection of specialties we call anesthesia in emergency medicine.

2. Airway

Glenn S. Vanstrum

Even in the best of hands, airway management can be a challenge. The interaction of the pathologic process, pharmacology, and anatomy preclude a pure "cookbook" approach to successful management. Of course, the basics of such maneuvers as jaw thrust, placement of airway adjuncts, and skillful intubation are prerequisites. Technical knowledge of procedures, however, will not prevent over- or undertreatment for a given clinical airway management situation, of which there are dozens. Treatment for respiratory arrest in a patient with terminal bronchoconstrictive disease is different from treatment for the same dire circumstance in a patient with severe coronary disease, just as a patient with unusual airway anatomy often requires a different approach than that used for a patient with airway trauma.

Because airway management requires synthesis of knowledge of pharmacology, trauma, pulmonary physiology, and cardiac function, many aspects of this topic will be considered throughout this volume. To facilitate direct consideration of this complex subject, this chapter is organized into three parts. The first part involves the forethought and examination that precede intervention. Thus, airway goals will be outlined, followed by a discussion of assessment techniques. The second part will include initial airway management and intubation. The third part is a discussion of a number of clinical scenarios.

An old adage states, "Experience is having made that mistake once before." In managing a difficult airway, experience is paid for dearly. Most major malpractice suits in anesthesiology involve hypoxia and the airway [1]. While this is not the case in emergency medicine, in which missed diagnoses take the top malpractice honors [2], all physicians should take heed that overconfidence in this aspect of medicine is a dangerous liability. Let us consider two cases in which experience was gained the hard way.

Victim of Cardiogenic Shock

A 66-year-old man is undergoing coronary catheterization. As angioplasty is attempted, he becomes increasingly restless, and his blood pressure and cardiac output fall. His breathing is labored. The cardiologist requests assistance. As a nasotracheal intubation is begun, the patient resists and develops epistaxis. Suddenly, he vomits.

Discussion. This is a situation in which a failing heart is faced with the oxygen demands of catecholamine release from a traumatic intubation. Underlying this acute stress is the increased work of breathing from pulmonary vascular congestion. Smooth use of muscle relaxants with cricoid pressure and rapid oral endotracheal intubation might, assuming skilled technique with adequate precautions, be a safer route of airway management.

Combative Trauma Patient

A 22-year-old woman with a lateral cranial hematoma and facial injury is brought to the hospital by paramedics. She was reported to have been riding as a passenger on the back seat of a motorcycle. Vital signs are blood pressure 180/90, heart rate 110, respirations 12 and ataxic. Four nurses are barely able to restrain her for a cervical spine film. Because a CT scan is needed and the patient is so combative, 10 mg IV pancuronium is injected to assist intubation. Despite multiple attempts at laryngoscopy, the larynx cannot be visualized, nor can the trachea be intubated.

Discussion. This case shows the downside of overzealous use of muscle relaxants. Although such drugs may have been warranted, many clinical questions need to be considered. Did the patient have a short jaw and squat neck, which could predispose to difficult intubation? Were adequate preparations made for intubation prior to injection of the muscle relaxant? How was the patient ventilating on her own, prior to intervention? Was pancuronium a good choice, or should a different induction technique using sodium thiopental and succinylcholine have been considered? Were cervical spine and antiregurgitation precautions implemented? Given that the drug was injected and intubation failed, now what? Should cricothyroidotomy be performed? Should the practitioner mask ventilate and call for help?

Although this patient survived, her course was complicated by a severe mediastinitis, resulting either from the traumatic intubation attempts or the ensuing cricothyroidotomy. The cardiac patient, however, deteriorated and developed ventricular fibrillation that ultimately proved refractory to all therapy including surgery. Both cases reiterate the point that airway management is not always straightforward, and the price paid for mistakes can be high.

AIRWAY MANAGEMENT: GOALS AND ASSESSMENT

GOALS IN AIRWAY MANAGEMENT

A multitude of therapeutic options are available for airway management, including oxygen delivery systems, various adjuncts and tubes, and a variety of techniques of placing those adjuncts. Before one can choose the optimal plan of attack, one must first decide on the desired goal of such treatment. We might outline such goals as follows.

PRIMUM NON NOCERE

Above all, do no harm. Five areas are especially dangerous for the unwary physician.

Protecting the cervical spine is a high priority. This means avoidance of all neck motion, especially neck flexion. The method of achieving such avoidance of motion during intubation is still controversial, and includes axial in-line traction or immobilization with gentle oral-tracheal intubation, nasotracheal intubation with immobilization, or cricothyroidotomy. A complete discussion of this topic, including the rationale for the author's preference for the first modality, is presented in Chapter 12. The topic is further discussed in the context of head trauma in Chapter 13.

Aspiration is another complication that is often avoidable and is sometimes iatrogenic. If a physician at any time gives a muscle relaxant to a patient with a full stomach, 15 to 20 mmHg digital pressure on the cricoid cartilage or Sellick's maneuver [3] must be applied until the tracheal cuff is inflated. Aspiration in this circumstance without use of this technique can only be considered iatrogenic. A *full stomach* is defined as solid food of any kind within 8 hours, or liquids within 6 hours. Some recent work has questioned whether this is not too conservative an estimate for liquids [4, 5], but the efficacy of Sellick's maneuver in preventing aspiration, whether due to passive regurgitation or active vomiting, has been well documented [3, 6]. This maneuver can withstand an esophageal pressure of at least 100 cm of water and is easily accomplished. It should be noted that this maneuver must be done correctly by the assistant, placing pressure on the cricoid and not the thyroid cartilage and maintaining a pressure no matter what difficulties the intubator is having [6]. A maternity mortality study from England noted that in 7 of 11 cases of aspiration, the assistant applied the cricoid pressure inappropriately or released it prematurely [7].

It should be obvious, then, that in a trauma patient with a probable full stomach and possible cervical spine fracture, the airway specialist must have two other individuals assisting prior to endotracheal intubation, one to provide immobilization or axial traction and the other to provide cricoid pressure (Fig. 2-1).

A common but more mundane iatrogenic problem in airway management involves dental damage [8]. About 15 percent of anesthesia malpractice claims arise from such problems [9], whether due to laryngoscopy or to the patient biting down on a hard oral airway. Although proper technique does decrease the incidence of this sort of damage, a difficult emergency intubation can result in damage if the upper incisors are not protected, either with a folded gauze pad or a commercial tooth protector. If a tooth is found to be missing, one must obtain a chest radiograph to rule out an aspirated tooth and to prevent the serious anaerobic infections associated with such an event.

One must also consider iatrogenic damage of the physiologic sort. If an isolated head injury patient, for example, is intubated in the emergency department without a pharmacologic attempt to ameliorate the resulting hyperdynamic storm, existing intracranial hemorrhage may be increased,

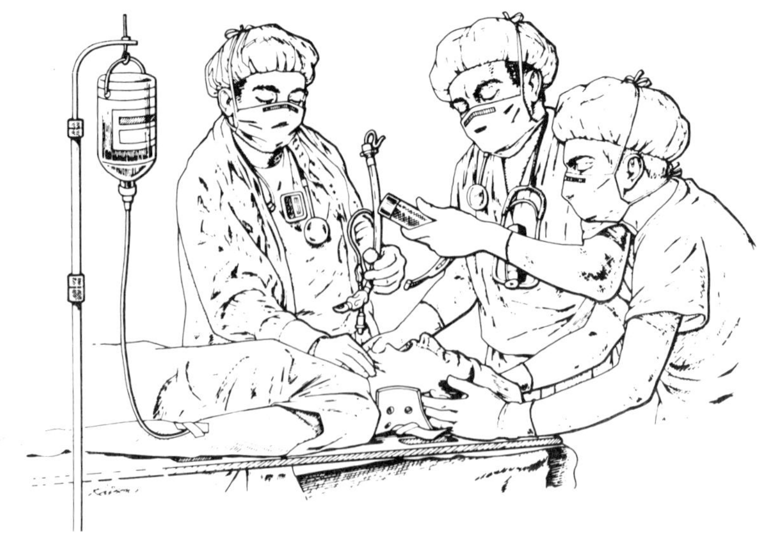

Fig. 2-1. Technique for oral intubation in a trauma patient. Patient is supine on spine board with semirigid collar in place. Drugs are given as needed (see text). Before paralyzing the patient, the anterior half of the collar is removed, and cricoid pressure is applied as another assistant holds the head in neutral position with or without in-line traction. Positive pressure ventilation is applied with bag, mask, and oxygen to ensure ability to ventilate the patient before neuromuscular paralysis. Cricoid pressure will keep gas out of the stomach. A rapid-acting IV neuromuscular blocking drug is given, and ventilation is continued. When the patient is relaxed, oral intubation with laryngoscope and endotracheal tube is performed, while assistant holding head maintains immobilization and possibly in-line traction. Cricoid pressure is maintained until the cuff on the endotracheal tube is inflated and auscultation both in the axilla and over the epigastrium confirms tracheal intubation and rules out esophageal intubation. The cervical collar is reapplied, the tube is taped, an oral airway or bite block is inserted, and positive pressure ventilation is continued. (From J. H. Siegal. *Trauma.* New York: Churchill Livingstone, 1987. With permission.)

with rise in intracranial pressure and possibly catastrophic results. The other side of the coin is that excessive intravenous sodium thiopental (the usual and most efficacious agent used to treat such hyperdynamic sequelae) can cause marked hypotension and even death in a patient with occult volume depletion.

A final primum non nocere warning must be given in regard to muscle relaxants. Although indisputably invaluable in assisting with intubation (as in the cardiogenic shock patient described above), inability to intubate after paralysis can, of course, lead to asphyxiation and death. Preoxygenation by positive ventilation with a bag and mask is often required prior to intubation if a patient is apneic or has ineffective respirations. It should be done in conjunction with cricoid pressure, to limit gastric inflation. If one cannot ventilate a patient with bag and mask, one should make preparations for cricothyroidotomy prior to administering muscle relaxants. In the majority of cases, even if intubation is difficult, one can ventilate by bag and mask effectively after paralysis is achieved. The efficacious use of such a simple device is, paradoxically, more difficult to master than endotracheal intubation [10], yet it is a prerequisite skill for anyone who intends to use muscle relaxants.

The use of paralytic agents by emergency physicians in the emergency department was retrospectively reviewed by a group from Hennepin County Medical Center in Minneapolis [11, 12]. In spite of carefully constructed protocols and training, they had intubation failure rates of 10 percent (4 of 40 patients) in the 1986 study and 12.5 percent (6 of 48 patients) in the 1982 study. All but one of the failures required cricothyroidotomy. It would be interesting to see a study comparing failure rates in similar patients in whom anesthesiologists used the muscle relaxants and performed intubation. This author suspects that failure rates might be lower, both because anesthesiologists use such agents daily and because in aggressive emergency departments there is a tendency, if intubation is difficult, to move very quickly (and often appropriately) to surgical procedures such as cricothyroidotomy. Bag-mask ventilation, with equipment that can generate enough positive pressure to ventilate past an upper airway obstruction, is the usual course adopted by anesthesiologists in a paralyzed patient who cannot be intubated after a first attempt. Such an option was not considered in either of the Minneapolis studies. Nevertheless, adequate patient selection, positioning, equipment, and experience are prerequisite to the safe use by any physician of muscle relaxants, and it should be recognized that there are many instances when their use is contraindicated or when cricothyroidotomy may be needed as a backup.

Use of muscle relaxants has not been limited to the ED but has even been extended to the prehospital phase of care. Hedges and associates report on the use of succinylcholine by paramedics to assist intubation [13]. Paramedics, after demonstrating proven field experience in intubation and completing extensive OR training in the use of paralyzing agents, successfully intubated 95 patients using the drug, with no esophageal intubations or failures requiring cricothyroidotomy.

One must weigh the risks and benefits in using a depolarizing agent such as succinylcholine, which has a rapid onset and is rapidly metabolized (usually) by pseudocholinesterase but can trigger fatal potassium release in patients with neurologic injury or crush injury, and can cause painful muscle fasciculations, malignant hyperthermia, or dysrhythmias. Nondepolarizing muscle relaxants have both a longer duration of action and a longer onset, even with priming doses, and present a different set of problems. Further pharmacologic considerations involving these drugs will be discussed in Chapters 5, 12, and 13. Only careful prior consideration of these risks and benefits will lead to the right decision in the stressful and urgent setting of impending airway obstruction.

VENTILATION

Excretion of carbon dioxide and prevention of respiratory acidosis are obvious goals of airway management. Most of the acidosis that occurs in acute cardiopulmonary arrest is due to the respiratory component, and excessive sodium bicarbonate administration is deleterious (see Chapters 3 and 4). Thus there are no pharmacologic shortcuts to elimination of carbon dioxide, and one should treat lack of ventilation with ventilation, not with bicarbonate [14].

OXYGENATION

The importance of aerobic metabolism needs no added emphasis in these pages. There are a number of causes of hypoxia [15]; they include low ambient oxygen (altitude and the like), diffusion abnormalities, hypoventilation (at an FIO_2 of 0.21, increased carbon dioxide does not leave "room" in the alveoli for oxygen molecules), and shunt and ventilation/perfusion abnormalities. Many of these problems are not treated simply by increasing FIO_2, but by modalities that include pharmacologic treatment of drug depression and pulmonary edema, positive end-expiratory pressure (PEEP), bronchoscopy, and removal of mucous plugs, or a return to sea level.

PROTECTION

Even though the cuff on an endotracheal tube is not to be relied on completely, it does offer protection against aspiration. Similarly, double-lumen endobronchial tubes are absolutely indicated for unilateral pulmonary hemorrhage or for operation on a lung abscess [16].

WORK OF BREATHING

Normally less than 3 percent of the body's total energy expenditure, work of breathing may rise precipitously with exercise or in disease states such as asthma or congestive heart failure [17]. Decreasing the work of breathing at times makes the difference between a stable patient and one with an impending arrest. As lung compliance deteriorates, greater and greater inspiratory pressures must be generated for a given volume, and increasing energy expenditure is required. On the other hand, the negative inspiratory pressure of spontaneous ventilation is often an important factor in assisting venous return, especially in conditions in which venous return is severely impeded. These include pericardial tamponade, pediatric cardiovascular postoperative states in which the right ventricle is bypassed (Fontan procedure), and patients with vascular compromise by tumor [18].

MECHANICS OF BREATHING

Airway management must include consideration of the state of the chest wall and diaphragm, which, in combination with the neurologic breathing apparatus, forms the bellows mechanism that moves gas in and out. Flail chest or multiple rib fractures may be managed without intubation by advanced pain control techniques such as epidural narcotic drip (see Chapter 7), or they may require intubation and positive pressure support. A newborn with lobar emphysema, on the other hand, can deteriorate rapidly with positive pressure ventilation, as the abnormal lung tissue expands with a ball valve effect at the expense of normal lung tissue. A similar adverse mechanical situation exists in a patient with a tension pneumothorax. Neurologic control of the lung bellows must also be intact, just as an electric bellows requires a functioning electrical system. Thus, patients with Guillain-Barré, periodic familial hypokalemia, and other diseases may require temporary pulmonary support.

AIRWAY ASSESSMENT

HISTORY

If a patient can complain that he or she cannot breathe, *dyspnea,* the unpleasant sensation of abnormal breathing, is present, but intubation may not be indicated. In acute airway management, many patients are too ill to converse well. Many physicians use a truncated history in such situations, based on the mnemonic AMPLE.

> A = Allergies?
>
> M = Medicines? (or drugs?)
>
> P = Past medical problems? (key organ systems are the heart, lung, liver, kidney, brain)
>
> L = Last time patient had anything to eat or drink?
>
> E = Events? (what happened?)

A careful history from paramedic personnel or family can be invaluable in the emergency airway situation. The presence or suspicion of drug abuse, the appearance of a vehicle after an accident, the need for prolonged extrication times—these can all be valuable clues to management. For example, the existence of a bent or fractured steering column indicates that the mechanism of injury was severe and that the possibility of occult chest trauma exists. Empty bottles of oxycodone and aspirin pills brought in by a family member or roommate can offer an explanation (aspirin overdose superimposed on narcotic overdose) for a patient with an otherwise unfathomable combined respiratory alkalosis and metabolic acidosis. A history of Addison's disease is a vital clue that no resuscitation effort will be effective until the patient is given steroid supplementation.

INSPECTION

Anatomy

Large protruding upper incisors, a recessed mandible, or a shortened distance between the mentum of the jaw and the thyroid cartilage (see below, The Difficult Intubation) all serve as warnings that airway management will be difficult. Morbid obesity, previous neck operation or cervical spine operation, or perioral trauma are other factors that will complicate airway management and influence decision making on therapy. One must be wary, for example, of using long-acting muscle relaxants in such patients before verifying that the patient can be ventilated. Finally, it is wise (although not always possible) to test the patient's ability to open the mouth prior to taking over airway management. Some individuals are unable to open their mouths adequately to permit, for example, the passage of both laryngoscope blade and endotracheal tube.

Color

A rapidly noted and important physical sign is cyanosis of the mucous membranes. Generally, it requires 5 gm of reduced hemoglobin per 100 ml of blood to produce cyanosis [19]. Thus a cyanotic patient with polycythemia from smoking, chronic obstructive pulmonary disease, chronic altitude exposure, or right-to-left cardiac shunt may in fact still have a sufficient amount of oxidized hemoglobin to ensure sufficient cellular delivery of oxygen. (As little as 1.5 gm methemoglobin per 100 ml of blood or 0.5 gm sulfhemoglobin per 100 ml of blood is sufficient to produce cyanosis [19].) However, cyanosis may not be present in other dire situations: Carboxyhemoglobin produces a characteristic cherry red flush of skin and mucous membranes, whereas cyanide poisoning may cause fatal cellular hypoxic conditions by binding to cytochrome oxidase but preserves the normal skin color. In spite of these considerations, the presence or absence of cyanosis is an important physical finding.

Rate

Normal respiratory rate is generally between 6 and 20 breaths per minute. Bradypnea is a sign of hypothermia, hypothyroidism, or, more commonly, narcosis, and is used by some to gauge the effect of narcotic administration. Interestingly, patients with narcotic ventilatory depression and resultant bradypnea may retain reasonably good tidal volumes, e.g., 8 to 10 ml/kg [20]. Tachypnea (>20 beats per minute [bpm]) is a sign of pain, impending respiratory disaster, increased metabolism coupled with increased carbon dioxide production (e.g., malignant hyperthermia), or volatile anesthetic therapy [20]. The latter, unlike narcotic therapy, leads to small tidal volumes. Ataxic breathing is seen with profound neurologic disaster or with inadequate reversal of muscle relaxants.

Depth

Depth of respiration reveals much about the mechanical problems of breathing. A patient with flail chest and painful broken ribs will be unable to muster normal (5 to 10 ml/kg) tidal volumes. The effects of narcotics and volatile anesthetic agents were mentioned above. A patient who is hyperventilating may have a normal rate but a 25 to 30 ml/kg tidal volume.

Use of Accessory Musculature

The patient with increased work of breathing, whether due to upper airway obstruction or to increased compliance from an intraparenchymal problem, may need extremely high negative intrathoracic pressures. Simple diaphragmatic motion may not generate this, and the intercostal, sternocleidomastoid, and trapezius musculature may be called into play. The wary clinician can spot this type of breathing "from across the room," and it usually dictates prompt action.

Tracheal Tug

A byproduct of increased intrathoracic negative pressure in conjunction with upper airway obstruction, this characteristic sign is seen as the inspiratory indentation of the space over the trachea bounded by the sternal notch and the insertion of the sternal heads of the sternocleidomastoid musculature. A patient with this sign demands treatment, whether by placement of an oral airway (if the patient is obtunded), by a nasal trumpet (if the gag reflex is intact), or by endotracheal intubation and positive pressure intubation. Usually the former treatment or extension of the patient's head in combination with jaw thrust will alleviate the problem (Fig. 2-2).

Paradoxical Chest Motion

There are two types of paradoxical chest motion. In a patient with upper airway obstruction, depression of the diaphragm without air ingress to the chest will produce a characteristic "rocking" motion of the patient's chest and abdomen. This sign is often seen in conjunction with tracheal tug. In normal inspiration both the chest and the abdomen expand together. The

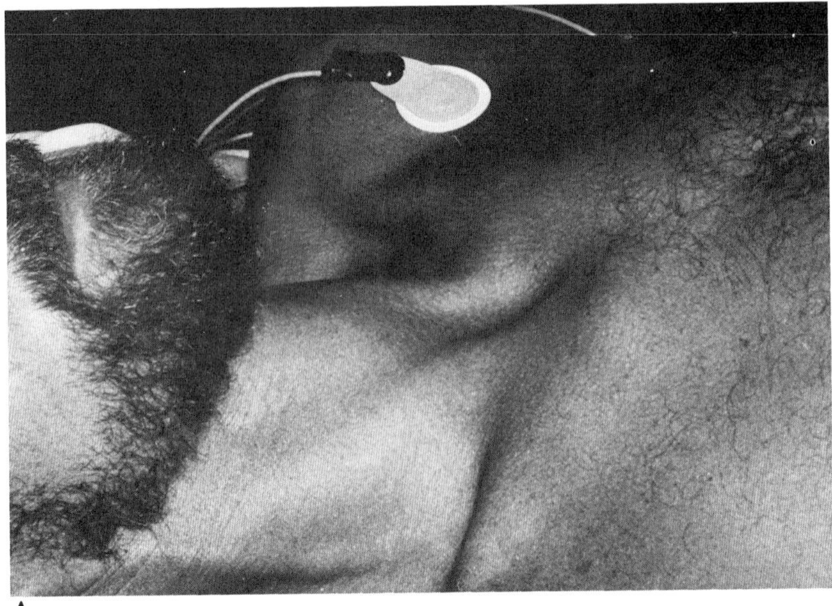

A

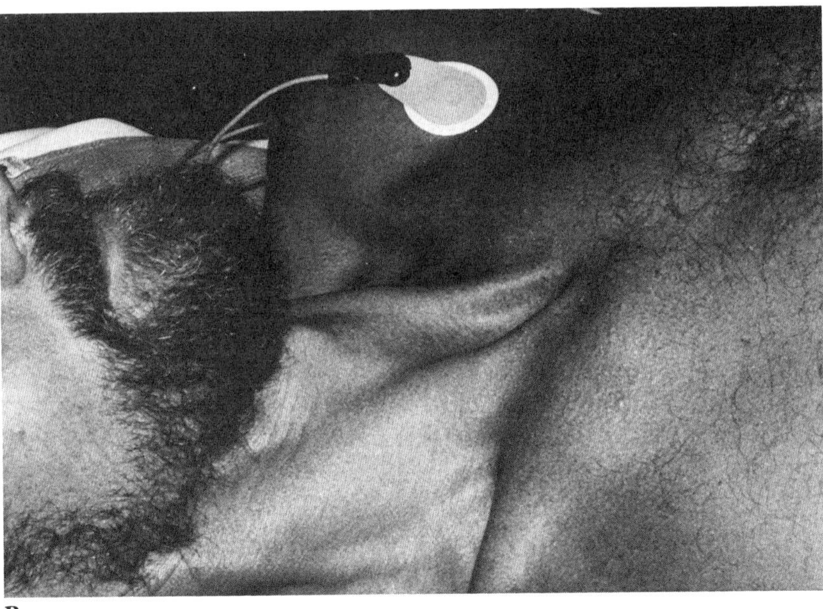

B

Fig. 2-2. Tracheal tug. *A.* Patient is in relaxed state. *B.* Inspiratory effort without an open airway produces marked indentation between the heads of the sternocleidomastoid in the neck overlying the trachea. Abnormal contraction of the thorax during the inspiratory attempt is often seen in conjunction with tracheal tug.

second type of abnormal motion is observed in patients with multiple rib fractures or flail chest. Normal chest expansion is replaced by retraction with inspiration over the affected segment.

Jugular Venous Pressure

A patient with true tension pneumothorax or cardiac tamponade will have the classic engorgement of the external jugular veins, in addition to other signs of respiratory and circulatory failure. Such a sign is helpful when it is present, but it may also simply portend volume overload or right ventricular heart failure. Absence of the sign does not necessarily preclude either of the aforementioned disasters because they may occur in conjunction with hypovolemia.

Evidence of Head Trauma

In evaluation of the airway, signs of facial or head trauma may alter one's management plan and set off certain warning signals. For example, jaw trauma should lead one to suspect an aspirated tooth. Signs of significant head trauma, such as depressed skull fracture or hematoma with corresponding neurologic deficit may lead one away from temporizing measures to rapid, aggressive airway management (keeping the possibility of cervical spine injury and full stomach in mind, of course).

Endotracheal Tube

If one is called to evaluate a patient who is already intubated, one must check for moisture with expiration and the depth of tube placement (20 to 21 cm at the maxillary tooth line for adult females, 22 to 23 cm for adult males, and "age plus 10 cm" for pediatric patients) as well as performing the usual stethoscopic auscultation of the thorax (see below under Auscultation). Is the cuff expanded but not rock hard? Are breath sounds greater in the epigastrium than over the thorax? Children (see Chapter 8) are notorious for presenting ambivalent examination results to the stethoscopist—sounds are transmitted so efficiently that "ventilation" of the stomach can masquerade as "full, bilateral breath sounds."

Ventilator

If the patient is on a mechanical ventilator, what are the inspiratory pressures? Is a manually operated bag available? One must check tidal volumes, pressures, and FIO_2 immediately, and, if one is unfamiliar with a certain ventilator, it may be better to ventilate the patient by hand with a bag-valve system—sometimes in an emergent situation the experienced hand can relay much more information than a forest of abstruse dials. Generally, an intubated patient with an acute inability to ventilate has one of the following conditions: tension pneumothorax, mucous plug, faulty ventilator, inadvertent extubation, trismus without a bite block, combative nonacceptance of the ventilated state, or simply a continuation of the disease process.

PALPATION

Crepitus

The unmistakable crackling sensation that is felt when palpating tissue containing subcutaneous air is a sign that can either be of little significance (rarely) or the first clue of impending disaster (more often). In a patient with deteriorating blood pressure, obtunded neck veins, and a history of having undergone a recent central venous pressure (CVP) catheter insertion by the subclavian route, the finding of crepitus on physical examination is more than sufficient evidence to decompress the patient's pleural space emergently. Withholding treatment while awaiting confirmatory chest radiographs in this situation is unwise. Crepitus in a patient who has suffered vehicular trauma, has neck or chest trauma, and requires high inspiratory pressures may well signify tracheal or bronchial fracture and deserves, at the very least, early bronchoscopy and, most probably, definitive surgical repair. On the other hand, crepitus in certain thoracic postsurgical states can present an alarming appearance yet not require any specific treatment and resolve spontaneously. A final cause of crepitus is the presence of air-forming bacteria (*Clostridium perfringens*) in a surgical wound.

Tracheal Shift

A classic sign of tension pneumothorax, lateral tracheal shift may also result from scarring due to radiation or radical neck dissections. Observation of external tracheal position is often helpful in permitting intubation in a patient in whom initial laryngoscopy reveals an absence of normal landmarks.

Cervical Spine

Gentle palpation of the posterior cervical spinous processes may reveal abnormal bony extrusions, stepoffs, and other clues to the presence of a cervical spine fracture in a trauma patient. If a patient is awake and communicative, his or her response to the examination can be valuable as well. Cervical fractures are painful, and it has been shown that in alert patients with normal neurologic responses on examination and no neck pain or tenderness, significant cervical spine injury can be excluded without the use of radiographs [21].

Abdominal Distention

If this finding is noted, one must be prepared for an increased chance of vomiting and aspiration. Often unskilled personnel using a bag-valve mask during a cardiopulmonary arrest will pump air into the stomach rather than open the airway and ventilate the lungs. The legacy of such treatment, a stomach full of air, can be managed by evacuation using nasogastric suction after careful endotracheal intubation with cricoid pressure.

Percussion

This physical sign, often delegated to the realm of internal medicine, can prove valuable in airway management, both in the diagnosis of pneumothorax, in which one finds increased resonance on the afflicted side, and in the diagnosis of hepatomegaly, which is an indicator of right heart failure and pulmonary hypertension.

AUSCULTATION

Stethoscopy and Abnormal Breath Sounds

Rales, the crackling sound similar to crumpled cellophane, usually represents alveolar filling or pulmonary edema. One should try to define the extent to which the rales involve the lung fields—i.e., basilar, or one-third or two-thirds of the thorax. *Rhonchi,* the coarse sounds produced by mucus in the large airways, hint of the need for cough and suctioning. *Wheezing* implies bronchospasm, and recording its presence on examination can be supplemented by an attempt to quantify the inspiratory-expiratory ratio. Wheezing can also be caused by mechanical obstruction of an airway system, such as a kinked endotracheal tube or a tube blocked by secretions. Bowel sounds in the chest might indicate to the wary clinician a diagnosis of ruptured diaphragm, a diagnosis that is often delayed.

Stethoscopy and Cardiac Sounds

The S_3 heart sound is a common but nonspecific sign of elevated left ventricular filling pressures [22]. Quiet surroundings make its detection more feasible. A loud pansystolic murmur in a patient with an acute myocardial infarction, hypoxia, and pulmonary edema may be caused by acute papillary muscle rupture or acute ventricular septal defect. A patient with an irregular apical sound and dyspnea may have mitral stenosis with decompensation because of acute atrial fibrillation. The classic diastolic rumble of mitral stenosis is not easily heard and often requires optimal stethoscopic conditions and lateral positioning. A patient with the classic diamond-shaped systolic ejection murmur of aortic stenosis often has a hypertrophied, volume-dependent left ventricle. Such a patient will be extremely sensitive to any agent that causes venodilation (e.g., sodium thiopental).

Stridor

Inspiratory stridor often indicates obstruction of the supraglottic or glottic larynx (at or above the vocal cords). Expiratory stridor is associated with subglottic obstruction [23].

BLOOD GAS TENSIONS

Arterial Blood Gas Tensions

Thorough evaluation of a patient's airway, if time permits, should include measurement of arterial blood gas (ABG) tensions. One should not withhold prompt positive pressure ventilation and intubation from a patient who has marked acute respiratory distress while ABG tensions are measured, nor should one withhold extubation pending ABG measurement from a patient who is bucking and coughing on the endotracheal tube and who can fulfill standard criteria [24] for extubation.

Given that there is still an important place for ABG measurement in evaluating the efficacy of a patient's airway, several key points deserve attention. The decision to intubate and ventilate a patient is a clinical one, based in part on the patient's level of exhaustion, prognosis, and prospect of improvement from concurrent therapy and in part on the PCO_2 and PO_2 levels. Generally, a PCO_2 greater than 50 mm Hg or a PO_2 less than 60 mm Hg on 50 percent mask oxygen, in the presence of worsening clinical conditions is an indication for intubation. On the other hand, one might withhold intubation without proof of marked deterioration in a patient with chronic obstructive pulmonary disease who, in spite of a PCO_2 of, say, 52, has a high serum bicarbonate level and a pH of 7.34. Thus, one must be wary in following CO_2 strictly as a marker of hypoventilation. A better notion of normalcy than a PCO_2 measurement of 40 is a pH of 7.40; thus, increasing nonrespiratory-compensated acidosis may be a sounder physiologic reason to assist ventilation. This author has found the Advanced Cardiac Life Support (ACLS) Golden Rules invaluable in assessing ABGs [25]. They state:

1. For every increase in PCO_2 of 10 mm Hg, the pH will decrease 0.08. Thus, a patient with a PCO_2 of 53 should have a pH of about 7.30. Any pH change less than this implies chronic hypoventilation with retention of bicarbonate. Hyperventilation will produce similar changes in a reverse direction.
2. For every increase or decrease in base excess of 10 meq (with normal bicarbonate levels defined as 25 meq/100 ml blood), the pH, after correction by Golden Rule 1 to a PCO_2 of 40, will increase or decrease by 0.15. Thus, a patient whose ABGs demonstrate a pH of 7.33 and a PCO_2 of 30 will have a base deficit of approximately 10 meq.

3. To correct a base deficit with bicarbonate, one needs to take the base deficit, multiply by the patient's weight, and then multiply by 0.25 (the approximation of the extracellular space). Then one would administer one-half that amount in meq of bicarbonate [25].

4. The final rule is not without some controversy. Because of evidence that excessive bicarbonate treatment may be deleterious, the ACLS standards have been modified and now suggest that clinicians "consider" the use of the drug [26]. This topic is addressed further in Chapter 4.

NONINVASIVE AIRWAY MONITORING

Oxygen Saturation

First developed by the Japanese bioengineer Takao Aoyagi and adapted for practical use by Dr. William New of the United States, the measurement of oxygen saturation has revolutionized monitoring of the pulmonary system, just as availability of the electrocardiogram revolutionized monitoring of the cardiac system. These monitors work by measuring the differential absorption of two frequencies of light, one in the red visible and the other in the infrared range. As varying amounts of oxyhemoglobin or deoxyhemoglobin absorb the light, comparisons are made with previously measured absorptions at known oxygen saturations. Fundamental to the technique is pulse sensing, by which artifacts from skin and other tissue are deleted from the data. A small sensor that projects and measures light absorption is attached to the fingertip, nose, or ear (Fig. 2-3).

Oxygen saturation monitors are currently produced by a number of companies, and refinements in accuracy, especially at low levels of saturation, are constantly being made. Clinically, one sees rapid changes during a second-to-second time frame as a patient's oxygenation status changes. For example, one may see rapid desaturation during a prolonged intubation attempt long before changes appear on the electrocardiogram. Conversely, in a patient who has been adequately preoxygenated, one may use an unhurried approach in a difficult intubation attempt because the saturation monitor will demonstrate whether the oxygen supply in the functional residual capacity (FRC) portion of the lung will keep the patient's blood well saturated. Patients who have diminished FRC, such as the morbidly obese, or patients with high metabolic demands proportionate to their FRC, such as those in the pediatric age group, will rapidly become desaturated, even with adequate preoxygenation.

These monitors do not provide accurate data in the presence of methemoglobinemia [27, 28] and carboxyhemoglobinemia [29, 30], however. Until third and fourth frequencies are added to the two light frequencies in use, one must be aware that these conditions will result in misleading oxygen saturation data.

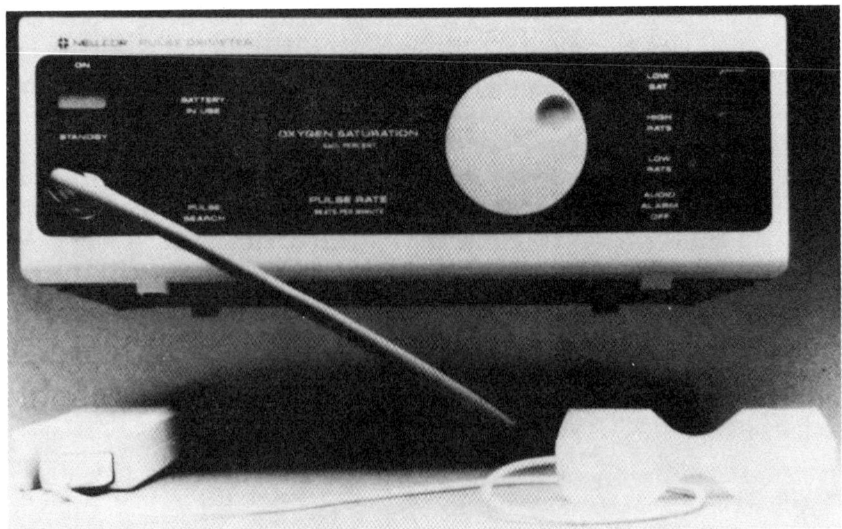

Fig. 2-3. Transcutaneous oxygen saturation device and finger probe. (From S. M. Shnider and G. Levinson [eds.], *Anesthesia for Obstetrics.* Baltimore: Williams & Wilkins, 1987. With permission.)

Oxygen saturation monitors have quickly become the near-standard of care in the operating room. They are used more and more frequently outside the operating room and will have an important place in the emergency department [31]. A recent evaluation of pulse oximetry in prehospital care showed it to be of invaluable benefit in identifying unsuspected, treatable hypoxia [32].

End-Tidal Carbon Dioxide Monitors

The monitoring technique of end-tidal carbon dioxide monitoring, also known as *capnometry,* is also rapidly becoming indispensable in the operating room because it provides a noninvasive means of quantifying the adequacy of ventilation. Most systems function by the aspiration of approximately 100 cc of gas per minute via a small (1- to 2-mm) catheter attached near the endotracheal tube. Carbon dioxide is measured by infrared absorption spectrophotometry, and a graphic wave form is printed. Because of the Bohr equation, one must be cognizant that anatomic or alveolar dead space will lower the mixed expired carbon dioxide, and its related value, the end-tidal carbon dioxide measurement, significantly from the desired value, the arterial carbon dioxide gas tension. Here is a simplified form of Enghoff's modification of the Bohr equation:

$$V_D/V_T = \frac{PaCO_2 - P\bar{E}CO_2}{PaCO_2}$$

where V_D = volume of dead space
     V_T = tidal volume
  $PaCO_2$ = pulmonary arterial carbon dioxide
  $P\bar{E}CO_2$ = pulmonary mixed-expired carbon dioxide

Capnography is a valuable adjunct for monitoring hyperventilation in a head-injured patient who has increased intracranial pressure. As such, it deserves a place in the computed tomography suite as well as the emergency department. Elevation or depression of arterial carbon dioxide levels from the ideal hyperventilatory range of 25 to 30 mm Hg can be detrimental due to either increased cerebral blood flow with high PCO_2 or decreased cerebral blood flow to the point of ischemia with reduced PCO_2 [33]. This monitor enables close, noninvasive adjustment of ventilation. It also provides rapid determination of esophageal intubation [34]. (See Chapter 3 for further discussion of this topic.)

Although both O_2 saturation monitors and end-tidal CO_2 monitors have proved invaluable, it must be understood that, as discussed above, they do at times give false-positive or false-negative information. Information gleaned from such technology must be weighed in light of the clinical situation and considered with a recognition of the limitations of technology. For example, a poor end-tidal CO_2 tracing post intubation could be due to esophageal intubation, or it could be due to severe bronchospasm with proper tube placement. Roizen has cautioned against making new technology the "standard of care" prematurely [35], and a Harvard standards study did fall short of making these types of newly popular monitoring the "standard of practice" for similar reasons [36].

ASSESSMENT SUMMARY

After the initial evaluation one must ask whether a problem exists. False alarms do occur, and one must be wary of them to avoid overtreatment. If a problem exists, one must try to define the anatomic source of the problem. Is there upper airway obstruction? Is there a lack of neurologic respiratory impulse due to drugs, neurologic catastrophe, or muscle weakness? Is there a large airway problem due to excretions, or a small airway problem due to bronchospasm? Is a parenchymal process such as alveolar filling responsible for the problem? Is there a mechanical problem with the breathing bellows mechanism? Once the anatomic site has been confirmed, one can work on the differential diagnosis for that part of the respiratory tree. It is conceded that when an airway expert is called to a respiratory emergency, the needed course of action is often a 10-second examination followed by cricoid pressure, mask ventilation, and immediate endotracheal intubation. There are enough situations that require a different approach, however, to make one pause and think before routinely rushing into such a procedure.

INITIAL MANAGEMENT AND INTUBATION

INITIAL MANAGEMENT

MODALITIES THAT OPEN THE AIRWAY

Positioning

One may divide consideration of positioning into four categories. First, there is positioning that optimizes opening of the upper airway, i.e., the jaw, tongue, and soft palate. The maneuvers of anterior jaw thrust and chin lift are well described in the ACLS manual [37].

Second, there is positioning that optimizes visualization for endotracheal intubation. Establishment of the "sniffing" position is the best single technique for lining up the axes of the mouth, soft palate, and trachea (Fig. 2-4). Just as one instinctively flexes the neck on the chest and extends the head on the neck to savor an odor, so the airway is optimally opened for intubation. In a patient with a suspected cervical spine injury, movement of the neck is contraindicated. Children, with their proportionately larger heads, often assume the sniffing position spontaneously and consequently do not need any positioning other than a simple flat surface on which to lie supine. The intubation of most adults will be facilitated dramatically, however, by the placement of a 5-cm-thick towel or headrest under the occiput. Often well-meaning but uninformed persons attempt to assist intubation by putting a towel under the neck, but this leads only to excessive hypertension and makes visualization of the cords more difficult. Obese patients may require elevation of the chest in addition to the occiput (Fig. 2-5).

A third aspect of positioning involves the mechanics of respiration. The supine position leads to decreased FRC, increased ventilation-perfusion inequality, and increased pulmonary shunting, all of which contribute to poor oxygenation [24]. Consequently, if a patient's cardiovascular status will tolerate some degree of the sitting position, the supine position is to be avoided in patients with compromised ventilation, especially obese patients.

A final aspect of positioning involves the prevention and management of aspiration. Many would add the sitting position to the usual recommendations for rapid sequence induction in a patient with a full stomach. Such positioning requires active regurgitation with a pressure difference at least equal to the vertical distance between the glottis and the lower esophageal sphincter. Once active vomiting or passive regurgitation has occurred, treatment includes placing the patient initially in a head-down or Trendelenburg position, active suctioning, positioning for endotracheal intubation, suctioning through the endotracheal tube, and finally, intubation and inflation of the endotracheal cuff.

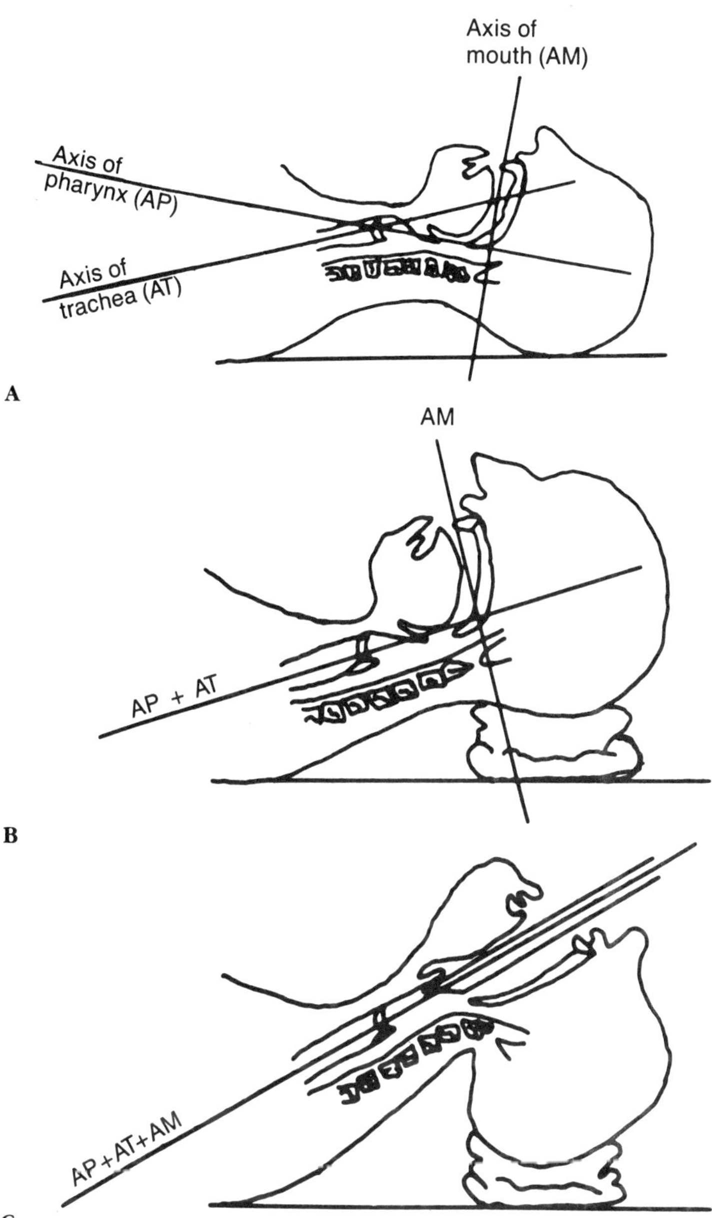

Fig. 2-4. Anatomic considerations for laryngoscopy and tracheal intubation. *A.* Axes of the mouth, pharynx, and trachea are shown with head in the customary neutral position. *B.* Axes of the pharynx and trachea are superimposed with the head resting on a firm pad or folded sheet. *C.* All three axes are aligned by flexion of the cervical spine and extension at the atlanto-occipital joint (sniffing position). (From F. K. Orkin and L. H. Cooperman [eds.], *Complications in Anesthesiology.* Philadelphia: Lippincott, 1983. With permission.)

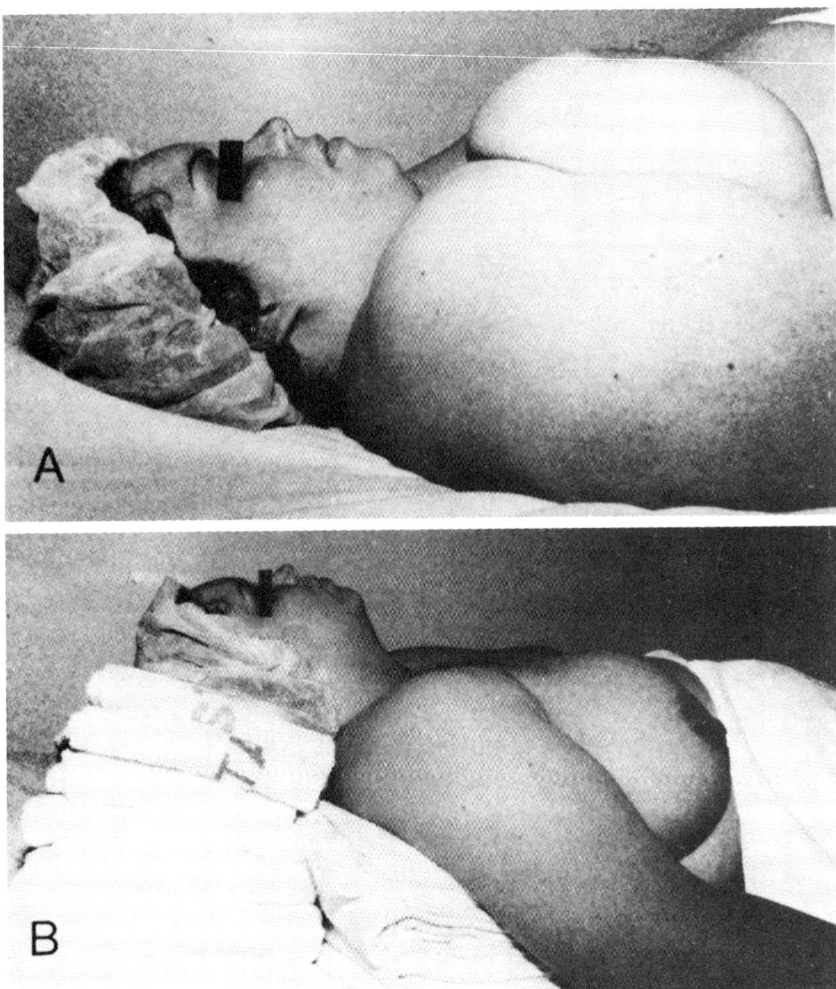

Fig. 2-5. *A.* Obese pregnant woman in the supine position. The atlanto-occipital gap is obliterated by fat, and access with a laryngoscope is hindered by large breasts. *B.* The same patient positioned with the shoulders elevated and the occiput further elevated so that the head assumes the "sniffing" position. Access to the airway is greatly facilitated. (From S. M. Shnider and G. Levinson [eds.], *Anesthesia for Obstetrics.* Baltimore: Williams & Wilkins, 1987. With permission.)

Nasal Airways

Also known as nasal trumpets, these devices are invaluable in maintaining upper airway patency in a patient with minimal to moderate obstruction. They are well tolerated by awake or sedated patients with an intact gag reflex, although skillful insertion is prerequisite. Plentiful lubrication with or without local anesthetic gel and an initial insertion angle parallel to the turbinates make insertion and patient acceptance much easier. Less than skillful technique can result in epistaxis, which is not a complication one desires in a patient who already has a compromised airway. Unfortunately, the more pliable, less traumatic nasal airways also tend to be less efficacious in keeping the upper airway open, whereas other, stiffer types are more likely to cause epistaxis.

Oral Airways

Oral airways, as adjuncts to airway management, are indispensable, and for several reasons. First, they markedly facilitate ventilation in many patients who have lost the gag reflex and also have obstructing relaxation of the tongue and soft palate. This problem is increased in the edentulous patient. Mask ventilation is much facilitated by insertion of an oral airway. A second use for these airways is prevention of unrestrained trismus and resulting occlusion of the soft endotracheal tube. The author is aware of an unreported case in which a young, powerful patient who required intubation and was not provided with a tooth guard or oral airway bit down so forcefully that he severed the tube, suffered an obstruction of the airway, and failed to survive the resulting efforts at resuscitation and cricothyroidotomy. The author has also seen a patient receive needle aspiration of both lung fields for suspected tension pneumothorax, which was postulated as the cause of a sudden cessation of ability to ventilate. After bilateral pneumothoraces were in fact created, it was discovered that the patient had simply developed trismus that had occluded the tube orally. The dangers of oral airway use involve precipitation of laryngospasm (discussed below), vomiting, and tooth breakage.

Endotracheal Intubation

Surely the mainstay in acute or chronic airway management, endotracheal intubation should be considered early in the course of a difficult resuscitation attempt. The benefits of intubation include protection from aspiration, the ability to ventilate a patient safely mechanically while performing other vital tasks, provision of a route for the administration of drugs when intravenous access is lacking (lidocaine, epinephrine, atropine, and naloxone [LEAN]), and facilitation of oxygenation by the ability to give 100 percent oxygen and positive end-expiratory pressure (PEEP). The risks include failure of the patient to ventilate while intubation is attempted, intubation of the esophagus (uniformly fatal if not discovered), tissue damage to the oropharynx from improper technique (leading to edema or infection), and tracheomalacia secondary to prolonged exposure of the trachea to cuff pressures that exceed capillary tissue perfusion pressures. A more complete discussion of endotracheal intubation follows.

Esophageal Obturator Airway

The esophageal obturator airway (EOA), which enables field personnel to ventilate the lungs by obstructing the esophagus with a 30-ml occluding balloon and subsequently using mask ventilation of the oropharynx, has suffered from a recent fall in popularity [38]. This lack of popularity is due both to intrinsic problems with the modality and to the increased training and experience of prehospital personnel in performing endotracheal intubation. Advantages of the EOA technique include the ability to position the esophageal obturator rapidly and blindly and the lack of need to alter cervical spine position. Disadvantages include, most prominently, a common failure to ventilate the patient adequately [39], an increased propensity for stomach inflation, inadvertent endotracheal intubation, and rare but devastating esophageal trauma. A newer modification with a port for nasogastric suctioning has been developed, the esophageal gastric tube airway (EGTA). The ACLS has taught that one must intubate endotracheally with the esophageal obturator in place because vomiting or regurgitation often occurs, even with the EGTA and prior suctioning, on removal of the device [26]. Although one cannot argue with the veracity of this warning, intubation is made extremely difficult by the obstruction of the oropharynx created by the large diameter of the EOA. Often one must disregard the ACLS warning, remove the EOA, and trust to cricoid pressure to lessen the risk of vomiting because intubation is impossible, with the EOA in place. Some would argue that it is better to take the time and effort to train and monitor paramedic personnel in techniques of safe endotracheal intubation, thus bypassing use of the EOA altogether [38]. Performance of intubation in the presence of cervical spine trauma is still controversial, however, and for that reason, the EOA may be with us for some time. A recent study comparing outcome in patients managed by both modalities showed no significant difference [29]. Other studies, however, have shown that inadequate ventilation results from the use of EOA [40, 41].

Cricothyroidotomy

When ventilation is impossible by oral means, placement of an airway via the cricothyroid membrane becomes necessary. This may be accomplished in one of three ways: needle ventilation, cricothyrotome insertion, or surgical incision and placement of a tracheotomy tube or endotracheal tube. Needle ventilation can be performed using a 14-gauge intravenous catheter attached to the hub from a 3.0 mm pediatric endotracheal tube. One can then inflate the lungs using a 55-psi oxygen jet ventilator with a pressure gauge attached to prevent traumatic pneumothorax. Care must be taken to allow adequate exhalation by means of frequent disconnection or use of a three-way stopcock, especially if total upper airway obstruction exists and high-flow oxygen sources are used. Use of the various cricothyrotomes is straightforward; a small incision with a scalpel is sometimes required. Combination of the needle ventilation-cricothyrotome technique has been reported using the Seldinger guidewire technique, dilators, and transtracheal insertion of a 8.5 Fr catheter as the airway [42]. Performance of cricothyroidotomy (see Chapter 12) can be done quickly and easily with a scalpel, a clamp, and a tracheostomy tube in the great majority of patients. When there is marked swelling in the cervical region, it becomes more difficult. The reader is referred to several excellent reviews on the subject [13, 43].

Probably the primary controversy in assesesing cricothyroidotomy techniques revolves around indications and associated risks. As mentioned previously, the American College of Surgeons and ATLS have changed their initial approach of insisting that the operation be performed if a patient has had possible cervical spine trauma and the choice for airway management has been narrowed to a choice between oral endotracheal intubation and cricothyroidotomy [29]. David Gens, a surgeon at the Maryland Institute for Emergency Medical Service Systems (formerly the Shock Trauma Center) recommends a single attempt at orotracheal intubation in the case of neck injury and then proceeding to cricothyroidotomy [44]. Certainly there are risks involved in the performance of cricothyroidotomy, especially when it is performed by physicians who are not surgeons. These include hemorrhage, aspiration, failure to place the airway accurately, and long-term sequelae such as tracheomalacia and vocal cord changes. Nevertheless, when there has been severe oral-facial trauma and normal landmarks are grossly distorted, orotracheal intubation may not be possible, and rapid cricothyroidotomy may well be lifesaving.

OXYGEN DELIVERY SYSTEMS

Patients with Good Respiratory Effort

Nasal prongs deliver only modest increases in supplemental oxygen but are well tolerated and useful for patients with stable myocardial infarction, stable trauma conditions, and the like. Mist masks deliver 30 to 40 percent FiO_2 and are useful in an intermediate class of patients. If a patient is dependent on the hypoxic drive of ventilation, Venturi masks, which entrain air by the Bernoulli principle, can deliver known concentrations of oxygen. Masks with rebreather bags can deliver up to 60 percent FiO_2 and are a last step before endotracheal intubation. Masks that can maintain constant positive pressure (CPAP) ventilation are available and are useful at times.

Patients with Doubtful or Absent Respiratory Effort

Positive pressure ventilation is implied in this group of patients, as opposed to those in whom negative intrathoracic pressure allows ventilation. Options for providing such ventilation are as follows:

1. *Bag-valve systems.* These systems employ nonrebreathing valves of various types and deliver fresh gas (oxygen) to the patient, releasing exhaled gas to the atmosphere or to a scavenging system. An excellent description of these systems is found in Dorsch and Dorsch's *Understanding Anesthesia Equipment* [45].

To achieve effective mask ventilation, one traditionally uses the left hand to provide jaw thrust and mask seal while the right hand ventilates. Obviously, one may switch this right-left configuration. On difficult airways one person may hold the mask and the other may ventilate. In bearded individuals it may be necessary to spread a film of lubricant along the mask edge to provide a seal. Edentulous patients will require an oral airway or even small cotton rolls placed within the mouth on either side to promote a seal. There is a learned skill in "working" the breath into the patient's lungs. Simple forceful squeezing of the bag will often result in "ventilating" the stomach (Fig. 2-6).

2. *Semi-open anesthesia circuits.* These systems, also known as the Mapleson systems [46], are familiar to most anesthesiologists from their pediatric experiences. The most commonly used apparatus, the Jackson-Rees modification of the Ayres T-piece, has a fresh gas flow input near the patient connection (which has the standard 15-mm internal diameter and 22-mm external diameter attachment), a short length of corrugated tubing, a reservoir bag, and a simple valve on the end of the bag. This system is lightweight, simple to use, and very easy to troubleshoot. It does require fresh gas flows that equal two times the patient's minute volume (usually 100 cc/kg) [45], and there is a concomitant increased loss of humidification and temperature. Because they allow an experienced operator to feel lung compliance accurately and to control inspiratory pressures, they are preferred by many anesthesiologists in a resuscitative or transport situation in lieu of the above bag-valve systems. They are especially useful when a pressure manometer is placed in line, thus quantitating inspiratory pressures that the experienced hand can only estimate (Fig. 2-7).

3. *Mechanical ventilators.* The mainstays of the intensive care unit (ICU) are volume- and time-cycled ventilator systems. Pressure-cycled ventilators, such as the Ohio ventilator, can produce varying tidal volumes because the patient's chest wall and lung compliance varies. Because of their compact size and simplicity, these ventilators have been used extensively in the past on anesthetic machines and are still in use both in the United States and in the rest of the world. They require constant monitoring of tidal volume.

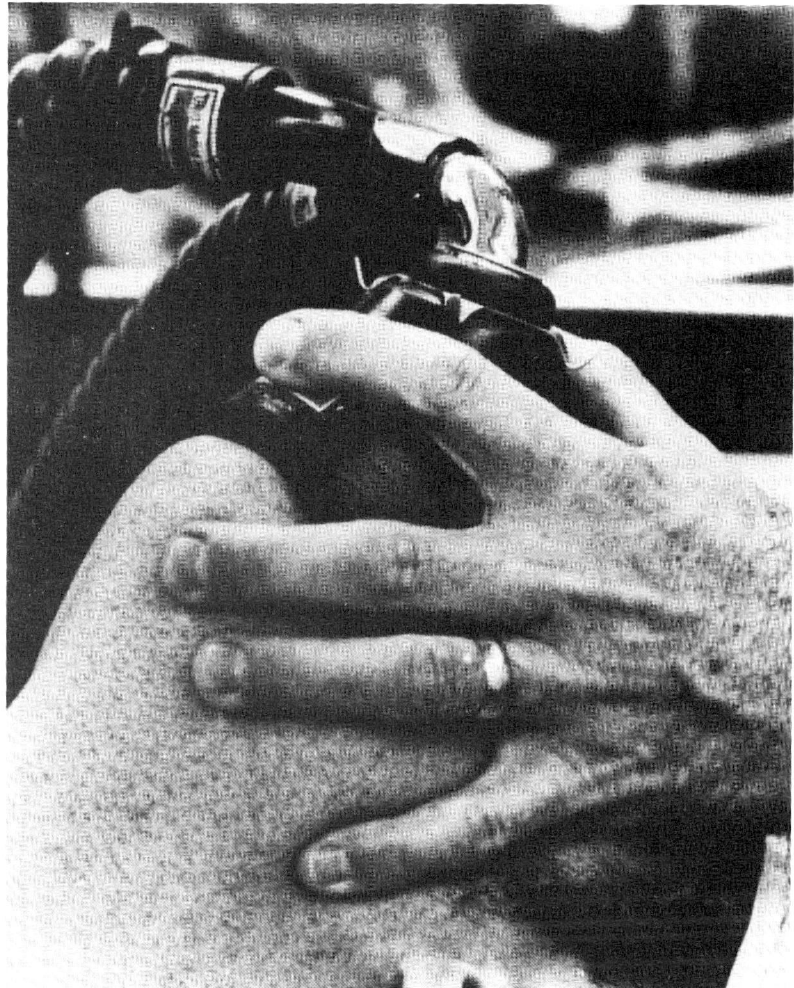

Fig. 2-6. Holding the mask with one hand, the third, fourth, and fifth fingers serve to provide jaw extension and oppose pressure from the index and thumb to provide a seal. (From J. A. Dorsch and S. E. Dorsch. *Understanding Anesthesia Equipment.* Baltimore: Williams & Wilkins, 1984. With permission.)

4. *High-frequency ventilators.* Although these devices initially had great promise, there are few indications for their use. Included among these are ventilation of premature infants [47] and other situations in which conventional ventilation is impossible. The use of high-frequency ventilation in bronchopleural fistulas has been called into question [48].

5. *Cardiopulmonary bypass–extracorporeal membrane oxygenation.* Although these modalities can no doubt be considered heroic, there are still

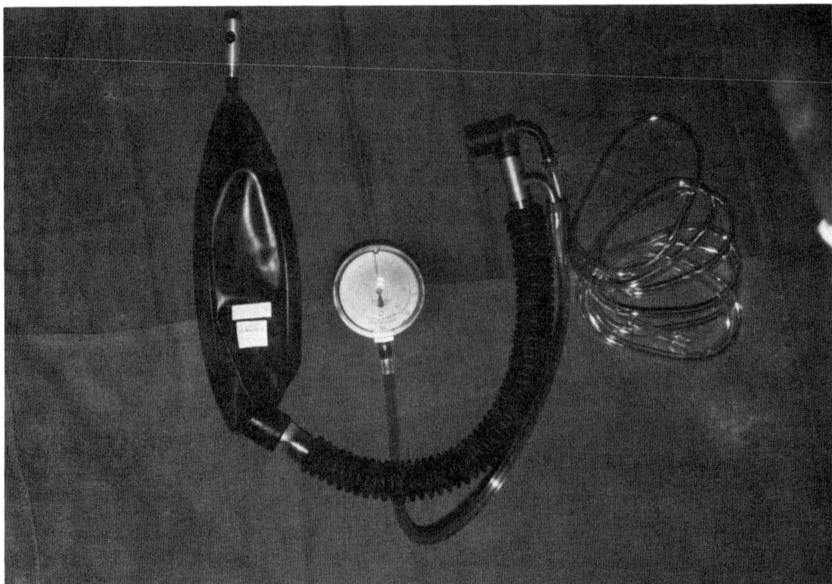

Fig. 2-7. Jackson-Rees modification of Ayres T-piece. This bag-mask arrangement has a simple valve at the end of the bag and provides manual "feel" of ventilations, unlike many bag-valve mask systems. The pressure gauge is especially useful in patients susceptible to barotrauma, i.e., pediatric patients.

some indications for such systems, which essentially bypass the lungs. Cardiopulmonary bypass (CPB) has been used with some success in treating severe hypothermia, while extracorporeal membrane oxygenation (ECMO), which failed to gain acceptance when used with adults, is experiencing a resurgence of use in pediatric patients with severe pulmonary problems that are reversible [49].

Patients with Good Respiratory Effort But with Dyspnea, Hypotension, and Pathologic Elevation of Central Venous Pressure

The differential diagnosis here is limited to tension pneumothorax, cardiac tamponade, and right heart failure secondary to pulmonary hypertension. Needle aspiration and pericardiocentesis are temporizing measures for the former two conditions; definitive treatment includes tube toracostomy and pericardiotomy by thoracotomy (see Chapter 12). The latter condition does not, unfortunately, have such straightforward treatment options. Pulmonary hypertension is aggravated by hypercarbia and hypoxia, and these should be relieved by the above modalities. More aggressive treatment utilizing vasodilators is discussed in Chapter 4.

ENDOTRACHEAL INTUBATION

Today endotracheal intubation is routinely and safely practiced by anesthesiologists, emergency physicians, and oral surgeons, and, more recently, by paramedics and emergency flight nurses. It has an excellent track record of safety yet can still result in devastating and even fatal complications. Currently, there are many intubating techniques as well as a large number of mechanical and pharmacologic adjuncts, attesting to the fact that establishing a patent and stable airway is not the easiest task, for if it were, there would be but one superior method.

ANATOMY

The anatomy of the airway has three axes, the oral axis, the pharyngeal axis, and the tracheal axis [50]. Successful visualization and intubation are facilitated by the alignment of these three axes, which, to repeat, is best accomplished by placing the head in the sniffing position (neck flexed, occiput raised 5 to 10 cm). The larynx is formed by the thyroid cartilage anteriorly, the arytenoid, corniculate, and cuneiform cartilages posteriorly, the epiglottal cartilate superiorly, and the cricoid cartilage inferiorly and posteriorly. The cricoid cartilage, which is shaped like a backward signet ring, with the broad portion posteriorly, is the only cartilaginous structure in the larynx or trachea that is unbroken by ligament. This fact is the foundation for the success of Sellick's maneuver, or cricoid pressure, in occluding the esophagus and preventing aspiration. The narrow portion of the cricoid cartilage anteriorly provides room for the cricothyroid membrane and, as a result, space for emergent surgical intubation.

The vocal folds are located just behind the laryngeal prominence of the thyroid cartilage or Adam's apple at the level of C5 in adults. They are composed of the thickened upper edges of the cricothyroid ligament, and they extend to the paired and mobile arytenoid cartilages [51]. Because the vocal folds are subjected to repeated trauma during phonation (and intubation), a layer of stratified squamous epithelium covers the mucous membrane, which in turn covers all the internal structure of the larynx. During cricothyroidotomy, the folds or cords are just above the surgically created opening in the anterior part of the cricothyroid ligament.

Motor nerve supply to the larynx is provided principally by the recurrent laryngeal branches of the vagus nerve, with the exception of the cricothyroid muscle, a vocal cord tensor, which is innervated by the superior laryngeal branch of the vagus. The recurrent nerve runs submucosally on the medial aspects of the thyroid lamina, where it is susceptible to compression by a cuff near the cords. Such compression may produce merely vocal cord dysfunction, caused by unilateral or incomplete damage, or catastrophic respiratory embarrassment, caused by bilateral nerve damage, with resultant bilateral abduction of both vocal cords [52].

Sensory innervation to the structures above the vocal folds is provided by the superior branch of the recurrent laryngeal nerve. This nerve can be anesthetized prior to awake intubation by injecting 2 to 3 ml of 2 percent lidocaine through a needle inserted perpendicularly between the hyoid cornu and the thyroid cornu [53].

Sensory innervation at and below the vocal folds is provided by the recurrent laryngeal nerves. Anesthesia for awake intubation here is best provided by cricothyroid membrane puncture, aspiration of air, and injection of 2 to 3 ml of 2 percent lidocaine as a topical anesthetic [50].

ENDOTRACHEAL TUBES

Ideal Endotracheal Tube

The ideal endotracheal tube would be nonkinkable, nonreactive to tissue, very thin (to minimize external diameter and tissue compression and to maximize internal diameter and minimize flow resistance), and nonflammable when exposed to laser radiation. It would have a cuff that would prevent any secretions or stomach contents from reaching the pulmonary parenchema and yet be harmless to the sensitive tracheal mucosa. Such an ideal cuff would also be able to withstand the needed application of forceps, such as the Magill forceps, without tearing and leaking. Best of all, this mythical tube would have a sensor that would unswervingly guide itself into the glottic space, and a CO_2 sensor that would reassure the practitioner that it was successfully placed, not in the esophagus, but in the trachea.

Obviously, we have a long way to go in developing such a tube, but current tubes have improved markedly from earlier models. Most tubes today are made of polyvinyl chloride. This substance is nonirritating and soft and limits tubes to a single use, because many sterilization procedures cause dangerous reaction products [45]. Other tubes are made of silicone, Teflon, rubber, polyethylene, or metal. The best available test for tissue reactivity involves implantation of a portion of a tube in a laboratory animal, along with known positive and negative controls. After a period of time, the animal (usually a rabbit) is sacrificed and histologic testing performed for signs of reaction. Tubes that have passed such tests and are found to be nontoxic are imprinted with the letters IT (implantation testing) or the more cryptic code Z-79.

Many special tubes exist, including nasal and oral Ring-Adair-Elwyn (RAE) tubes, spiral embedded tubes, special tubes for jet ventilation, Endotrol cable flexing tubes, and foil-wrapped tubes for use with laser surgical techniques. Dorsch and Dorsch have presented an excellent review of the entire inventory [45].

Key aspects of endotracheal tubes, beyond manufacturing materials, include the internal diameter, which is the convention used for labeling tubes, length, which is longer than needed in the standard tube and invites shortening after a tube is placed, and type of cuff (i.e., high or low pressure). Because the resistance of a gas is inversely proportionate to the fourth power of the radius, the diameter of the tube is the principal determinate of airway resistance. A rule of thumb is to use a 7-mm tube in an adult female, and an 8-mm tube in an adult male. In the pediatric age group, 3.0-mm tubes are used in premature infants, and 3.5 mm tubes in newborns. A general rule for older ages is to use the formula:

$$4 + \frac{age}{4} = \text{tube diameter in millimeters}$$

As further discussed in Chapter 8, one must vary pediatric tubes according to the patient. Uncuffed tubes, used in children under 6, require the onset of leak at 25 to 30 mm Hg of inspiratory pressure. If a tube is so large that it will not permit any leak at these pressures, the next smaller tube should be used. Many physicians also estimate the initial tube size by comparing their tube with the diameter of the child's little finger. Regardless of the formula, table, or technique used, the above leakage rule must be kept in mind because too large a tube will predispose to mucosal ulceration, tracheal swelling, and postextubation croup, whereas too small a tube will predispose to aspiration and make effective positive pressure ventilation difficult.

Although most use the new high-volume (5 to 10 cc), low-pressure cuffs, some physicians still prefer low-volume, high-pressure cuffs. The tradeoff is the lessened risk of tracheal ulceration in the former for the greater protection from aspiration in the latter. Because capillary pressure in the tracheal wall is about 30 mm Hg [50], cuff pressures approaching this figure will predispose the patient to ulceration and such complications as granuloma formation, stenosis, and membrane formation [54]. Few would advocate using high-pressure cuffs for prolonged (more than 2 hours) intubation. On the other hand, there are frequent reports of aspiration occurring with the low-pressure variety [45], and improper overinflation of these cuffs can also cause tracheal damage. Low-pressure cuffs will probably remain the mainstay of current usage, but their limitations are best remembered. In any case, it is important for all physicians to remember that endotracheal tube cuffs are designed to produce a seal in the trachea, not in the larynx, where damage to the anterior branch of the recurrent laryngeal nerve may result [55].

Laryngoscopes

A wide variety of direct laryngoscope blades and handles have been developed. The two most popular are the curved blade, or Macintosh blade, and the straight blade with a slight curve on the tip, or Miller blade (Fig. 2-8). It behooves any person who would perform endotracheal intubation to be-

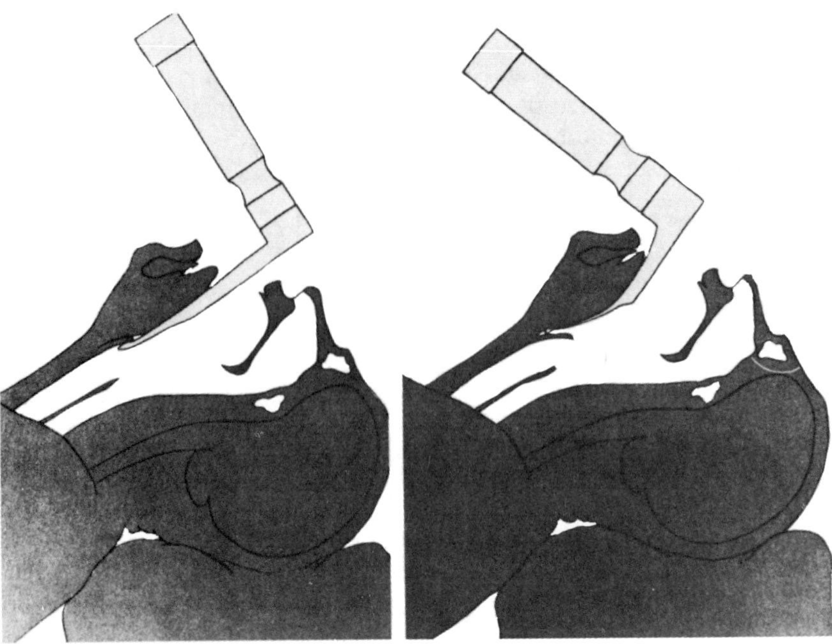

Fig. 2-8. Intubation with straight and curved laryngoscope blades. *Left,* the straight blade picks up the epiglottis and offers a better view of the larynx but causes increased stimulation and less opening of the oral and pharyngeal structures. *Right,* the curved blade is inserted in the vallecula. It offers greater widening of soft tissue structures and less stimulus, but the view may be obstructed by the epiglottis. In pediatric patients, the straight blade tip is placed in the vallecula—i.e., it is used as a curved blade. (From J. A. Dorsch and S. E. Dorsch. *Understanding Anesthesia Equipment.* Baltimore: Williams & Wilkins, 1984. With permission.)

come familiar with both of these blades. Both have advantages and disadvantages, and each offers a different approach to a potentially difficult intubation. The curved blade, the tip of which is placed in the vallecula anterior to the epiglottis, offers a wider separation of both the oral and soft palate tissues, thus giving the laryngoscopist more room to manipulate a large tube such as a double-lumen tube, or to use a device such as the Magill forceps to remove foreign bodies or place a nasotracheal tube. A drawback in using this blade is that one does not often get a good view of the vocal folds but rather only a glimpse of the arytenoid and corniculate cartilage.

The straight blade with a curved tip, the Miller blade, is placed beneath the epiglottis so that the epiglottis is actually lifted to expose the vocal cords. Although this maneuver may stimulate the glottis more than the Macintosh blade, it does offer the advantage of enabling one consistently to observe the tube pass through the cords. A disadvantage in the use of this blade is that it tends to provide a smaller opening through the soft tissue of the mouth and soft palate. Thus one may have the frustrating experience of being able to visualize the glottis well but unable to manipulate the tube into it. In pediatric patients this blade is often used in the same manner as the curved blade, i.e., it is placed in the vallecula, and the epiglottis is raised indirectly.

Both blades come in different sizes. Often the large sizes (Miller 4 or Macintosh 4) are useful in obese patients. A Miller 0 is used in infants, and a Miller 2 is often used in all patients over 1 year of age.

The inventory of laryngoscope blades is not limited to those mentioned above. There are straight blades with a curved tip, left-handed blades (used in the right hand), blades with mirrors for the anterior larynx, blades with prisms (used also for the difficult, anterior larynx), and blades with a multitude of different angles and curves. Dorsch and Dorsch [45] present an excellent review of this subject. Handles are also manufactured in a variety of styles, one of the most useful being the short handle, which can be efficacious in the patient who is extremely obese.

INTUBATION TECHNIQUE

Preparation

Fundamental to successful intubation is adequate preparation. A mnemonic useful to consider (at 4 A.M., when one is at the nadir of one's daily endogenous cortisol cycle and a combative, head-injured patient must be paralyzed and intubated) is the following: SOAP ME.

> S = Suction. Have suction ready with a tonsil or Yankauer tip. Often the few minutes it takes to assemble can mean the difference between harmless vomiting and fatal aspiration.

> O = Oxygen. Oxygen supplies should be checked and passive preoxygenation provided, which will fill the functional residual capacity of the lungs and give the patient a safety margin while the intubation takes place. Avoid positive pressure preoxygenation unless absolutely necessary, because masking a patient will predispose to increasing the stomach air bubble and subsequent vomiting. Make sure there is a modality with which positive pressure ventilation can be initiated. If one is using "E" cylinder oxygen, it must be remembered that 2200 psi = 625 liters of oxygen and that a tank with less than 500 psi will empty rapidly at 8 or 10 liters per minute.

> A = Airway. Ensure that a functioning laryngoscope (if the light fails, consider a loose bulb first, batteries second) and a properly sized endotracheal tube with a nonprotruding stylet and 10 cc syringe attached are available. Make sure the patient is

in the sniffing position if no cervical spine injury is suspected. If a cervical spine injury is suspected, keep the patient in a neutral position, and have an assistant provide either immobilization or about 10 pounds of axial traction. Finally, assuming that the patient has a full stomach, have a second assistant provide firm but nondistorting cricoid pressure.

P = Pharmacology. If one is using succinylcholine, consider a defasciculation dose of a nondepolarizing drug (see Chapters 5 and 13). Consider the patient's volume status and neurologic status, and weigh the need for sodium thiopental, narcotics, lidocaine, or ketamine. If one is using a nondepolarizing muscle relaxant such as vecuronium, it is best not to give simultaneous thiopental with it because the two form a tenacious precipitate.

ME = Monitoring Equipment. Is the ECG working? Is the O_2 saturation monitor attached (if one is available)? Is a stethoscope ready?

Orotracheal Intubation

Once preparation is complete, the patient is preoxygenated. This may be done by having the patient breathe a high FIO_2 mixture spontaneously or by gently mask-ventilating the patient with cricoid pressure to prevent stomach distention and vomiting.

At this point preparation for the extreme stimulus of laryngoscopy is considered. If the patient is awake, topical anesthesia is then administered. If the patient is combative, intravenous muscle relaxants, lidocaine, narcotics, and/or an appropriate dose of barbiturate (see Chapter 5) can be given. If the patient is in extremis or in full arrest, of course, these steps are superfluous.

Just before intubation, one should put gloves on (see Chapter 11), place a tooth guard if needed, and open the jaw with the right thumb and middle finger crisscrossed (thumb on mandibular teeth, middle finger on maxillary teeth). One then gently slides the laryngoscope blade into the right side of the mouth, sweeps the tongue to the left, places the tip of the blade either in the vallecula or under the epiglottis, depending on the blade used, and applies force upward and outward in a vector forming a 45- to 55-degree angle with the patient's trachea. After visualizing the glottic opening, the tube is gently passed, with the right hand, through the cords, the stylet is removed, the balloon inflated, and positive ventilation begun. Only when stethoscopic examination or, preferably, end-tidal CO_2 readings confirm the intratracheal position of the tube is cricoid pressure released.

Nasotracheal Intubation

There are two ways to perform intubation using this route. The first is indirect nasotracheal intubation, which normally requires a spontaneously breathing patient, although it has been done in apneic patients. Often it is facilitated by the following factors:

1. Lubrication of the nasal passage by placement of a well-lubricated nasal trumpet. If a lidocaine gel is used, nasal analgesia will also result. Gentle technique is essential even with good lubrication.
2. Administration of a vasoconstrictor, such as 1 ml of either 0.25 percent phenylephrine or 4 percent cocaine.
3. Superior laryngeal nerve blocks and topical laryngeal blocks as described in Chapter 6 (if a patient is awake and has adequate airway reflexes).

Intubation is achieved, after adequate preoxygenation and cervical spine and aspiration control measures have been instituted, by gently passing a well-lubricated tube and hearing or feeling breath sounds. When the sounds reach a maximum, the tube is passed through the cords on inspiration. If one is unable to pass the tube, the tube may be rotated, or, if the cervical spine is normal, the neck can be flexed to make the tube pass more posteriorly or extended to make it pass more anteriorly.

A second mode of nasotracheal intubation is direct laryngoscopy used in a paralyzed patient, the tube guided under direct vision with or without the aid of Magill forceps. One is admonished not to grasp the cuff with those forceps because most low-pressure cuffs are easily torn.

Nasal intubation is not without risks, the major one being failure. Although success improves with skill, apneic or near-apneic patients, those who need intubation the most, are the most difficult to intubate reliably with blind nasotracheal intubation. Other problems include initiation of gagging and vomiting, placement of the tube intracranially in a patient with craniofacial instability, epistaxis, and the eventual sequelae of maxillary or ethmoid sinusitis. Epistaxis may be especially troublesome, occurs most commonly in the presence of coagulopathy, and may be treated mechanically by compression around the tube if the intubation was successful or by withdrawing the tube and inflating the cuff in the nasal passage if it was unsuccessful. Most emergency physicians are familiar with the various balloons on the market for the control of posterior epistaxis. These can be useful for obstinate epistaxis but often require parenteral antibiotic and analgesic coverage. Treatment of coagulopathy is reviewed in Chapter 12.

A final consideration regarding nasotracheal intubation is the prevention and recognition of infectious sequelae secondary to the procedure. One reason this form of intubation is still in favor with many acute care physicians is that they do not have an opportunity to see these devastating if more chronic sequelae. Maxillary sinusitis or ethmoid sinusitis have both been associated with even modest periods of nasal intubation, especially in severely traumatized, critically ill patients [56]. Such patients are immunologically compromised, and sinusitis can rapidly lead to meningitis, cerebral venous thrombosis, and other feared sequelae if the complication is not suspected, diagnosed, and treated. Diagnosis involves unexplained fever, purulent drainage, headache, tenderness to localized facial percussion, and fluid collections noted on sinus radiographs or computed tomography (CT). Treatment includes antibiotic coverage that offers penetration of the blood-brain barrier (i.e., third-generation, not first-generation cephalosporins, aminoglycosides, or ampicillin and chloramphenicol) and replacement of the nasal tube with an oral tube or a tracheostomy.

Securing an Endotracheal Tube

Several points are important in securing a nasal or oral endotracheal tube. First, in a cardiac arrest situation, one must be very cognizant of what auxiliary personnel are doing to the tube if one has delegated taping and fixation while going on to some other more immediate task. Invariably, the tube, which should be taped at 21 cm of depth at the maxillary tooth line in females and 23 cm in males, will mysteriously migrate deeper as one is concentrating on the CVP or cardiotonic drips. The resulting endobronchial intubation can lead to severe shunting and hypoxemia. For this reason the author always tapes tubes personally. Second, an oral tube should not be fixed to the mandible, which, of course, is mobile and can thus change the depth of the tube. Third, be extremely wary of cervical circumferential fixation techniques, especially in patients in whom there is a possibility of development of increased intracranial pressure (ICP). Such fixation can restrict venous drainage and increase ICP markedly. Finally, when taping a tube in an emergent situation, the author prefers to keep the tape on the roll and hold the roll close to the skin surface as the tape is unwound. This technique is similar to the technique used in orthopedics with cast rolls and avoids tangling and confusion, both of which lose valuable time. Many prefer the newer varieties of one-half-inch plastic tape that are strong, do not slip, and yet do not form a permanent bond with the patient's skin. Use of adhesive tape is contraindicated in the geriatric population for this reason because their skin is easily traumatized.

Changing an Endotracheal Tube

In the event of cuff damage, one must often change an endotracheal tube to allow positive pressure ventilation and prevent aspiration. This can best be accomplished in the adult by using a 60-cm flexible stylet (Fig. 2-9). These devices are passed through the existing tube after adequate preoxy-

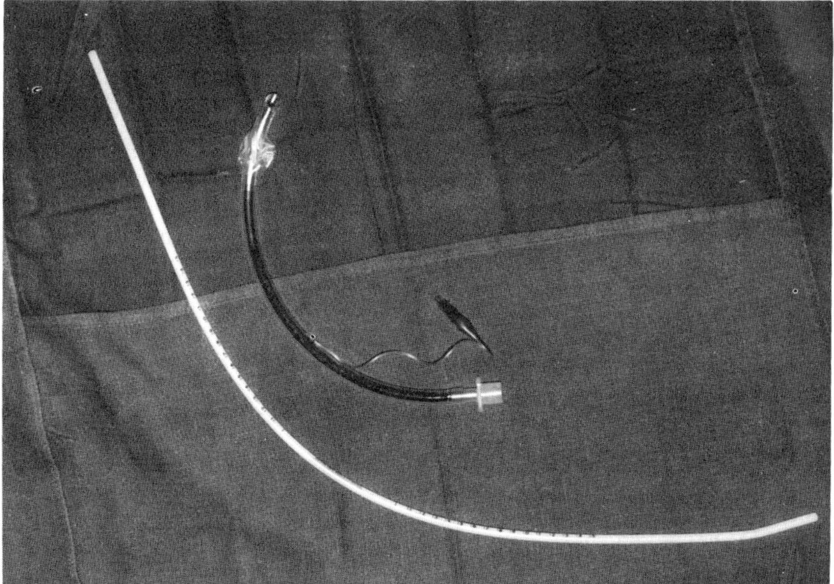

Fig. 2-9. Flexible stylet used for changing an endotracheal tube with a damaged cuff or for a difficult intubation. Shown with standard low-pressure "implantation tested" endotracheal tube.

genation, suctioning, and appropriate pharmacologic blunting of hyperadrenergic reflexes with intravenous lidocaine, narcotics, and/or sodium thiopental. The existing tube is then removed with the stylet left in place, and the new tube is passed over the stylet. Use of muscle relaxants can be helpful with this procedure. One must be prepared to perform laryngoscopy should problems occur, and aspiration prevention measures must be scrupulously followed.

Placement Verification

The gold standard of proper positioning of an endotracheal tube in the trachea, as opposed to the esophagus, is verification of CO_2 production on the end-tidal CO_2 monitor or mass spectrometer [34]. Visualization of the passage of the tube through the vocal cords (more easily done with the straight blade than the curved blade) is also confirmatory, as is visualization of tracheal rings and the carina as viewed through the flexible bronchoscope. Note well that auscultation of the precordium, while not to be neglected, is not always reliable insurance against endobronchial intubation, especially in children, in whom the small chest transmits sound from stomach ventilation very well [57], or in the obese, in whom very little sound is transmitted from any cavity. Similarly, visualization of water vapor with exhalation and "the feel of the bag" cannot be relied on. If one must rely on auscultation, it is imperative to auscultate the epigastrium as well as the precordium. One may place the stethoscope bell behind the pectoralis major muscle in the axilla because this area of the precordium has less chest wall mass and can better differentiate endobronchial intubation. If there is any doubt about the location of the tube, it is better to extubate and ventilate by mask than to wait for deoxygenation, bradycardia, and irreversible cardiopulmonary arrest. Failure to intubate the trachea is still the leading cause of major injury and death in anesthesiology [58]. Obviously, this fact makes a case for having oxygen saturation monitors available, which will show desaturation over several minutes if esophageal intubation has occurred, or, better yet, end-tidal CO_2 monitors, which will manifest failure to intubate the trachea in the space of several breaths. The electrocardiogram is *not* an adequate indicator because improper intubation will not show cardiac changes until an arrest situation has developed.

Extubation

Although the emphasis in emergency medicine centers on intubation criteria, it behooves emergency physicians also to be cognizant of safe parameters for extubation because the clinical picture may change rapidly, and continued intubation may not be in a patient's best interest. In cases of head trauma, for example, one is often faced with a choice between an extubated patient who may or may not be ventilating adequately and a paralyzed, intubated patient in whom an adequate neurologic examination is impossible. Because the middle ground of an awake, nonparalyzed intubated patient who is straining and bucking on the tube is not usually tenable, the latter scenario usually develops. But suppose that one is faced with a patient who was intubated and is now awake, has normal CT scan results, is alert, and follows commands. What are safe criteria for extubation? Consider the following parameters [24]:

1. Vital capacity of 15 ml/kg or greater (1050 ml in a 70-kg patient).
2. Minimum inspiratory negative pressure of 25 mm Hg or greater.
3. Ability to sustain head lift above the pillow for 5 seconds.
4. Ability to maintain a pH of 7.38 or greater without respirator assistance. (Note that PCO_2 is not the blood gas parameter that is necessarily followed.)
5. Absence of major organ system dysfunction, such as cardiogenic shock, renal failure, or neurologic dysfunction.

Once the decision to extubate has been reached, the patient should be preoxygenated with 100 percent oxygen for at least 3 minutes, suctioned around the tube, and extubated with exhalation. If a bag-mask setup is available, it is useful to extubate after giving a large tidal volume because mucus within the tube will be expelled with the resulting cough. Alternatively, one may suction sterilely within the tube just prior to extubation. Such suctioning can cause marked increases in heart rate, blood pressure, and intracranial pressure [59, 60]. One can ameliorate these and not impede respiratory effort greatly by administering 1 mg/kg of lidocaine intravenously just prior to the procedure.

Complication Prevention

The most common serious complication associated with endotracheal intubation, namely, failure to recognize esophageal intubation, has been discussed above. A more uncommon but potentially fatal complication is perforation of the pharynx with resultant mediastrinitis [61, 62] or perforation of the trachea with massive subcutaneous emphysema [63]. This can best be prevented by gentle technique and early abandonment of a difficult intubation attempt.

Hyperdynamic sequelae of laryngoscopy and intubation, which include tachycardia, hypertension, and increased intracranial pressure, can lead to myocardial infarction, pulmonary edema, or cerebrovascular disaster [64]. These are best prevented by adeqeuate pharmacologic preparation for intubation, for which a number of agents have been examined and used. These include sodium thiopental [65], hydralazine [66], lidocaine, either intravenous or laryngotracheal [67], beta blockers [68], including the new short-acting drug esmolol [69], nitroglycerin [70], and fentanyl [71]. Probably the safest drug among these is lidocaine; unfortunately, it is also probably the least efficacious [72].

Laryngospasm, in which both vocal folds—the "false cords"—are adducted, allowing no passage of ventilation, can result from laryngoscopy in a patient who has been inadequately anesthetized (Fig. 2-10). It probably represents a teleologic attempt on the organism's part to prevent aspiration. If one forces a tube through, one can create dangerous hemorrhage and future dangerous sequelae (granuloma, laryngeal edema, laryngotracheal membrane, and so on). Laryngospasm can be treated by patient, steady, positive pressure by mask. It is most efficaciously treated by the expeditious use of succinylcholine, 0.5 mg/kg intravenously, or 2 mg/kg intramuscularly, if no intravenous line is available. If succinylcholine is contraindicated (see Chapters 5 and 13) one might use vecuronium, 0.05 to 0.1 mg/kg. Just as some surgeons say, with gallows humor, "All bleeding stops, eventually," anesthesiologists might also say, "All laryngospasm stops, eventually." Persistence in waiting for the spasm to pass may well lead to cardiopulmonary arrest, however, and it is therefore best to treat this disorder rapidly.

Other common serious sequelae of intubation include vomiting and aspiration, and spinal cord damage in the cervical–spine fractured patient.

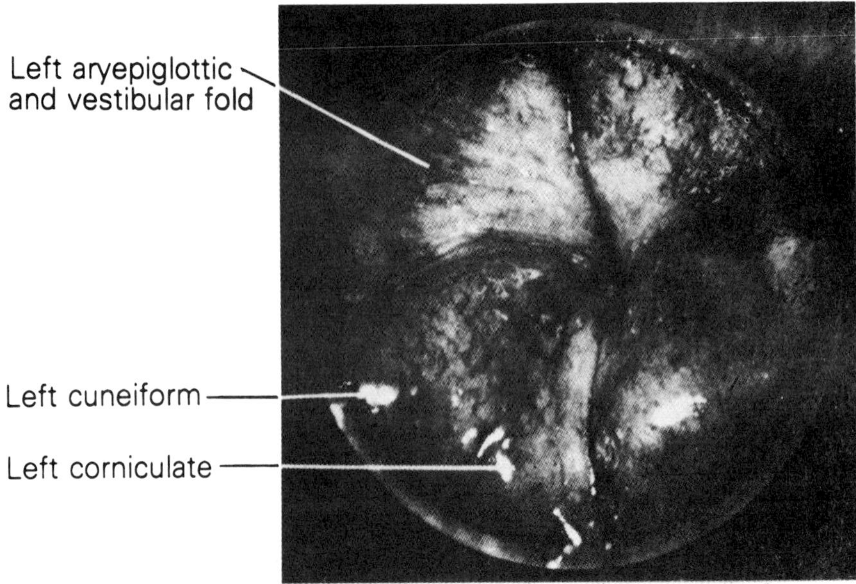

Fig. 2-10. Laryngeal spasm is shown in a photograph of the closed laryngeal entrance. The tubercle of the epiglottic cartilage has been forced up out of the picture by the laryngoscope. (From W. Becker, R. A. Buckingham, P. H. Holinger, et al. [eds.], *Atlas of Otorhinolaryngology and Bronchoesophagoscopy.* Stuttgart: G. Thieme, 1969. Photograph by Dr. Paul Holinger. Used with permission.)

Prevention of these problems was addressed above and includes axial traction or immobilization and cricoid pressure during the intubation sequence.

There remain a host of other complications from endotracheal intubation, including bacteremia, bronchial obstruction, foreign body aspiration, tracheal dilatation, meteorism (massive gastric dilatation), laryngitis, airway edema, vocal cord dysfunction and granuloma (Fig. 2-11), tracheal stenosis, laryngotracheal membrane, and subglottic cysts. These have been reviewed [73–75] elsewhere. Generally speaking, adequate training and technique, meticulous attention to positioning of the tube, and avoidance of overinflation of the cuff can avoid most of these complications. One must bear in mind that failure to intubate expeditiously can also be disastrous, as can the performance of cricothyroidotomy (see below).

THE DIFFICULT INTUBATION

Assessment

Often it is helpful to have prior warning that a patient has an anatomic or physiologic predisposition to difficult intubation. For example, if a patient has an extremely short mandible and large upper incisors, one might want

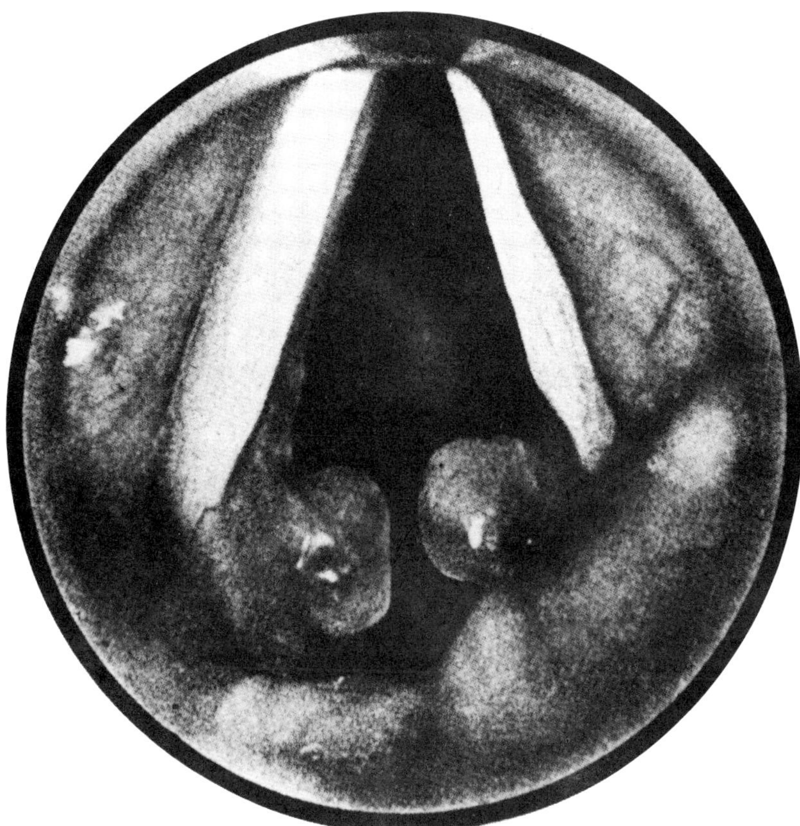

Fig. 2-11. Postintubation granulomas of the vocal folds. Their position at the junction of the ligamentous (white) and cartilaginous portions of the folds is typical. (From W. Becker, R. A. Buckingham, P. H. Holinger, et al. [eds.], *Atlas of Otorhinolaryngology and Bronchoesophagoscopy.* Stuttgart: G. Thieme, 1969. With permission.)

to use a muscle relaxant that is very short acting (e.g., succinylcholine) rather than a longer acting drug such as vecuronium. In this way the patient can be returned more quickly to spontaneous respiration should intubation prove impossible. Thus careful assessment, if possible, is necessary prior to any active intervention. Airway physical examination and evaluation should include the following areas:

1. Dentition. Protruding incisors, loose teeth that may be dislodged and aspirated, and chipped teeth should all be noted. Edentulous patients with dentures are uniformly easier to intubate and more difficult to mask ventilate. They usually require the insertion of an oral airway prior to mask ventilation.

2. Mandible. Many patients with seemingly normal appearing facies have an inability to open the jaw more than a centimeter. Such patients, if asked, will often say that their dentist complains about how difficult it is to gain intraoral access. One might consider the use of awake nasal intubation or fiberoptic bronchoscopic assistance in such patients.

Other patients have micrognathia and a very short distance between the tip of the mandible and the prominent protrusion of the thyroid cartilage or Adam's apple. Normally this distance is at least 6.5 cm or four fingertips. Should one be able to fit only three or fewer fingertips between the jaw tip and the thyroid cartilage, a difficult visualizataion of the glottis almost certainly awaits the intubating physician. One should evaluate a patient's face not just *en face* but also from the lateral aspect. This view is more apt to reveal a potential problem (Fig. 2-12).

Pediatric syndromes such as Pierre Robin syndrome (macroglossia and micrognathia) or Treacher Collins syndrome (hypoplasia of the facial, malar, and mandibular bony structures) also predispose to difficult intubation (see Chapter 8). In such patients muscle relaxants are relatively contraindicated. In adults, severe rheumatoid arthritis, burn contractures, or acromegaly can make intubation exceedingly difficult.

3. Presence of prior surgery or trauma. Following radical neck operation, burns, and other occurrences one can expect the glottal opening to be shifted by the contraction process of scar formation. A patient with a tracheostomy may or may not be intubatable from above. Usually it is best to use the tracheostomy stoma for airway management. If a tracheostomy scar is present, one should find out the reason for the procedure and consider using a smaller endotracheal tube than usual.

4. Cervical spine mobility. Limitation or instability of the cervical spine may make intubation difficult or dangerous. Patients with rheumatoid arthritis often have atlantoaxial instability, and one should try to find the limits of neck movement and whether or not such movement causes neurologic symptoms prior to intubation.

5. Presence of stridor. The hallmark of large airway obstruction, stridor should lead one to consider the presence of a foreign body (and to have Magill forceps ready) or epiglotitis or croup. Stridor plus the presence of neck trauma should alert the physician to the possibility that the airway will be edematous on laryngoscopy, and that cricothyroidotomy may be necessary.

Treatment Corollaries

As a rule, if a difficult intubation is suspected based on one's assessment, it is wisest to avoid muscle relaxants. Unfortunately for the decision-making process, they do facilitate a difficult intubation and must be considered as a treatment option. Thus they must at times be used, but one is advised to

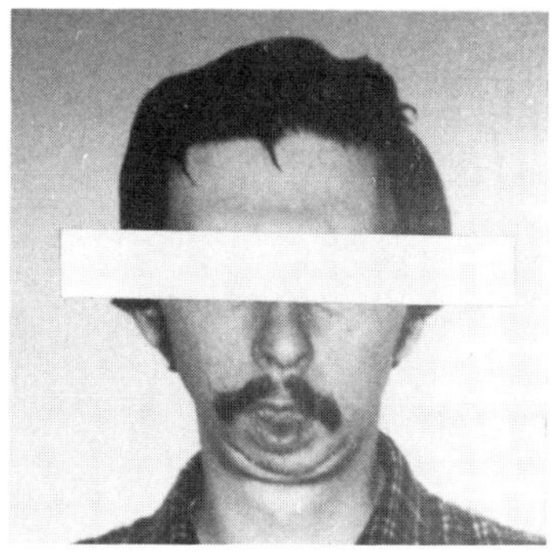 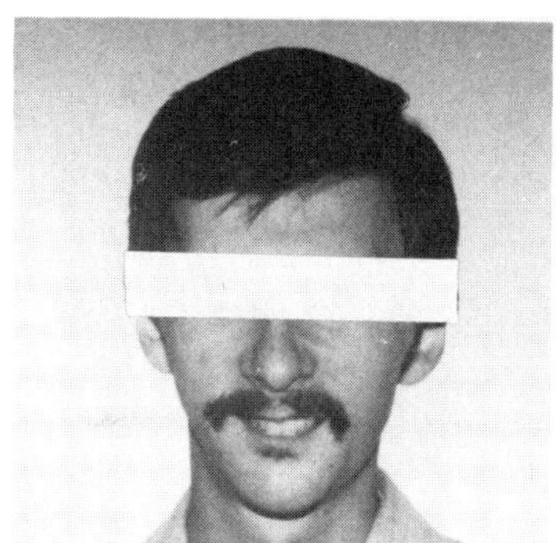

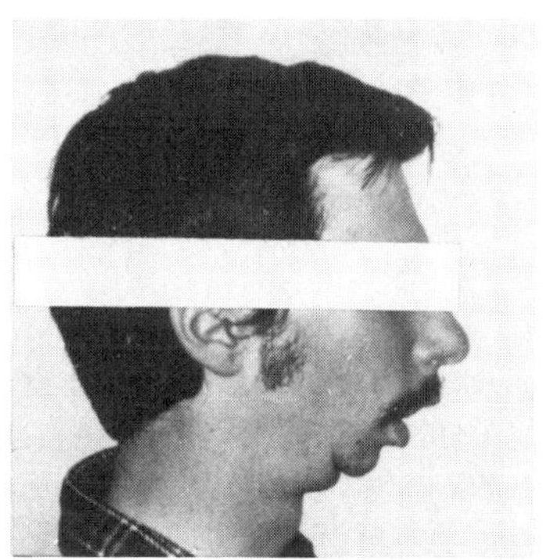 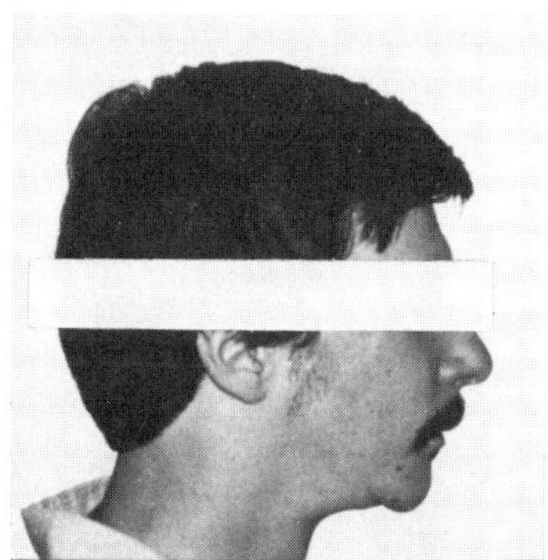

Fig. 2-12. In this patient, who had reconstructive facial surgery, the preoperative facial anatomy (*left*) demonstrates maxillary overbite and a shortened mentum-thyroid cartilage relationship. These abnormalities, which are classic representations of anatomy that predisposes to difficult intubation, are best appreciated by lateral inspection of the facies (*lower left*) and may be contrasted with the postsurgical result (*right*). Nasotracheal intubation with the patient awake was initially unsuccessful during anesthetic induction, but the airway was secured by a retrograde intubation technique (see text). (Photographs courtesy of Dr. Joel Berger, San Diego, California.)

avoid long-acting nondepolarizing agents (see Chapters 5 and 13) in such circumstances. Awake nasal, or even oral, intubation, with or without sedation and local block, is often an excellent option. A wary physician will be judicious in the use of sedatives in such patients because partial obstruction and hypoxia can lead to agitation, adding to the management difficulties. Some would use ketamine in these patients because it is a milder respiratory depressant than narcotics such as morphine [76], and many airway reflexes are retained with moderate doses (1 mg/kg). Ketamine, through release of endogenous catecholamines, also maintains blood pressure, but, unfortunately, it stimulates and increases cerebral blood flow (see Chapter

5). If neither oral intubation in the standard manner with or without muscle relaxants nor awake nasal intubation seems appropriate, one of the techniques listed below may be helpful in intubating and ventilating the patient with a difficult airway.

ALTERNATE TECHNIQUES OF INTUBATION AND VENTILATION

Fiberoptic Laryngoscopy

Although this technique takes some practice to master, it can be of great utility in intubating a patient with abnormal airway anatomy in an atraumatic fashion. It is valuable for urgent intubation but not as applicable for emergent intubation. A recent study by Delaney and Hessler showed that time requirements for successful fiberoptic laryngoscopy in the ED demonstrated a marked learning curve [77]. Initially, one should practice its use with a mannekin and then proceed to elective intubations before attempting to use the technique in a patient with abnormal anatomy. The technique is performed as follows:

1. Pretreat the patient with an antisialogogue such as glycopyrrolate, 0.2 mg IV. Prepare the fiberoptic laryngoscope by slipping a lubricated endotracheal tube over the end, focusing on an inanimate object, and verifying that the attached suction, light source, and oxygen supply are functioning. Apply antifogging solution to the scope's end, or warm the scope in warm water. Lubricate the scope, paying scrupulous attention to keeping the optical area clean.

2. Administer a superior laryngeal nerve block and laryngeal nerve block if the patient does not have a full stomach. Alternatively, topical lidocaine can be sprayed into the patient's oropharynx. Mild sedation is also helpful. Sodium thiopental and muscle relaxants are advisable only if a qualified assistant is available.

3. Pass the scope into the patient's nose or mouth (the former will show the glottis at a less acute angle) and find the epiglottis. If there is too much collapse of tissue for adequate visualization, either from oversedation or muscle relaxation, have an assistant extend the jaw or place a laryngoscope in the usual place and apply force outward at a 45 degree angle. This maneuver can usually be avoided if the patient is breathing normally.

4. Maneuver the scope through the vocal folds, check to visualize the distinctive tracheal rings, and pass the endotracheal tube to a position above the carina.

Common reasons for failure include inadequate planning and inexperience. Often a more rapid in and out motion will help the endoscopist find the landmarks. If one sees only "red," often the scope may be jammed into

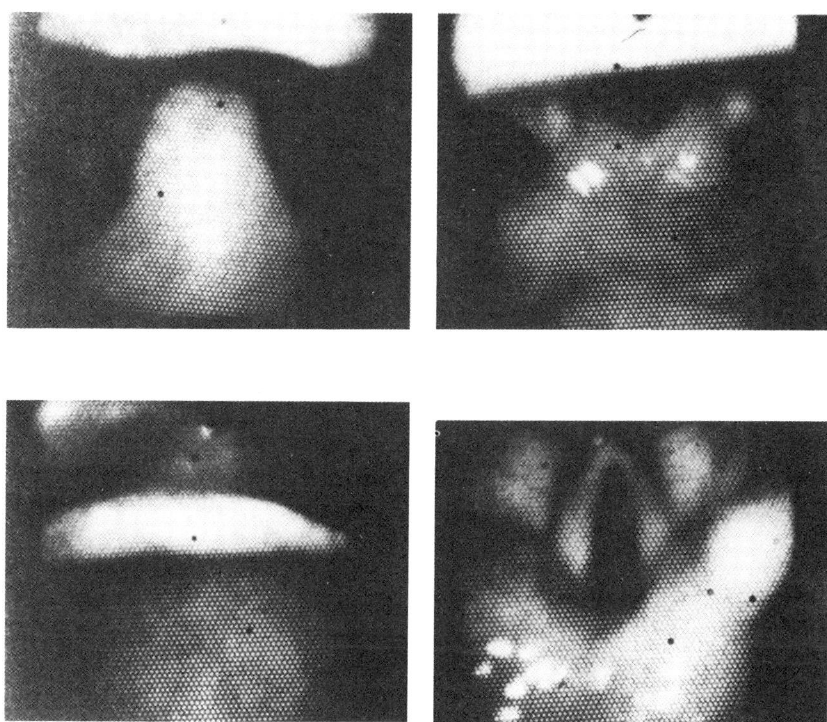

Fig. 2-13. Views of the oropharynx as seen during fiberoptic intubation sequence. In the *upper left* photograph the upper surface of the tongue and uvula are seen. As the laryngoscope enters further, the free edge of the epiglottis is seen (*lower left*), and the epiglottis, arytenoid cartilages, and posterior half of the glottis become visible (*upper right*). Finally, the glottis, with the arytenoids and vocal folds, are clearly seen (*lower right*). (From T. H. Witton. An introduction to the fiberoptic laryngoscope. *Can. J. Anaesth.* 28:475, 1981. With permission.)

the pyriform fossa. Patil et al. have prepared an excellent book on this topic [78] (Figs. 2-13 and 2-14).

Flexible or Fiberoptic Stylet

The fiberoptic stylet, with or without fiberoptic lighting, can be invaluable in a difficult intubation. In its simplest form, one simply uses the flexible stylet described earlier for changing an endotracheal tube and passes this into the glottic opening. This is a good technique to use in the glottis that can be visualized but where lack of mandibular mobility, teeth, or edema make insertion of a large tube impossible. Once the stylet is in place, it is usually a simple matter to pass over a lubricated standard endotracheal tube.

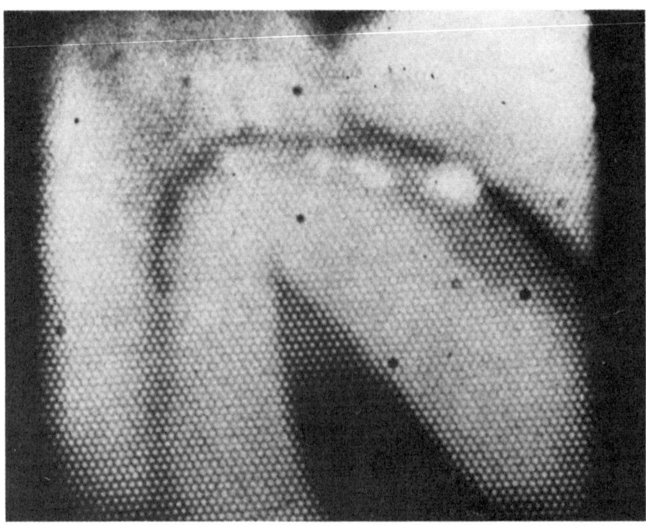

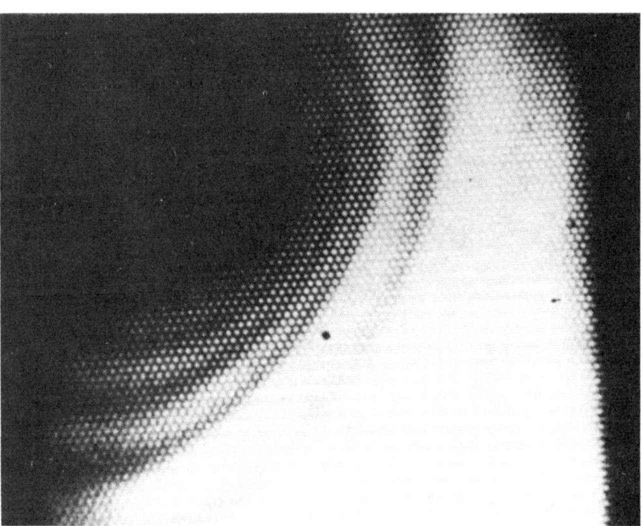

Fig. 2-14. As the fiberoptic laryngoscope is passed through the glottis, the vocal folds are seen just before the trachea is entered (*top*), and the cartilaginous rings of the trachea are visible (*bottom*). At this point in the intubation sequence, the endotracheal tube is gently threaded into the trachea and positioned above the carina confirmed, and the fiberoptic laryngoscope is removed. (From T. H. Witton. An introduction to the fiberoptic laryngoscope. *Can. J. Anaesth.* 28:475, 1981.)

Stylets with fiberoptic lighting are also manufactured and can be passed without laryngoscopy into the oropharynx. Obvious transillumination can be observed when the stylet has entered the larynx, and an endotracheal tube can be threaded as above [31, 79].

Digital Techniques

This technique, the original mode of endotracheal tube placement, has been rediscovered, especially in field use. It involves placing one's gloved index and middle fingers with the volar surface next to the patient's tongue. One simply lifts the tongue forward, palpates the epiglottis, and guides the endotracheal tube into the glottis [31, 80]. It is preferable that the patient have a bite block in place prior to performing this maneuver, and afterward, auscultation to ensure tracheal placement is a necessity.

Invasive Techniques

Techniques that involve establishing access to the airway by direct penetration through the neck into the trachea were discussed above. Obviously, when making the decision to use these techniques one must weigh the risks of hemorrhage, infection, failure of technique, and long-term sequelae such as tracheal stenosis with the risks of failure to intubate or mask ventilate (i.e., anoxic brain injury or death). These risks are outlined below. One must recognize that the decision to establish an airway invasively is extremely difficult and depends on the clinical situation as well as on the available personnel, experience, training, and equipment.

Chevalier Jackson, one of the founding fathers of otolaryngology, led the condemnation of cricothyroidotomy with his classic article in 1921, in which he warned of the sequela of subglottic stenosis [81]. In a study of 655 elective cricothyroidotomies by Brantigan and Grow in 1976 [82], not a single instance of subglottic stenosis was reported, although a 6.1 percent complication rate was reported, including 14 patients with hemorrhage. Several papers followed this report, praising the use of cricothyroidotomy in emergencies [43, 83]. The literature seems to agree that the procedure is contraindicated if previous laryngeal pathology exists because this predisposes to subglottic stenosis [84] or if the patient is a child less than 10 years of age [85]. A third obvious contraindication is a patient in whom endotracheal intubation is possible [43]. To this author's knowledge, a controlled study that compares short- and long-term outcomes in skillful initial use of oral endotracheal intubation with cricothyroidotomy in emergency patients with facial trauma, cervical spine fracture, or facial and cervical traumatic swelling has not yet been performed. In its absence, it is safe to recommend, after mask ventilation, a careful attempt at endotracheal intubation in such patients with suctioning, cervical traction, and cricoid pressure [31, 44]. If success seems unlikely, ventilation of the patient should be continued by mask if possible (realizing that distention of the stomach with air will predispose to vomiting), and percutaneous cricothyroidotomy should be performed by one of the three modalities listed above.

Retrograde Technique

A variation on the cricothyroidotomy technique involves passing a 0.21-inch central venous pressure (CVP)-type flexible guidewire or a pediatric endotracheal tube stylet through a needle placed in the cricothyroid space. This is threaded up to the oropharynx, where it is grasped and used to guide an endotracheal tube past the cords and into the trachea [86]. If severe swelling prohibits visualization of the guidewire, an 8-inch CVP catheter may be passed over the wire, and air injection can facilitate oral location.

Helium

In situations in which upper airway edema severely restricts ventilation, the use of helium as an oxygen diluent can be beneficial. This technique is based on the lesser density of helium as opposed to nitrogen [87]. Specific clinical situations in which this procedure may be considered include epiglottitis and traumatic tracheal injuries. The use of helium, however, can be considered only temporizing, and it requires maintaining inventory of a rarely used gas and prevents use of a high FiO_2. Nevertheless, its use can effect dramatic improvement in ventilation and buy valuable time for more definitive measures.

WHO SHALL INTUBATE—AND WHERE

Controversy exists when the question of airway management in prehospital care arises. As the art and science of cardiopulmonary resuscitation has advanced, there has been a trend away from the prehospital use of the esophageal obturator airway toward endotracheal intubation by paramedics in the field [88] (see Chapter 1). The stated advantages of EOA/EGTA placement are ease of insertion, lesser requirements for training and time of performance, lack of need for a laryngoscope, and safer insertion in patients with cervical trauma [89, 90]. Disadvantages include inadequate ventilation, trauma to the esophagus, and tracheal placement [47]. Endotracheal intubation offers the advantages of optimal ventilation, protection from aspiration, and placement of a route for both suctioning secretions and administering drugs [91]. Disadvantages include the greater expense and time needed for both the training and maintenance of skills in paramedic personnel, the risk of inadvertent esophageal placement, and, worse, failure to recognize such placement [92].

Although there is no question that paramedics can become skilled intubators with sufficient practice [91], it must be recognized that field conditions are much more difficult than hospital conditions, with bright daylight often making visualization difficult, and street noises making auscultation difficult. The uncontrolled positioning often found by paramedics in the victims also adds to the problem [93]. Thus it becomes obvious that intensive training in the more "benign" environment of the operating room (some anesthesiologists would argue about the benignity of the OR) is necessary to prevent patients with esophageal intubations paying for the learning curve of paramedics. Such training programs have ben successfully established [94, 95], but unrecognized esophageal intubations still occur.

Whether these risks are balanced by the increased efficacy of oxygenation achieved with the endotracheal tube remains to be shown. Goldenberg and others in St. Paul, in the first prospective, controlled, randomized study comparing field endotracheal intubation with EOA/EGTA intubation, were unable to show any real advantage in outcome between the two modalities [92]. One can look at this study in two ways, either agreeing with the authors that the EOA is really better because it is cheaper in terms of training and maintenance of skills in personnel, or, on the other hand, believing that with time, as paramedic skills and training programs improve, the known advantages of the successfully placed endotracheal tube will eventually improve outcome. Obviously, other trials need to be conducted. In the meantime, this author believes that a wise approach would be to keep the EOA/EGTA in the prehospital armamentarium and to continue to train paramedics in the use of *both* modalities. All authors agree that for a paramedic endotracheal intubation program to succeed, it is essential to maintain skills and monitor abilities closely. Supervisors must periodically ensure that excessive time is not wasted on field intubation attempts, that esophageal intubation is persistently sought with epigastic as well as precordial auscultation, and that other airway modalities such as the EOA/EGTA are used when appropriate.

As discussed in the first part of this chapter, some more innovative prehospital programs have initiated use of succinylcholine by paramedics [13]. The risk-benefit ratios of such programs await further clinical research.

CASE STUDIES

The following case studies represent some clinical airway management problems. The suggested protocols represent the author's approach to very difficult clinical problems and are not the only acceptable treatment modalities. The protocols do assume possession of certain skills and equipment. Appropriate management of seemingly similar clinical situations may require different approaches, based on local conditions and a given practitioner's experience and training. Many of the procedures and drugs discussed here will be reviewed in detail in later chapters in this volume.

TRAUMA AIRWAY PROBLEMS

Isolated Head Injury

A 22-year-old man is brought by paramedics to the ED after crashing his motorcycle. No helmet was noted at the scene. Initial vital signs were heart rate (HR) 104, blood pressure (BP) 145/94, respiratory rate (RR) 15, but on admission to the ED his pulse decreased and his blood pressure mounted. His Glasgow Coma Score (see Chapter 13) was initially 14, but he soon stopped localizing pain, would not open his eyes to any stimulus, and stopped muttering. His neck is in a stiff cervical collar. Screening physical examination reveals no other injury sites other than a large frontal hematoma, and the airway anatomy appears normal. Two large-bore intravenous lines are running wide open.

Treatment Options. Nasotracheal intubation, oral intubation with in-line traction, cricothyroidotomy.

Suggested Approach. Apply electrocardiogram (ECG) O_2 saturation monitors, and automatic blood pressure cuff. Let patient breathe high-flow O_2 spontaneously as suction and intubation materials are prepared. After one assistant applies cricoid pressure and another applies gentle in-line traction, administer 0.1 to 0.2 mg/kg of vecuronium IV, wait 10 seconds (to avoid precipitation in IV line), and give 2 to 3 mg/kg sodium thiopental IV. Slow IV fluid infusion in this patient with normal hemodynamics and wait 60 seconds. Intubate gently using Macintosh blade (to provide room for suctioning and removal of foreign material). Do not let assistant release cricoid pressure until cuff is inflated and CO_2 is noted on end-tidal CO_2 monitor. Hyperventilate and prepare for transport to CT scan area or OR. Insert an arterial line.

Blunt Multiple Trauma

A 30-year-old woman is brought to the hospital by paramedics after a motor vehicle accident that involved a fatality, a 30-minute extrication time, and a crushed steering column. The patient's vital signs are BP 80/60, HR 140, RR 24 and shallow. A MAST suit is inflated, and two IVs have been inserted. Screening examination shows head, chest, and abdominal injuries.

Treatment Options. Nasotracheal intubation, oral intubation with in-line traction, cricothyroidotomy.

Suggested Approach. Prepare patient as above. Omit sodium thiopental. Use succinylcholine 1 mg/kg IV to facilitate oral intubation if necessary or consider a nasotracheal intubation if airway anatomy appears abnormal. Do not fail to use cricoid pressure or cervical immobilization or in-line axial traction. Contraindications to the use of succinylcholine include crush injury or neurologic injury (potassium release), history of malignant hyperthermia (succinylcholine is a trigger agent), severe bradycardia (vagomimetic effect), or open eye injury (fasciculations increase intraocular pressure). This patient will need an arterial line and a CVP line. A pulmonary artery (PA) catheter may be needed depending on the extent of the thoracic injuries.

Tracheobronchial Trauma with Hemoptysis

A 28-year-old male has crashed his hang glider. Paramedics intubated the patient at the scene as he was "drowning in his secretions." As they bring the patient into the trauma room, copious blood without gastric contents is noted in the endotracheal tube. Vital signs are BP 70/50, HR 130. Physical examination shows breath sounds that are tubular and noisy bilaterally but increased on the right. There is extensive crepitus around the neck. No breath sounds are apparent in the epigastrium. Right-sided thoracic and extremity injuries predominate. Large-bore peripheral IVs have been inserted.

Treatment Options. Endobronchial intubation with present tube (which blocks the left lung field), endobronchial intubation of left lung with Robert Shaw double-lumen tube (which allows either main stem bronchus to be blocked), bronchoscopy, bilateral tube thorocostomies, emergent thoracotomy.

Suggested Approach. Suction the existing tube and pass it from the 23-cm mark at upper incisors to the 27-cm mark (to intubate the right main stem bronchus). If no change in bleeding is noted, place Macintosh blade to vallecula and examine glottis (patient is pre-arrest and may not need muscle relaxants). If unable to do so because of muscle tone, give vecuronium IV 0.1 mg/kg. While visualizing glottis, remove existing tube and place double-lumen tube in left main stem bronchus (OR training is required for safe use of double-lumen tubes). Inflate distal balloon and preferentially ventilate right lung field. If bleeding is diminished, proceed with appropriate surgical intervention (probably thoracotomy but at least tube thoracostomies and bronchoscopy). If bleeding persists (bilateral lung contusion), reintubate the patient with standard endotracheal tube and apply PEEP as tolerated. Rapid arterial line placement is essential. CVP placement is also indicated. Massive volume replacement is, of course, a sine qua non.

Penetrating Trauma

A 30-year-old male is brought to the ED with an upper chest stab wound. He is pulseless and apneic, has distended neck veins, and is warm to the touch.

Treatment Options. Orotracheal intubation, nasotracheal intubation, pericardiocentesis, tube thoracostomy, thoracotomy.

Suggested Approach. Expeditiously intubate the patient orotracheally. Check breath sounds bilaterally. Have assistants ventilate with 100 percent O_2 and begin massive intravenous volume replacement. If breath sounds are clear bilaterally, assist surgeon (if present) or perform left thoracotomy, place rib spreader, and incise pericardium (avoiding phrenic nerve—see Chapter 12). Collect intrathoracic blood in an autotransfusion device. Obtain hemostasis, suturing with pledgets if a cardiorrhaphy is indicated. If breath sounds are unilaterally diminished, decompress pneumothorax and reevaluate. Place arterial line immediately if possible, then place CVP line. Transfer to OR for definitive surgical repair.

Known Cervical Spine Fracture

An 18-year-old male is brought to the hospital by paramedics after a diving accident. He is unable to move arms or legs and has shallow ventilation; his vital signs are BP 90/60, HR 55, RR 30, and temperature (T) 33.8°C. His color is cyanotic, but diaphragmatic movement is apparent.

Treatment Options. Supply O_2, but do not ventilate. Nasotracheal versus orotracheal intubation. Cricothyroidotomy.

Suggested Treatment. In a patient with probable cervical spine fracture and cord lesion, intubation is indicated if ventilation is inadequate or if other factors demand it. In this case near-drowning is an additional diagnosis. Thus, this author would preoxygenate, support the circulation with IV fluids, and attempt nasotracheal intubation with cricoid pressure and in-line traction. Should this prove difficult, one could attempt a gentle intubation orotracheally without paralytic agents. If necessary, a drug such as vecuronium may be given with immobilization or axial in-line traction. Cricothyroidotomy would be considered a last resort in this situation. Although the slow pulse rate implies neurogenic hypotension, this author would not use sodium thiopental prior to intubation in the face of hypothermia and hypotension. Arterial line placement will also be needed.

Maxillofacial Trauma

A 50-year-old woman was the passenger in a head-on motor vehicle accident. She suffered severe maxillofacial injuries. Paramedics have placed an EOA. Vital signs are BP 110/60, HR 110, RR 24. Physical examination shows a semicomatose woman with a Le Fort III fracture and a tympanitic abdomen. The airway is bloody and partially obstructed.

Treatment Options. Orotracheal intubation, nasotracheal intubation, cricothyroidotomy, retrograde intubation.

Suggested Treatment. After the usual preparations, including preparation of suction, preoxygenation, muscle relaxants, and IV lidocaine (vital signs are ambiguous—patient may have occult abdominal or thoracic injury; thus use of sodium thiopental is dangerous despite the head injury), attempt orotracheal intubation with cricoid pressure and axial traction without muscle relaxants. If patient struggles and intubation is unsuccessful, administer 1 mg/kg succinylcholine and reattempt intubation while cricothyroidotomy tray is readied. Remove EOA after intubation and gastric suctioning. Make no more than one attempt at oral intubation if landmarks are unrecognizable and mask ventilation is difficult with succinylcholine. Perform cricothyroidotomy if the attempt fails. Nasal intubation is, of course, contraindicated with such facial injuries.

Hanging Victim

An 18-year-old man is brought to the ED after attempted suicide by hanging. His facies is cyanotic and swollen. Vital signs are BP 100/60, HR 60, and RR 4. A necktie rope is still around his neck. Paramedics have instituted cervical spine stabilization and O_2 by mask.

Treatment Options. Orotracheal intubation with cervical spine traction, nasotracheal intubation, cricothyroidotomy.

Suggested Treatment. After the usual preparation, this author would intubate orotracheally with gentle axial traction. The usual fracture found with this injury is a C2 laminar fracture with dislocation of the C2 vertebral body on C3 [96]. The cause of death in hanging is not usually cervical cord injury but asphyxiation [97]. (Captain Kidd required three hangings before his executioners were successful in achieving their desired result.) Because the mechanism of injury is fairly clear and cerebral anoxia and elevated ICP are probable, one should use sodium thiopental in a modest dose (1 to 2 mg/kg) to ameliorate any ICP rise of intubation.

MEDICAL PROBLEMS

Cardiogenic Shock

A 67-year-old man is admitted to the emergency department. Paramedics state that he was complaining of severe chest pain. They were unable to give nitroglycerin or morphine because of hypotension. Vital signs are BP 90/50, HR 110, RR 30. He is on high-flow mask oxygen and a lidocaine drip. Physical examination shows respiratory distress, frothy pink sputum, and elevated neck veins.

Treatment Options. Awake nasotracheal intubation, awake oral intubation, rapid sequence oral intubation with muscle relaxants.

Suggested Approach. This is an extremely difficult situation because cardiogenic shock patients at this stage have a very high mortality. One approach would be to continue to preoxygenate, pass a nasal trumpet with lidocaine ointment, and gently attempt an awake nasotracheal intubation. If the attempt is unsuccessful and the patient becomes agitated and unrestrainable, as is often the case in patients with hypoxia, this author would have an assistant apply cricoid pressure, give vecuronium 0.1 mg/kg, and perform orotracheal intubation. One should be wary of giving sodium thiopental or ketamine (see Chapter 5) in this situation.

Asthmatic

A 14-year-old female, observed in the ED for several hours, shows deteriorating arterial blood gas tensions. Her PCO_2 has risen from 38 to 48 mm Hg. She looks fatigued. She has had IV aminophylline bolus and drip, three beta-2 agonist aerosol treatments, subcutaneous epinephrine, steroids, anticholinergics, and oxygen therapy, all to no avail. Vital signs are BP 130/90, HR 140, RR 18 with prolonged expiratory phase.

Treatment Options. Nasotracheal intubation, awake oral intubation with or without IV agents.

Suggested Approach. Once the difficult decision to intubate has been made, the stress of the procedure in this teenager with extreme catecholamine release probably ought to be ameliorated. The author would prepare as usual for a rapid-sequence induction (SOAP ME), continue preoxygenation, use a defasciculating dose of nondepolarizing muscle relaxant (3 mg of curare, or 0.5 mg of vecuronium), and give 1 mg/kg of ketamine, followed by 1 mg/kg of succinylcholine and intubation within 60 seconds. The use of histamine-releasing drugs, such as curare or metocurine, or drugs with sulfhydryl groups, such as thiopental, is not recommended in asthmatics. Following intubation and the institution of positive pressure ventilation, one should consider the use of, first, a depolarizing muscle relaxant that has minimal histamine release, such as vecuronium, and second, an intratracheal aerosolized bronchodilating agent. Should the patient's condition continue to worsen and attempts to ventilate become more difficult, consider a transfer to the OR and use of a volatile anesthetic agent such as halothane.

Laryngeal Tumor

A 58-year-old man with a history of laryngeal tumor presents to the ED with inspiratory stridor. He is unable to speak. He is scheduled for his first radiation treatment tomorrow. Vital signs are BP 150/100, HR 100, RR 28.

Treatment Options. Attempt naso- or orotracheal intubation with or without muscle relaxants. Ventilate with helium/oxygen by mask, pending surgical assistance from the patient's ENT surgeon. Perform "stat" cricothyroidotomy.

Suggested Approach. One should be wary of intubation or any respiratory depressant drug use in this man. There is a high probability that one will be unable to force a tube past the tumor, and once a muscle relaxant, for example, is given, an unplanned and uncontrolled cricothyroidotomy might become the only method of ventilation. Because these tumors enlarge slowly over time, one could use the helium mixture, if available, and temporize, pending formal tracheostomy. Of course, if the patient acutely decompensates and become apneic, one should intubate the patient with a small diameter tube. Cricothyroidotomy could prove very difficult in such a patient with distorted anatomy but may be a last resort.

Mildly Lethargic Overdose Patient Without Gag Reflex

A 23-year-old female is admitted to the ED with a diagnosis of ingestion of a large number of diazepam pills. Her roommate states that she has been depressed and is taking some antidepressant medication. She is lethargic and is barely able to hold her head up. No gag reflex is present. Vital signs: BP 100/60, HR 78 with frequent PVCs, RR 10.

Treatment Options. Ipecac, PO. Awake intubation. Orotracheal intubation with pharmacologic support.

Suggested Approach. Obviously, intubation and tube gastric lavage is indicated. The history and premature ventricular contractions (PVCs) suggest tricyclic overdose and make any potentially myocardial depressant pharmacologic intervention dangerous. The author would go ahead with the nasotracheal intubation and hyperventilate the patient post intubation. One should perform the usual treatment for such an overdose, including gastric lavage, activated charcoal, cathartics, IV bicarbonate, and phenytoin for dysrhythmias. One should consider use of physostigmine if the above measures are not successful and the patient continues to deteriorate.

ANATOMIC PROBLEMS

Acromegalic Patient in Arrest

A 56-year-old male is found by the graveyard nursing shift to be in full arrest on the metabolic ward. He carries the diagnosis of acromegaly. Although personnel from respiratory therapy are attempting to mask the patient, they are unable to get a mask to fit. Despite numerous pages, no physician is in the house but the emergency physicians. The ED is temporarily slow, and the ED physician responds to the arrest. Despite multiple attempts at intubation, the glottis is not visible and the trachea is not intubated.

Treatment Options. Cricothyroidotomy, fiberoptic laryngoscopy, stylet intubation, retrograde intubation.

Suggested Approach. Although fiberoptic laryngoscopy, stylet intubation followed by the threading of an endotracheal tube, and retrograde intubation are all good ways to intubate such a patient in a nonemergent circumstance, such as during elective induction of anesthesia in the operating room, all these techniques require either special equipment or extra time. For a patient in cardiac arrest on the ward, such luxuries are not feasible. Consequently, in this situation this author would take one shot at an oral blind endotracheal intubation, using the largest laryngoscope blade available. If this failed, he would proceed immediately with cricothyroidotomy. The author would use a smaller tube than usual because the mucous membrane hypertrophy common to acromegaly makes the glottal opening small. Because of this patient's unusual diagnosis, metabolic causes for the arrest such as potassium imbalance, acute corticosteroid, deficiency, or hypoglycemia should be sought for and treated. See Chapter 1 for a discussion of appropriate response to cardiac arrest.

Obese Pregnant Patient

A 270-pound, 5-foot 2-inch term pregnant patient is admitted to the ED with massive vaginal hemorrhage. Her vital signs are BP 80/60, HR 130, RR 30. Paramedics have begun IV resuscitation through two large-bore IV lines. Fetal heart tones are not obtainable.

Treatment Options. Transfer to the obstetric OR. Do not transfer; resuscitate first.

Suggested Approach. This patient needs an immediate cesarean section because her bleeding is most probably due either to placenta previa or abruptio placentae. Place the patient in the left uterine tilt position to decompress her vena cava and her aorta (see Chapter 9), let her breathe oxygen spontaneously via a 100 percent rebreather mask, and take her, if possible, to the obstetric OR.

If she suffers a cardiac arrest in the ED, the standard ACLS routine must be altered as follows. Provide uterine tilt. Establish cricoid pressure immediately. Do not mask ventilate if possible because such patients are at extreme risk of aspiration. Intubate without relaxants if possible, or use succinylcholine as needed. Use a large laryngoscope blade; if unable to place the blade due to the patient's chest, use a short-handled blade, place the blade in the mouth before attaching the handle, or turn the handle laterally before inserting the blade [98]. If unable to intubate initially, mask ventilate while the assistant maintains cricoid pressure. Proceed with cesarean section if volume replacement and cardiopulmonary resuscitation (CPR) are unsuccessful in restoring vital signs (see Chapter 9).

Tracheoinnominate Fistula

A Code Blue is called overhead. On arrival at the bedside, one sees a male nurse providing vigorous CPR. The patient is on the ventilator and has had a tracheostomy. Blood is pouring into the ventilator tubing with each chest compression. No vital signs are available.

Treatment Options. Perform thoracotomy. Adjust the tracheostomy tube balloon. Perform digital compression of the innominate artery.

Suggested Approach. Bedside lateral thoracotomy in the situation of tracheoinnominate artery fistula is useless. Definitive therapy will require median strenotomy and repair or resection of the innominate artery, but to keep the patient alive pending this procedure, one can either expand the tracheostomy tube balloon to occlude the artery or perform an Utley maneuver [99]. This involves dissecting with one's finger over the trachea deep into the mediastinum, with the volar surface anterior, and then flexing the finger upward against the sternum, thereby occluding the innominate artery. Such a resuscitative measure can be highly successful, although because of the low incidence of this complication many are unaware of the diagnosis and proper treatment. In a series from Charity Hospital, ten patients had the complication in a 12-year period, and five survived, compared with only eight survivors documented prior to this in the world literature [100].

CONCLUSION

We have examined the airway and related aspects of breathing from the perspective of both the anesthesiologist and the emergency physician. In the ensuing chapters we will expand this perspective to include the organ systems and topics such as trauma, pain management, and pharmacology. In the final analysis, however, the maintenance of the airway is, and always shall be, of primary importance.

REFERENCES

1. Davis, D. D. An analysis of anesthetic mishaps from medical liability claims. *Int. Anesthesiol. Clin.* 22:31, 1984.
2. Fastow, J. Medical malpractice and emergency medicine: The crisis of the 80's. *Am. J. Emerg. Med.* 3:571–573, 1985.
3. Sellick, B. A. Cricoid pressure to control regurgitation of stomach contents during induction of anesthesia. *Lancet* 2:404, 1961.
4. Maltby, J. R., Sutherland, A. D., Sale, J. P., et al. Preoperative oral fluids: Is "NPO after midnight" justified? *Anesthesiology* 65:A244, 1986.
5. Sutherland, A. D., Maltby, J. R., Sale, J. P., et al. The effect of preoperative oral fluid and ranitidine on gastric fluid volume and pH. *Can. J. Anaesthesiol.* 34:117–121, 1987.
6. Gibbs, C. P., Modell, J. H. Aspiration Pneumonitis. In R. D. Miller (ed.), *Anesthesia* (2nd ed.). New York: Churchill Livingstone, 1986. P. 2041.
7. Tomkinson, J., Turnball, A., Robson, G., et al. Report on Confidential Enquiries into Maternal Deaths in England and Wales 1976–1978. London: Her Majesty's Stationery Office, 1982.
8. Lockhart, P., Felbau, E., and Gabel, R. Dental complications during and after tracheal intubation. *J. Am. Dent. Assoc.* 112:480–484, 1984.
9. Wood, M. D. Anesthesia claims decrease. *Anesthesia Patient Safety Foundation Newsletter.* Park Ridge, Ill. 1:23, 1986.
10. Bayne, C. G. Management of the Airway. In W. G. Baxt (ed.), *Trauma.* Norwalk, Conn.: Appleton-Century-Crofts, 1985.
11. Thompson, J. D., Fish, S., and Ruiz, E. Succinylcholine for endotracheal intubation. *Ann. Emerg. Med.* 11:526–529, 1982.
12. Roberts, D. J., Clinton, J. E., and Ruiz, E. Neuromuscular blockade for critical patients in the emergency department. *Ann. Emerg. Med.* 15:152–156, 1986.
13. Hedges, J. R., Dronen, S. C., Feero, S., et al. Succinylcholine-assisted intubations in prehospital care. *Ann. Emerg. Med.* 17:469–472, 1988.
14. Grogano, A. W. Acid-base balance. *Int. Anesthesiol. Clin.* 24:1, 1986.
15. West, J. B. *Ventilation/Blood Flow and Gas Exchange* (2nd ed.). Oxford: Blackwell, 1970.

16. Benumof, J. L., and Alfery, D. D. Anesthesia for Thoracic Surgery. In R. D. Miller (ed.), *Anesthesia.* New York: Churchill Livingstone, 1986. P. 1395.
17. Ganong, W. F. *Review of Medical Physiology* (11th ed.). Palo Alto: Lange, 1983. P. 527.
18. Sibert, K. S., Biondi, J. W., and Hirsch, N. P. Spontaneous respiration during thoracotomy in a patient with a mediastinal mass. *Anesth. Analg.* 66:904–907, 1987.
19. Braunwald, E. Cyanosis, Hypoxia and Polycythemia. In K. J. Isselbacher, et al. (eds.), *Harrison's Principles of Internal Medicine* (9th ed.). New York: McGraw-Hill, 1980. P. 166.
20. Benumof, J. L. Respiratory physiology and respiratory function during anesthesia. In R. D. Miller (ed.), *Anesthesia.* New York: Churchill Livingstone, 1986. P. 1143.
21. Fischer, R. P. Cervical radiographic evaluation of alert patients following blunt trauma. *Ann. Emerg. Med.* 13:905–907, 1984.
22. Braunwald, E. Heart Failure. In K. J. Isselbacher, et al. (eds.), *Harrison's Principles of Internal Medicine* (9th ed.). New York: McGraw-Hill, 1980. P. 1035.
23. Marlowe, F. I., and Aghamohamadi, A. Otolaryngologic Emergencies. In J. Tintinalli, R. J. Rothstein, R. L. Krome (eds.), *Emergency Medicine: A Comprehensive Study Guide.* New York: McGraw-Hill, 1985. P. 733.
24. Yao, F. S. Morbid Obesity. In F. S. Yao (ed.), *Anesthesiology.* Philadelphia: Lippincott, 1983. P. 451.
25. Sladen, A. Acid-Base Balance. In K. M. McIntyre and A. J. Lewis (eds.), *Textbook of Advanced Cardiac Life Support.* Dallas: American Heart Association, 1983. Pp. 135–140.
26. Revised standards for ACLS and CPR. *J.A.M.A.* 255:2933–2954, 1986.
27. Barker, S. J., Tremper, K. K. Hyatt, J., et al. Effects of methemoglobinemia on pulse oximetry and mixed venous oximetry. *Anesthesiology* 67:A171, 1987.
28. Eisenkraft, J. B. Pulse oximeter desaturation due to methemoglobinemia. *Anesthesiology* 68:279–282, 1988.
29. Barker, S. J. Carboxyhemoglobin and pulse oximetry. *Anesthesiology* 68:300, 1988.
30. Barker, S. J., and Tremper, K. K. The effect of carbon monoxide inhalation on pulse oximetry and transcutaneous PO_2. *Anesthesiology* 66:677–679, 1987.
31. Jones, J., Heiselman, D., Cannon, L., et al. Continuous emergency department monitoring of arterial saturation in adult patients with respiratory distress. *Ann. Emerg. Med.* 17:463–468, 1988.
32. McGuire, T. J., and Pointer, J. E. Evaluation of a pulse oximeter in the prehospital setting. *Ann. Emerg. Med.* 17:1058–1062, 1988.
33. Shapiro, H. M. Anesthesia Effects Upon Cerebral Blood Flow and Metabolism. In R. D. Miller (ed.), *Anesthesia.* New York: Churchill Livingstone, 1986. Pp. 1257–1258.
34. Birmingham, P. K. Cheney, F. W., and Ward, D. J. Esophageal intubation: A review of detection techniques. *Anesth. Analg.* 65:886–891, 1986.
35. Roizen, M. F. Smart tech, standards, egos, and the need for technology assessment. *J. Clin. Anesthesiol.* 1:51–54, 1988.
36. Eichhorn, J. H., Cooper, J. B., Cullen, D. J., et al. Anesthesia practice standards at Harvard: A review. *J. Clin. Anesthesiol.* 1:55–65, 1988.
37. White, R. D., Goldberg, A. H., and Montgomery, W. H. Adjuncts for Airway Control and Ventilation. In K. M. McIntyre and A. J. Lewis (eds.), *Textbook of Advanced Cardiac Life Support.* Dallas: American Heart Association, 1983. Pp. 39–48.

38. Paris, P. M. Airway intervention in the field. *Am. J. Emerg. Med.* 2:459–461, 1984.
39. Bass, R. R. The esophageal obturator airway: A reassessment of use by paramedics. *Ann. Emerg. Med.* 11:358–360, 1982.
40. Smith, J. P., et al. A field evaluation of the EOA. *J. Trauma* 23:317–321, 1983.
41. Auerbach, P. S., and Geehr, E. C. Inadequate oxygenation and ventilation using the esophageal gastric tube airway in the prehospital setting. *J.A.M.A.* 250:3067–3071, 1983.
42. Campbell, C. T., Harris, R. C., Cook, M. H., et al. A new device for emergency percutaneous transtracheal ventilation in partial and complete airway obstruction. *Ann. Emerg. Med.* 17:927–931, 1988.
43. Kress, T. D., and Balasubramaniam, S. Cricothyroidotomy. *Ann. Emerg. Med.* 11:197–201, 1982.
44. Gens, D. A. Cervical Soft Tissue Injuries. In R. A. Cowley, A. Conn, and C. M. Dunham (eds.), *Trauma Care.* Philadelphia: Lippincott, 1987. P. 90.
45. Dorsch, J. A., and Dorsch, S. E. *Understanding Anesthesia Equipment.* Baltimore: Williams & Wilkins, 1984.
46. Mapleson, W. W. The elimination of rebreathing in various semiclosed anesthetic systems. *Br. J. Anesthesiol.* 26:323–332, 1954.
47. Froese, A. B., Butler, P. O., Fletcher, W. A., et al. High-frequency oscillatory ventilation in premature infants with respiratory failure. *Anesth. Analg.* 66:814–824, 1987.
48. Bishop, M. J., Benson, M. S., Sato, P., et al. Comparison of high-frequency jet ventilation with conventional mechanical ventilation for bronchopleural fistulae. *Anesth. Analg.* 66:833–838, 1987.
49. Ortiz, R. M., Cilley, R. E., and Barlett, L. H. ECMO in pediatric respiratory failure. *Pediatr. Clin. North Am.* 34:39–46, 1987.
50. Stoelting, R. K. Endotracheal Intubation. In R. D. Miller (ed.), *Anesthesia.* New York: Churchill Livingstone, 1986: Pp. 523–552.
51. Snell, R. S. *Clinical Anatomy for Medical Students.* Boston: Little, Brown, 1973. Pp. 763–765.
52. Ellis, P. D. M., and Pallister, W. K. Recurrent laryngeal nerve palsy and endotracheal intubation. *J. Laryngol. Otolaryngol.* 89:823–826, 1975.
53. Katz, J. *Atlas of Regional Anesthesia.* Norwalk, Conn.: Appleton-Century-Crofts, 1985. Pp. 58–59.
54. Dobrin, P., and Canfield, T. Cuffed endotracheal tubes: Mucosal pressures and tracheal wall blood flow. *Am. J. Surg.* 133:562–568, 1987.
55. Mehta, S. Guided orotracheal intubation in the operating room using a lighted stylet. *Anesthesiology* 66:105, 1987.
56. Walsh, T. J., and Caplan, A. S. Use of antibiotics in the traumatized and critically ill patient. In R. A. Cowley, A. Conn, and C. M. Dunham (eds.), *Trauma Care: Medical Management.* Philadelphia: Lippincott, 1987. Pp. 51–70.
57. Uejima, T. Esophageal intubation (Letter). *Anesth. Analg.* 66:481–482, 1987.
58. Keehan, R. L., and Boyan, C. P. Cardiac arrest due to anesthesia: A study of incidence and causes. *J.A.M.A.* 253:2373–2377, 1985.
59. Rudy, E. B., Baun, M., Stone, K., et al. The relationship between endotracheal suctioning and changes in intracranial pressure: A review of the literature. *Heart Lung* 15:488–494, 1986.
60. White, P. F., Schlobohm, R. M., Pitts, L. H., et al. A randomized study of drugs for preventing increases in intracranial pressure during endotracheal suctioning. *Anesthesiology* 57:242–244, 1982.
61. O'Neill, J., Giffin, J., and Cottrell, J. Pharyngeal and esophageal performation following endotracheal intubation. *Anesthesiology* 60:487–488, 1984.

62. Johnson, K., and Hood, D. Esophageal perforation associated with endotracheal intubation. *Anesthesiology* 64:281–283, 1986.

63. Orta, D. A., Cousar, J. E., Yergin, B. M., et al. Tracheal laceration with massive subcutaneous emphysema. *Thorax* 34:655–669, 1979.

64. Fox, E. J., Sklar, G. S., Hill, C. H., et al. Complications related to the pressor response to endotracheal intubation. *Anesthesiology* 47:524–525, 1977.

65. Unni, V. K. N., Johnston, R. A., Young, H. S. A., et al. Prevention of intracranial hypertension during laryngoscopy and endotracheal intubation. *Br. J. Anaesthesiol.* 56:1219–1223, 1984.

66. Davies, M. J., Cronin, K. D., and Cowie, R. W. The prevention of hypertension at intubation. *Anaesthesia* 36:147–152, 1981.

67. Hamill, J. F., Bedford, R. F., Weaver, D. C., et al. Lidocaine before endotracheal intubation: Intravenous or laryngotracheal? *Anesthesiology* 55:578–581, 1981.

68. Farnon, D., and Curran, J. Beta-receptor blockade and tracheal intubation. *Anaesthesia* 36:803–805, 1981.

69. Murthy, V. S., Patel, K. D., Elangovan, R. G., et al. Cardiovascular and neuromuscular effects of esmolol during induction of anesthesia. *J. Clin. Pharmacol.* 26:351–357, 1986.

70. Hood, D. D., Dfwan, D. M., James, F. M., et al. The use of nitroglycerin in preventing the hypertensive response to tracheal intubation in severe preeclampsia. *Anesthesiology* 63:329–332, 1985.

71. Martin, D. E., Rosenberg, H., Aukberg, S. J., et al. Low-dose fentanyl blunts circulatory response to tracheal intubation. *Anesth. Analg.* 61:680–684, 1982.

72. Chraimmer-Jorgensen, B., Hoilung-Carlson, P. F., Marving, J., et al. Lack of effect of intravenous lidocaine on hemodynamic responses to rapid sequence induction of general anesthesia: A double-blind controlled clinical trial. *Anesth. Analg.* 65:1037–1041, 1986.

73. Blanc, V., and Tremblay, N. The complications of tracheal intubation: A new classification with a review of the literature. *Anesth. Analg.* 53:202–213, 1974.

74. Bishop, M., Meymuller, E., and Fink, B. Laryngeal effects of prolonged intubation. *Anesth. Analg.* 63:335–342, 1984.

75. Kastanos, N., et al. Laryngotracheal injury due to endotracheal intubation: Incidence, evolution and predisposing factors. *Crit. Care Med.* 11:362–367, 1983.

76. Bourke, D. L., Malit, L. A., and Smith, T. C. Respiratory interactions of ketamine and morphine. *Anesthesiology* 66:153–156, 1987.

77. Delaney, K. A., and Hessler, R. Emergency flexible fiberoptic nasotracheal intubation: A report of 60 cases. *Ann. Emerg. Med.* 17:919–926, 1988.

78. Patil, V. U., Stehling, L. C., and Zauder, H. L. *Fiberoptic Endoscopy in Anesthesia.* Chicago: Year Book, 1983.

79. Fox, D. J., Castro, T., and Rastrelli, A. J. Comparison of intubation techniques in the awake patient: The flexilum surgical light vs. blind nasal approach. *Anesthesiology* 66:69–71, 1987.

80. Stewart, R. D. Tactile orotracheal intubation. *Ann. Emerg. Med.* 13:175–178, 1984.

81. Jackson, C. High tracheotomy and other errors: The chief causes of chronic laryngeal stenosis. *Surg. Gynecol. Obstet.* 32:392–398, 1921.

82. Brantigan, C. O., and Grow, J. B. Cricothyroidotomy: Elective use in respiratory problems requiring tracheotomy. *J. Thorac. Cardiovasc. Surg.* 71:72, 1976.

83. Toye, F. J., and Weinstein, J. D. Clinical experience with percutaneous tracheostomy and cricothyroidotomy in 100 patients. *J. Trauma* 26:1034–1040, 1986.

84. Brantigan, C. O., and Grow, J. B. Subglottic stenosis after cricothyroidotomy. *Surgery* 91:217–221, 1982.

85. Sise, M. J., et al. Cricothyroidotomy for long-term tracheal access. *Ann. Surg.* 200:13–17, 1984.

86. Riou, B., Barriot, P., Bodenan, P., et al. Retrograde intubation in trauma patients. *Anesthesiology* 67:A130, 1987.

87. Benumof, J. L., and Alfery, D. D. Anesthesia for Thoracic Surgery. In R. D. Miller (ed.), *Anesthesia,* New York: Churchill Livingstone, 1986. P. 1444.

88. Smith, J. P., and Bodai, B. I. The urban paramedic's scope of practice. *J.A.M.A.* 253:544–548, 1985.

89. Meislin, H. W. The esophageal obturator airway: A study of respiratory effectiveness. *Ann. Emerg. Med.* 9:54–59, 1980.

90. Smith, J. P., Bodai, B. I., Seifkin, A., et al. The esophageal obturator airway. *J.A.M.A.* 250:1081–1084, 1983.

91. Pepe, P. E., Copass, M. K., and Joyce, T. H. Prehospital endotracheal intubation: Rationale for training emergency medical personnel. *Ann. Emerg. Med.* 14:1085–1092, 1985.

92. Goldenberg, I. F., Campion, B. C., Siebold, C. M., et al. Esophageal gastric tube airway vs endotracheal tube in prehospital cardiopulmonary arrest. *Chest* 90:90–96, 1986.

93. Mackey, J. A. New technique for field intubation. *Ann. Emerg. Med.* 12:408, 1983.

94. Guss, D. A., and Poslusky, M. Paramedic orotracheal intubation: A feasibility study. *Am. J. Emerg. Med.* 2:399–401, 1984.

95. Stewart, R. D., Paris, P. M., Pelton, G. H., et al. Effect of varied training techniques on field endotracheal intubation success rates. *Ann. Emerg. Med.* 13:1032–1036, 1984.

96. Schneider, R. C. High Cervical Injuries. In R. H. Wilkins and S. S. Rengachary (eds.), *Neurosurgery.* New York: McGraw-Hill, 1985. Pp. 1701–1708.

97. Boyarsky, A. H., Flancbaum, L., and Trooskin, S. Z. The suicidal jailhouse hanging. *Ann. Emerg. Med.* 17:537–539, 1988.

98. King, H. K., Wang, L. F., and Khan, A. K. A modification of laryngoscopy technique. *Anesthesiology* 65:566, 1986.

99. Utley, J. R., Singer, M. M., Roe, B. B., et al. Definitive management of innominate artery hemorrhage complicating tracheostomy. *J.A.M.A.* 220:557, 1972.

100. Jones, J. W., Reynolds, M., Hewitt, R. L., et al. Tracheo-innominate erosion: Successful surgical management of a devastating complication. *Ann. Surg.* 184:194–204, 1976.

3. Pulmonary Considerations

Thomas G. Karagianes

This chapter is predicated on the idea that knowledge of normal and pathologic pulmonary physiology, when coupled with an understanding of the effects of treatment, provides the optimal approach to the diagnosis and management of pulmonary disorders. An overview of clinically important physiology will be presented, focusing on the most vital function of the lungs, gas exchange. The first two sections will discuss hypoxemic and hypercarbic pulmonary dysfunction. Selected aspects of positive airway pressure and mechanical ventilation will follow. The final section offers an approach to specific clinical problems by utilizing the information on physiology provided in previous sections to demonstrate the correlation between the physiology and treatment of pulmonary disorders.

IMPAIRED OXYGENATION AND HYPOXEMIA

Abnormalities of gas exchange are best viewed as dysfunctions in oxygenation (hypoxemia) or ventilation (hypercarbia). Although both may coexist, the therapeutic approach is facilitated by separate assessment. The causative factors of impaired oxygenation and hypoxemia in general will be addressed.

LOW $\dot{V}/\dot{Q}$

The matching of ventilation ($\dot{V}$) and perfusion ($\dot{Q}$) is quite complex. A dynamic interplay between such factors as pulmonary compliance and resistance, transpulmonary pressure, gravity, cardiac output, pulmonary vascular characteristics, body position, mode of ventilation, and lung volumes determines the $\dot{V}/\dot{Q}$ ratio.

Ideally, ventilation and perfusion are matched with a homogeneous coupling of alveolar ventilation and pulmonary capillary perfusion ($\dot{V}/\dot{Q} = 1$). To a degree, $\dot{V}/\dot{Q}$ inequality exists in the normal lung, principally as a result of the gravitational dependence of both ventilation and perfusion. Relative hypoperfusion of the apices and hyperperfusion of the dependent lung regions exists in the upright position. At its two extremes, $\dot{V}/\dot{Q}$ mismatch will result in intrapulmonary shunt ($\dot{V}/\dot{Q} = 0$) or dead space ventilation ($\dot{V}/\dot{Q} = \infty$). Low $\dot{V}/\dot{Q}$ units ($\dot{V}/\dot{Q} < 1$) produce hypoxemia as a result of decreased ventilation relative to perfusion. Varying degrees of low $\dot{V}/\dot{Q}$ units and intrapulmonary shunt are present in almost all hypoxemic pulmonary disorders.

Lung volumes are an important determinant of $\dot{V}/\dot{Q}$ matching. Functional residual capacity (FRC) is the volume of the lung at end expiration. End-inspiratory volume (EIV) is the volume at the end of inspiration and represents the sum of the FRC and tidal volume ($\dot{V}_T$). Closing capacity (CC) is the sum of the residual volume of the lung and the closing volume and can be viewed as the volume below which airway closure occurs. Closing ca-

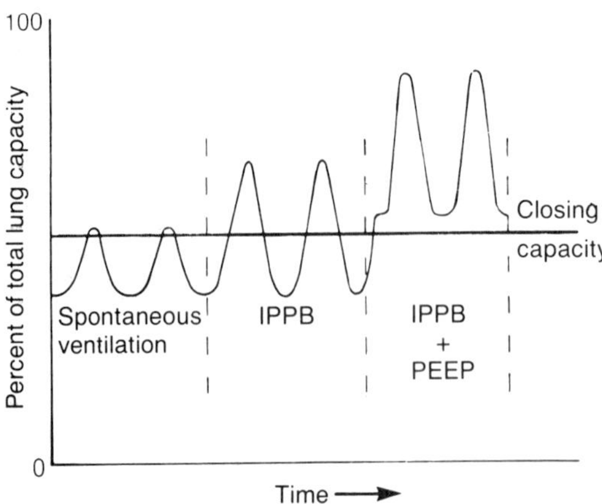

Fig. 3-1. Low $\dot{V}/\dot{Q}$ unit during spontaneous ventilation. Ventilation is improved as tidal volume is increased with intermittent positive pressure breathing (IPPB) or by mechanical ventilation in general. Positive end-expiratory pressure (PEEP) increases FRC to above closing capacity, establishing the normal relationship and allowing oxygen transfer during the entire respiratory cycle. (From J. L. Benumof. *Anesthesia for Thoracic Surgery.* Philadelphia: Saunders, 1987. With permission.)

pacity is increased by smoking, supine position, advanced age, and obesity. FRC is reduced in many situations (e.g., after general anesthesia) and many disorders (e.g., pulmonary edema). The relationship between FRC, EIV, and CC is crucial in determining ventilation, or gas flow into a certain lung region. Normally, FRC exceeds CC, and gas exchange will occur during the entire respiratory cycle. Low $\dot{V}/\dot{Q}$ units, typified by EIV > CC > FRC, spend only a portion of the respiratory cycle "open" (above CC), resulting in diminished ventilation (inadequate inspiratory oxygen delivery) relative to perfusion. This situation can be offset by an increased FiO_2 (fractional inspired oxygen concentration), which will maintain an adequate PaO_2 (partial pressure alveolar oxygen) for oxygen transfer until the next influx of oxygen. The number and severity of low $\dot{V}/\dot{Q}$ units will determine the degree of hypoxemia and consequently the level of FiO_2 required to correct it. If the EIV is below the CC, ventilation is absent, and an intrapulmonary shunt is present. Besides treatment of the underlying disease, therapy is aimed at increasing the FRC, possibly with the use of positive end-expiratory pressure (PEEP) or continuous positive airway pressure (CPAP). Increasing the tidal volume and reducing the closing capacity are further therapeutic objectives (Fig. 3-1).

Low $\dot{V}/\dot{Q}$ units are not exclusively a result of a reduced FRC. In chronic obstructive pulmonary disease (COPD) and asthma, FRC is typically increased above closing capacity. However, low $\dot{V}/\dot{Q}$ units are an important cause of hypoxemia in these patients. The inadequate ventilation arises primarily from an increased resistance secondary to bronchospasm or airway narrowing from secretions or chronic structural abnormalities. Application of CPAP or PEEP is usually not appropriate, and therapy is aimed at cautiously increasing the FIO_2, reducing airway resistance, and treating the acute decompensating event.

Hypoxic pulmonary vasoconstriction (HPV) is the lung's attempt to reduce perfusion to underventilated (inadequate PAO_2) regions by producing vasoconstriction in lung units with alveolar hypoxia. This results in better $\dot{V}/\dot{Q}$ matching and a higher PaO_2. Drugs known to inhibit HPV, thus potentially increasing $\dot{V}/\dot{Q}$ mismatching, include nitroprusside, nitroglycerin, calcium channel antagonists, beta agonists, and inhalational anesthetics. Pulmonary hypertension also reduces the effectiveness of HPV.

The gravitational influence on $\dot{V}/\dot{Q}$ matching can be exploited in patients with nonhomogeneous, typically unilateral, disease. For example, a patient with a left-sided pulmonary contusion would be expected to show improvement in PaO_2 when the noninjured right lung is placed in a dependent position. Pulmonary blood flow is increased much more than ventilation is reduced, thus shifting blood flow to the "good" lung and improving oxygenation.

INTRAPULMONARY SHUNT

Excluding the normal anatomic shunts (e.g, thebesian veins) and intracardiac shunts (e.g., cyanotic congenital heart disease), only the intrapulmonary shunt will be discussed. This shunt is the primary mechanism of hypoxemia in pneumonia, pulmonary edema, and atelectasis. Intrapulmonary shunt is that fraction of the cardiac output that is delivered to nonventilated ($\dot{V}/\dot{Q} = 0$) lung units and thus is not exposed to alveolar oxygen. Obviously, increasing the FIO_2 will not influence the PO_2 of the shunted fraction of blood. Indeed, the PaO_2 response to FIO_2 helps differentiate $\dot{V}/\dot{Q}$ mismatch from shunt. Figure 3-2 shows the PaO_2 response to increasing FIO_2 at varying degrees of shunt. Even small degrees of shunt have a pronounced effect on PaO_2, whereas the effect on $PaCO_2$ is minimal despite a shunt of 50 percent (Fig. 3-3). This disparity reflects the difference in dissociation curves between oxygen and carbon dioxide and explains the profound effect of a main stem intubation on PaO_2 but not $PaCO_2$.

ABNORMAL DIFFUSION

Abnormal diffusion of oxygen across the alveolar-capillary membrane is another cause of impaired oxygenation. Fick's law governing gas flow is:

$$\text{Gas flow} = D(P_1 - P_2)$$

where D is the diffusing capacity of the lung and P_1 and P_2 are the alveolar and pulmonary capillary oxygen partial pressures, respectively. Clinically,

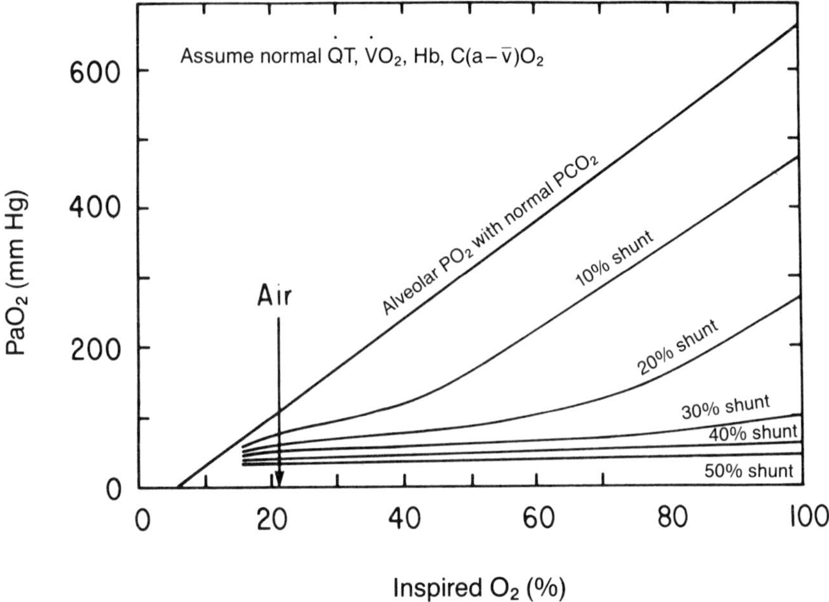

Fig. 3-2. Effect of changes in FiO$_2$ on PaO$_2$ for various degrees of pulmonary shunt. (From J. L. Benumof. *Anesthesia for Thoracic Surgery.* Philadelphia: Saunders, 1987. With permission.)

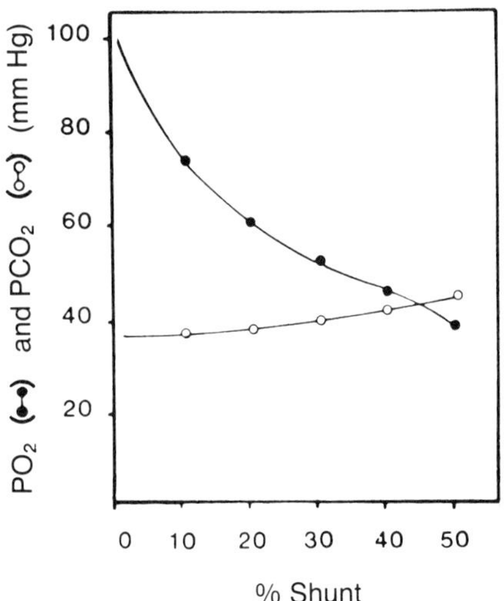

Fig. 3-3. Effect of increasing shunt on PaO$_2$ and PaCO$_2$. (From D. R. Dantzker. *Chronic Obstructive Pulmonary Disease.* New York: Churchill Livingstone, 1983. With permission.)

diffusion impairment is rare and of little importance, particularly in view of the ease of correction by increasing the FiO_2 (increased P_I).

REDUCED P_AO_2

P_AO_2 is derived from the simplified alveolar gas equation:

$$P_AO_2 = FiO_2(P_B - PH_2O) - P_ACO_2/R$$

where P_B = barometric pressure, PH_2O = water vapor pressure (47 mm Hg at 37°C), and R is the respiratory quotient and is typically 0.8. $PaCO_2$ may be substituted for P_ACO_2 (alveolar carbon dioxide partial pressure). Examination of the equation offers three possibilities for a reduced P_AO_2 and consequently hypoxemia. Alveolar hypercarbia secondary to hypoventilation will displace alveolar oxygen in accord with the alveolar gas equation. The P_AO_2 must decrease as the P_ACO_2 increases, resulting in a fall in PaO_2. The hallmark of this situation is hypercarbia and a normal alveolar-to-arterial oxygen difference indicative of unimpaired oxygenation. High altitude reduction in barometric pressure will reduce the P_AO_2, which can be mitigated by an increased FiO_2. Hypoxic gas mixtures ($FiO_2 < .21$) may result from equipment malfunction or the inadvertent breathing of an excessively high concentration of nitrous oxide.

NONPULMONARY CONTRIBUTION

The mixed venous blood that passes through the intrapulmonary shunt with no change in oxygen content mixes with that fraction of cardiac output exposed to alveolar oxygen. Mixed venous oxygen partial pressure ($P\bar{v}O_2$) will thus influence the PaO_2, the degree of which is directly proportional to the amount of shunt. $P\bar{v}O_2$ is a function of cardiac output, oxygen consumption, and arterial oxygen content. A reduction in PaO_2 may result from a reduced $P\bar{v}O_2$ and therefore will not reflect a worsening of pulmonary pathology. As a therapeutic corollary, PaO_2 can be increased in patients with a significant shunt by factors that increase the $P\bar{v}O_2$ such as an increase in cardiac output and arterial oxygen content or a reduction in oxygen consumption.

MONITORING

Arterial blood gas analysis remains the gold standard for assessment of oxygenation. However, noninvasive monitors have decreased the need for blood gases in many situations. Pulse oximetry has revolutionized oxygen saturation monitoring (see Chapter 2). Adjustments in FiO_2 or PEEP can be approached with greater safety by using pulse oximetry. The shape of the oxygen dissociation curve dictates that a major disturbance in oxygenation may go undetected during elevated FiO_2 breathing because saturation and not partial pressure of oxygen is measured.

Transcutaneous PO_2 ($tcPO_2$) monitoring is invaluable in monitoring neonates, in whom good correlation exists between $tcPO_2$ and PaO_2. Transcutaneous PO_2 is dependent on hyperemic dermal perfusion arising from local hyperthermia. Adults have thicker keratin layers and fewer dermal capillaries, both of which impair $tcPO_2$ accuracy. Since $tcPO_2$ is perfusion or flow dependent, any change in flow resulting from a reduction in cardiac output or local hyperemia will affect the measurement, thereby limiting its utility in tracking PaO_2 in critically ill adults.

Oxygenation Indices

It is clinically useful to have a means of quantifying the impairment in oxygenation and a method for comparing PaO_2 values obtained at different FiO_2 levels. For example, it is intuitively difficult to ascertain whether a PaO_2 of 87 at FiO_2 of 0.35 indicates a change in oxygenation when compared to a PaO_2 of 116 at FiO_2 of 0.5. Further, an index capable of estimating the PaO_2 when the FiO_2 is changed is useful.

The difference between alveolar and arterial oxygen partial pressures ($P(A-a)O_2$) is a time-honored approach to assessment of oxygenation. Its popularity has declined somewhat because it requires calculation of the alveolar gas equation and because as FiO_2 is increased, a significant artifactual increase in the gradient develops [1, 2].

A more accurate index of oxygenation is the PaO_2/PAO_2 ratio [1]. It remains fairly constant over a wide range of FiO_2 levels, although some inaccuracy occurs at FiO_2 levels below 0.3, particularly if significant areas of low $\dot{V}/\dot{Q}$ exist [3]. The normal ratio is greater than .75. The PaO_2/FiO_2 ratio has the advantage of being simple to calculate and more constant than $P(A-a)O_2$ as FiO_2 varies [2]. It ignores $PaCO_2$, but changes in $PaCO_2$ are typically small.

Oxygen consumption, cardiac output, and balance between shunt and low $\dot{V}/\dot{Q}$ regions are some of the factors that can affect these ratios, and therefore a change in the ratio is not always indicative of a change in oxygenation. It is important to stress that the ratios are not a substitute for documentation of an adequate PaO_2 after a change in FiO_2.

Shunt Fraction

Calculation of $\dot{Q}s/\dot{Q}T$ is an important assessment of impaired oxygenation. The shunt fraction is the percentage of the cardiac output not exposed to alveolar oxygen. If the measurements are obtained at FIO_2 levels below 1.0, low $\dot{V}/\dot{Q}$ regions will also contribute to the shunt value. $\dot{Q}s/\dot{Q}T$ is obtained from the equation:

$$\dot{Q}s/\dot{Q}T = \frac{CcO_2 - CaO_2}{CcO_2 - C\bar{v}O_2}$$

where

CcO_2 = pulmonary and capillary O_2 content,

CaO_2 = arterial O_2 content, and

$C\bar{v}O_2$ = mixed venous O_2 content

Oxygen content (CO_2), expressed as volumes percent (milliliters per deciliter), is obtained from the equation:

$$O_2 \text{ content} = 1.39 \times Hgb \times \% \text{ Sat} + 0.0031 \times PO_2$$

Pulmonary end-capillary oxygen content is calculated by inserting the PAO_2 obtained from the alveolar gas equation and the saturation obtained from the oxygen dissociation curve. Saturation of arterial and mixed venous blood is usually measured with a co-oximeter. This calculation requires sampling of mixed venous blood from the pulmonary artery, typically via the distal port of a pulmonary artery catheter, thereby limiting its use.

In summary, tracking response to therapy and estimating the PaO_2 as the FIO_2 is changed requires more than a comparison of PaO_2 values. The $\dot{Q}s/\dot{Q}T$ calculation is not practical in many clinical situations. $P(A-a)O_2$ and PaO_2/PAO_2 both require solving the alveolar gas equation; however, the latter is more accurate and stable over a wide range of FIO_2 levels. The PaO_2/FIO_2 ratio offers ease of calculation and good accuracy in most situations. If significant differences in $PaCO_2$ exist amongst the comparison points, then the PaO_2/PAO_2 ratio should be utilized.

By substituting the numbers given in the example cited above under Oxygenation Indices, the use of the PaO_2/FIO_2 ratio can be demonstrated:

$$87/0.35 = 249 \text{ and } 116/0.5 = 232$$

The smaller number indicates a decrement in oxygenation. The estimated PaO_2 after a change in FIO_2 can be obtained by rearranging the ratio to:

$$PaO_2 = \frac{\text{previous } PaO_2}{\text{previous } FIO_2} \times \text{present } FIO_2$$

VENTILATORY DYSFUNCTION AND HYPERCARBIA

Ventilatory or hypercarbic failure is generally viewed and defined as inadequate ventilation, or "not enough breathing," which is a major oversimplification of a complex situation. It is actually the dynamic interplay of the ventilatory capability, ventilatory requirement, and work of breathing that determines the adequacy of ventilation.

VENTILATORY CAPABILITY

Movement of inspiratory and expiratory gas volumes in the lungs (breathing) is necessary for CO_2 removal. Since the lungs themselves are incapable of moving gas in and out of the air spaces, a ventilatory pump exists to perform this function. The primary components of the ventilatory pump are the controller (medullary respiratory centers), the nervous system (spinal cord, phrenic and peripheral nerves), the muscles of ventilation (respiratory muscles), and the skeletal component (rib cage) (Table 3-1).

Abnormal control of breathing is manifested by a reduced ventilatory drive (typically, respiratory rate) in response to a potent stimulus (hypercarbia). The classic example is a narcotic overdose patient with a diminished respiratory rate secondary to a "right shifted" CO_2 response curve.

Loss of neural stimulation of the ventilatory muscles will reduce ventilatory capability. Acute spinal cord injury represents disruption of innervation to the ventilatory muscles, the degree of which is dependent on the level of the injury. Neurologic diseases such as amyotrophic lateral sclerosis, Guillain-Barré syndrome, and neuromuscular junction abnormalities typified by myasthenia gravis will predispose to ventilatory pump failure.

Thoracic skeletal abnormalities reduce ventilatory capability. Kyphoscoliosis impairs thoracic expansion and increases the work required for expansion. Flail chest represents an acute reduction in ventilatory pump function. Ventilatory muscle contraction normally results in the thorax "moving up and out," generating the negative pleural pressure necessary for inspiration. Since the flail segment is not fixed, it is incapable of providing the supporting structure for the respiratory muscles during inspiration, and it also demonstrates paradoxical inspiratory motion in response to negative pleural pressure.

Primary muscle diseases represent a rare cause of ventilatory failure. However, fatigue of the ventilatory muscles, which may be deconditioned, atrophic, or inefficient, is a very frequent cause of ventilatory failure. The diaphragm has an optimal length (stretch) that will produce the greatest tension [4] (Fig. 3-4). Under- or overstretching occurs with lung hyperinflation or abdominal distention, respectively, and will change the diaphragm configuration and stretch, thereby reducing its strength. Abdominal distention will also impair diaphragmatic excursion, further decreasing ventilatory capability and predisposing to fatigue.

Table 3-1. Components of the ventilatory pump with representative abnormalities

---

Medullary respiratory center
  Drugs
  Altered receptor input
Spinal cord
  Cervical cord injury
  Amyotrophic lateral sclerosis
Peripheral nervous system
  Guillain-Barré syndrome
  Phrenic nerve paresis
Neuromuscular junction
  Myasthenia gravis
  Muscle relaxants
Muscles
  Fatigue
  Nutritional depletion
  Suboptimal stretch
Thoracic skeleton
  Flail chest
  Kyphoscoliosis
Abdomen
  Distention
  Reduced compliance

See text for discussion.

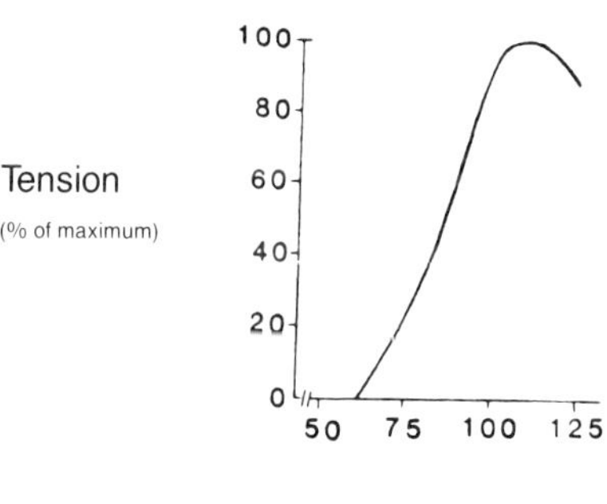

Fig. 3-4. Length-tension relationship of skeletal muscle (e.g., diaphragm). (From M. J. Tobin. Assessment of Pulmonary Function in Critically Ill Patients. In W. B. Shoemaker, et al. [eds.], *Textbook of Critical Care* [2nd ed.]. Philadelphia: Saunders, 1989. With permission.)

Evaluation of ventilatory muscle function is difficult and represents an area of increasing research. The commonly used bedside ventilatory parameters of vital capacity and maximal inspiratory pressure are subject to significant variation and represent only the situation at a "point in time." In weaning studies, little correlation is noted between successful weaning and the above parameters [5–7]. This result is not unexpected because such measurements partially evaluate only one of the three important determinants of a patient's ventilatory potential.

Observation of breathing patterns provides important information about the ventilatory pump and is frequently overlooked. During inspiration, the thorax and abdomen normally expand in a synchronous manner. Paradoxical motion of either is a clue to an abnormality of the pump. With intact thoracic innervation but phrenic nerve dysfunction, the abdomen paradoxically moves inward with inspiration and outward with expiration. Acute cervical cord injury that spares phrenic nerve function results in thoracic paradox, as the negative pleural pressure generated by the diaphragm moves the lax thorax inward. Thoracic paradox is also observed with upper airway obstruction as negative intrathoracic pressure is generated in an inspiratory effort. Associated with paradoxical thoracic motion is the "tracheal tug," in which the suprasternal trachea is "tugged" downward by the negative pleural pressure (see Fig. 2-2).

There is an ongoing search for better indicators of ventilatory muscle fatigue than tachypnea (sensitive, not specific) or the late (too late) point of hypercarbia. Use of the accessory muscles of ventilation implies a taxed ventilatory pump. Asynchronous thoracoabdominal movement and "respiratory alternans" (alternating thoracic/abdominal paradox) have been observed in patients with early muscle fatigue [8, 9]. The importance of the bedside evaluation of breathing patterns in providing valuable information cannot be overemphasized.

The ventilatory muscles perform the work of breathing. The chance of ventilatory muscle failure is a function of the interplay between (1) the amount of work, (2) the condition and efficiency of the muscles, and (3) the adequacy of oxygen and substrate delivery to the muscles.

Oxygen Demand and Supply

Normally, the ventilatory muscles require only 2 to 5 percent of the total oxygen consumed to perform the work of breathing. However, as the work and the frequency (minute ventilation) with which this work must be performed are increased, the oxygen cost of breathing may rise to 25 percent or greater of the total oxygen consumption [10]. In animal studies assessing blood flow to various vascular beds, it was noted that as cardiac output was decreased, the blood flow to other organs including the brain fell before blood flow to the diaphragm was reduced [11]. The implication is that in states of diminished oxygen delivery, usually resulting from a reduced cardiac output, some organs may experience inadequate oxygen delivery. Since total oxygen delivery is the product of cardiac output and arterial oxygen content, arterial desaturation and anemia will also act to decrease delivery. Other factors (e.g., intra-abdominal pressure) may also influence diaphragmatic blood flow. Inadequate oxygen supply and the resultant ventilatory muscle weakness may be a fairly common cause of acute ventilatory failure. Therapeutic extrapolations would lead to the institution of mechanical ventilation, thereby relieving the patient of the oxygen cost of breathing and increasing oxygen availability to other organs.

As the oxygen cost of breathing is increased, more cardiac work is necessary to deliver this oxygen. In patients with coronary artery disease, ischemia is directly linked to cardiac work. It has been noted that the degree of ventilatory support is inversely related to the degree of ST-segment depression in patients with coronary artery disease and acute respiratory failure [12]. This observation underscores the interplay between oxygen cost of breathing and oxygen delivery. The therapeutic advantage of performing the work of breathing via mechanical ventilation must be considered and counterbalanced with the hemodynamic effects of tracheal intubation and mechanical ventilation in certain cardiac conditions such as coronary artery disease and congestive heart failure.

VENTILATORY REQUIREMENT

The rate in liters per minute at which the ventilatory pump must move the gas volumes is the ventilatory requirement, i.e., the minute ventilation ($\dot{V}_E$). As $\dot{V}_E$ increases, the chance of ventilatory failure is enhanced. Increased CO_2 production ($\dot{V}CO_2$) or increased dead space ventilation ($\dot{V}_D$) will require a higher minute ventilation. This follows from the equations:

$$PaCO_2 = \frac{\dot{V}CO_2}{\dot{V}_A}$$

and

$$\dot{V}_A = \text{alveolar ventilation} = \dot{V}_E - \dot{V}_D$$

Isolating $\dot{V}_E$:

$$\dot{V}_E = \frac{\dot{V}CO_2}{PaCO_2} + \dot{V}_D$$

For a given $PaCO_2$, increases in $\dot{V}CO_2$ or $\dot{V}_D$ will elevate the necessary minute ventilation. The relationship between $\dot{V}_D$ and $\dot{V}_E$ for various $PaCO_2$ levels is shown in Figure 3-5.

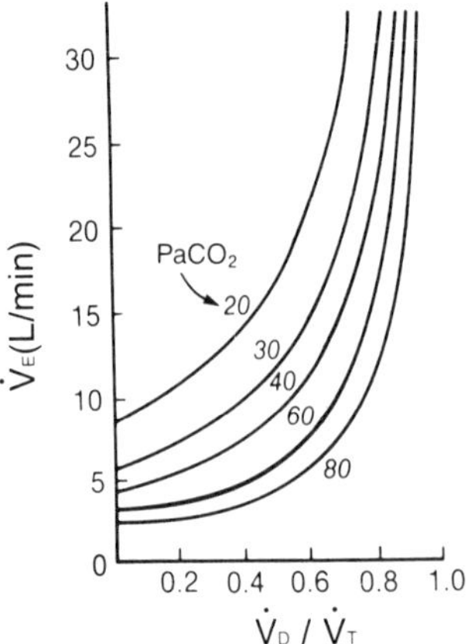

Fig. 3-5. Relationship between $\dot{V}_D/\dot{V}_T$ and $\dot{V}_E$ for various $PaCO_2$ levels. In patients with high $\dot{V}_D/\dot{V}_T$, a significantly lower $\dot{V}_E$ is necessary to maintain a higher $PaCO_2$, thus partially explaining the hypercarbia of advanced COPD. (From J. L. Benumof. *Anesthesia for Thoracic Surgery.* Philadelphia: Saunders, 1987. With permission.)

Dead Space Ventilation

Dead space ventilation does not participate in gas exchange and reflects that portion of the inspiratory volume in airways without alveoli or in alveoli with diminished or absent pulmonary capillary perfusion relative to ventilation (high $\dot{V}/\dot{Q}$ or $\dot{V}/\dot{Q} = \infty$). The relationship between airway pressure and pulmonary arterial and venous pressures will determine blood flow to a lung region and thus $\dot{V}/\dot{Q}$ matching. A reduction in pulmonary artery pressure will result in hypoperfusion of ventilated lung regions and accounts for the increased $\dot{V}_D$ associated with low cardiac output. If airway pressure is greater than pulmonary vascular pressures, then perfusion is limited and $\dot{V}_D$ will rise. A complete discussion of this topic (i.e., zones of the lung) is beyond the scope of this chapter.

The Bohr equation offers quantitation of dead space ventilation as the dead space to tidal volume ratio:

$$\dot{V}_D/\dot{V}_T = \frac{PaCO_2 - P_ECO_2}{PaCO_2}$$

where $PaCO_2$ is substituted for P_ACO_2 and P_ECO_2 is the partial pressure of mixed expired carbon dioxide. Substituting the partial pressure of end-tidal CO_2, ($PetCO_2$), which is usually obtained from a capnograph, for P_ECO_2 will lead to an approximation of physiologic dead space in most circumstances. An acute increase in the arterial to end-tidal PCO_2 difference ($P(a-et)CO_2$), which is normally less than 5 mm Hg, may be useful because it reflects increased physiologic dead space. This fall in $PetCO_2$ may be the first indication of an air embolus. Pulmonary emboli of any type will impair perfusion and thus increase physiologic dead space. There are, however, many other reasons for an increase in $P(a-et)CO_2$ (e.g., COPD), thereby reducing its specificity.

The correlation between the $PetCO_2$ and $PaCO_2$ is dependent on many variables, the most important of which are the degree of lung disease (e.g., high $\dot{V}/\dot{Q}$ units), airway pressures, and the cardiovascular status (pulmonary perfusion pressure). Care must be taken not to assume that $PaCO_2$ equals $PetCO_2$ or that a fixed difference between the two is constant (e.g., $PaCO_2 = PetCO_2 + 4$) and then adjust minute ventilation utilizing the $PetCO_2$ measurement. The correlation between $PaCO_2$ and $PetCO_2$ may be quite variable in patients with respiratory failure, and therefore, $PetCO_2$ is probably best utilized as an approximation of $\dot{V}D/\dot{V}T$ rather than $PaCO_2$ [13].

Carbon Dioxide Production

Carbon dioxide production is the other determinant of the ventilatory requirement; it increases for a number of reasons in acutely ill patients. Hyperthermia, agitation, increased muscular activity, and elevated "stress" hormone levels all elevate $\dot{V}CO_2$ and consequently $\dot{V}E$.

The volume of CO_2 produced ($\dot{V}CO_2$) per oxygen consumed ($\dot{V}O_2$) is reflected in the respiratory quotient, $R = \dot{V}CO_2/\dot{V}O_2$. The R values vary between carbohydrate (1), protein (0.8), and lipid (0.7). R in excess of 1 may result if carbohydrate is converted to lipid. A greater lipid to carbohydrate ratio in nutritional formulations will reduce CO_2 production, a benefit for patients with diminished alveolar ventilation [14].

WORK OF BREATHING

Work, defined as the product of force and distance, can be modified for ventilation work to the product of pressure times volume ($W = P \times V$). In other words, ventilation work equals the pressure change (transpulmonary pressure) necessary to move a volume of gas. The determinants of the work of breathing are the resistance to gas flow and the elasticity of the lungs and extrapulmonary structures (thorax and abdomen).

Resistance

Airway resistance is inversely related to the fourth power of the radius, making size of the airways the most important determinant of resistance. Resistance is also affected by flow rate and increases further as flow changes from laminar to turbulent. Total resistance is the sum of patient, ventilator, and circuit resistance.

Bronchial narrowing (e.g., bronchospasm) and secretions, by reducing airway caliber and causing turbulent flow, are the most important patient

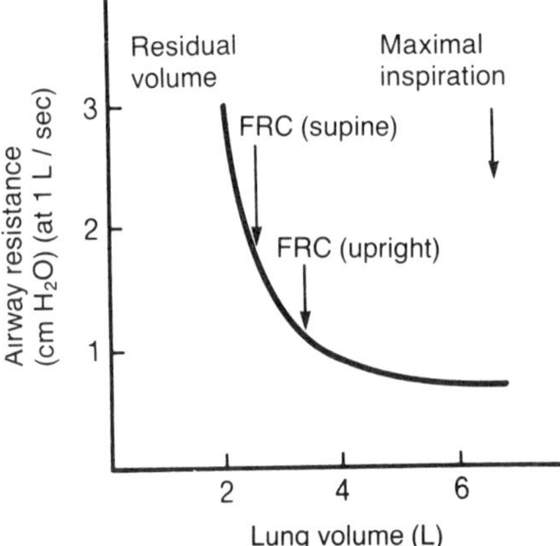

Fig. 3-6. Airway resistance is reduced as lung volumes are increased, as in changing from a supine to an upright position. (From J. L. Benumof. *Anesthesia for Thoracic Surgery.* Philadelphia: Saunders, 1987. With permission.)

causes of increased resistance. Small lung volumes also increase resistance (Fig. 3-6). Small endotracheal tubes or tubes that are partially occluded by secretions or kinking can significantly increase the work of breathing. The resistance of various endotracheal tubes as a function of flow rate is noted in Figure 3-7.

Compliance

Compliance, defined as the change in volume per change in pressure ($\Delta V/ \Delta P$), is a direct function of elastance and is the clinical estimate of the work necessary to overcome elastic forces of the lung and chest wall (total compliance). The more inelastic (less compliant) the lungs are, the greater will be the pressure necessary to inflate them (Fig. 3-8). Inelasticity of the extrapulmonary structures, chest wall, and abdomen, will also increase the work of breathing. In most clinical situations, it is the inelastic "stiff" lungs that increase the work of breathing, not inelastic extrapulmonary structures. However, this latter situation must be considered in certain clinical situations, such as marked chest wall edema, thoracic burn eschar, or significant abdominal distention. The separation of pulmonary from extrapulmonary compliance involves the measurement of pleural pressure.

Measurement

Work of breathing can be obtained from the integral, $W = \int PdV$; however, solving the equation requires the use of elaborate instrumentation. Oxygen cost of breathing, obtained by subtracting the $\dot{V}O_2$ with full ventilatory sup-

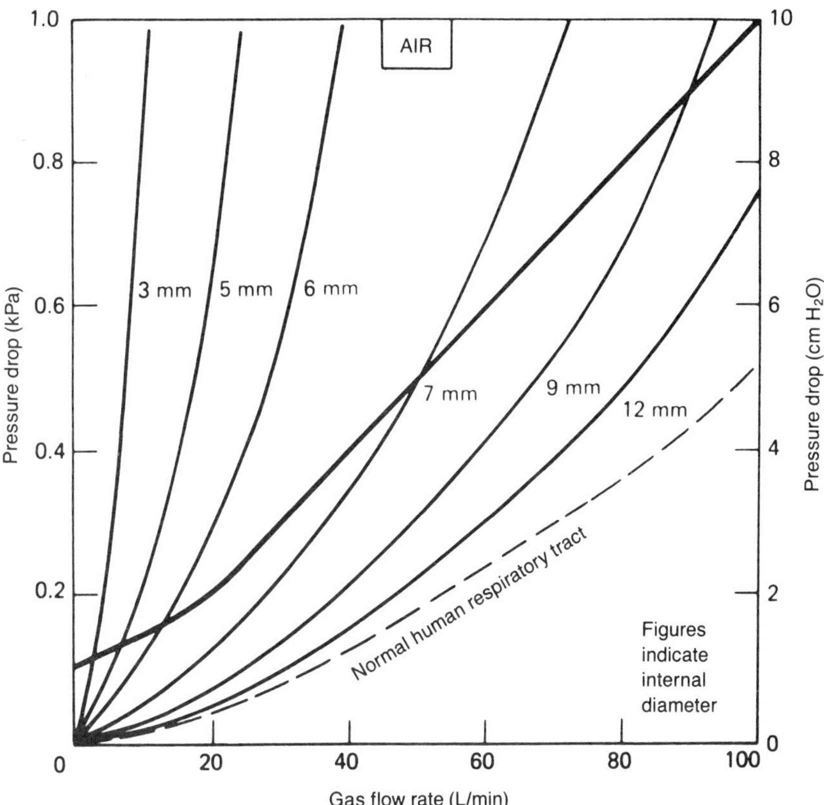

Fig. 3-7. Resistance of various endotracheal tubes can be obtained by dividing the pressure drop by the gas flow rate. Flow rate is commonly expressed in liters per second; therefore, the above flow rate may be divided by 60. The darkest line represents the suggested upper limit of resistance for adults. (From J. F. Nunn. *Applied Respiratory Physiology* [3rd ed.]. London: Butterworths, 1987. With permission.)

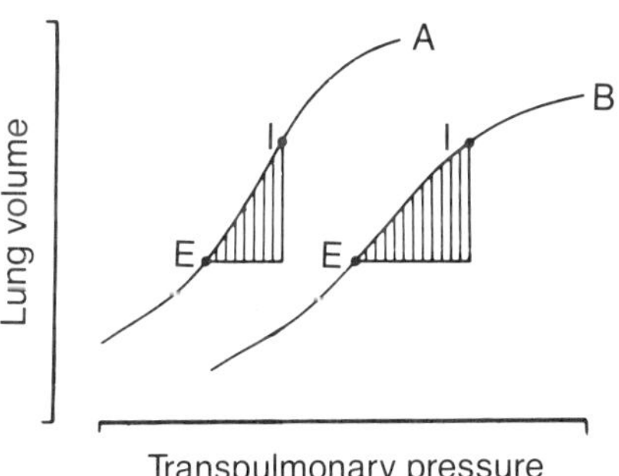

Fig. 3-8. Curve B represents a reduction in compliance such as might result from an acute lung injury. The amount of work involved in increasing the lung volume from the end exhalation volume (E) to the end inspiratory volume (I) is shown by the hatched area. (From J. B. Downs. Airway Pressure Support. In J. M. Civetta, R. W. Taylor, and R. R. Kirby, [eds.], *Critical Care.* Philadelphia: Lippincott, 1988. With permission.)

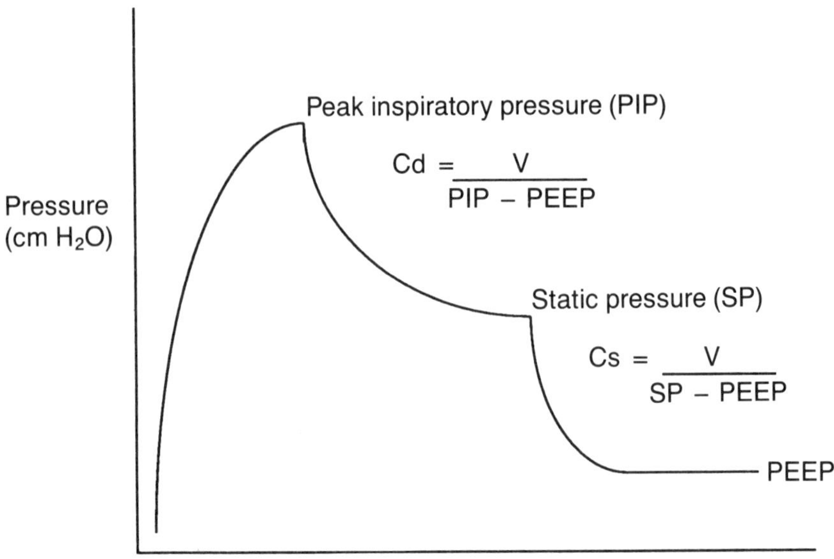

Fig. 3-9. Equations for dynamic (Cd) and static (Cs) compliance. See text for complete explanation. Normal static compliance for mechanically ventilated patients is about 50 to 85 ml per cm H_2O. The higher number reflects the use of muscle relaxants (i.e., by increasing chest wall compliance). Normal dynamic compliance is not firmly established; however, it averages about 60 ml per cm H_2O in anesthetized patients receiving muscle relaxants.

port from the $\dot{V}O_2$ during spontaneous ventilation, is also not practical for a number of reasons.

Fortunately, the work of breathing is rather easily estimated in mechanically ventilated patients. Calculation and comparison of dynamic and static compliances will approximate the work of breathing and allow separation into elastic and resistance work. The compliance equations, normal values, and a stylized airway pressure trace are noted in Figure 3-9. To obtain the static pressure (SP) measurement necessary for the static compliance calculation, the inspired volume is held in the lungs for at least 0.5 seconds by utilizing the inspiratory pause or plateau control on the ventilator or by occluding the expiratory limb of the circuit. The volume is the delivered tidal volume, not the set tidal volume on the ventilator, and is usually measured with a spirometer. Compression loss in expanding the ventilator circuit tubing prevents the use of the set tidal volume. Dynamic compliance is a function of both resistance and elastance, whereas static compliance is determined only by elastance. Therefore, the difference between the two is a function of increased resistance, provided peak flow rates are not elevated. The peak inspiratory pressure (PIP) to static pressure difference (PIP – SP) is an easy bedside estimate of resistance. If PIP and SP are both elevated, then reduced compliance is present; however, if only PIP is elevated, increased resistance is indicated. Resistance may also be calculated using the equation R = PIP − SP/flow. Flow must be constant during the measurement, necessitating square wave flow generation.

CONCLUSION

Ventilatory failure arises when the ventilatory pump is unable to provide adequate alveolar ventilation. As the ventilatory requirement and the work of breathing increase, the ventilatory pump is taxed. It is the interplay of these three factors that determine the risk of ventilatory failure. Therapy is directed at reducing resistance and elastic work, decreasing ventilatory requirement, and improving the capacity of the ventilatory pump, which may require mechanically supported ventilation to allow the pump to rest and provide time for implementation of other therapeutic interventions.

MECHANICAL VENTILATION, PEEP, AND CPAP

Mechanical ventilation is typically utilized to function as the ventilatory pump, but it will also improve oxygenation in many circumstances. PEEP and CPAP are commonly employed to improve FRC, compliance, and oxygenation. Defined goals and an understanding of the physiology and side effects of mechanical ventilation, PEEP, and CPAP are necessary for appropriate use of these modalities. A detailed discussion of mechanical ventilators is beyond the scope of this chapter, and therefore only a few clinically useful points will be addressed; pressure, time cycled, and high-frequency ventilators are excluded.

VENTILATOR MODE

The degree of ventilatory support desired is an important aspect in selecting the mode of ventilation. Is the goal complete rest of the ventilatory pump, or is partial support indicated? The control mode is full support, without a machine response to a patient's futile attempts at inspiration. Assist/control guarantees the set number of mechanical breaths and assists patient-initiated breaths with a set tidal volume. It provides a varying degree of ventilatory muscle rest, depending on patient inspiratory effort and ventilator characteristics. It has been demonstrated that in the assist mode, significant amounts of work are performed with each inspiratory effort [15]. Intermittent mandatory ventilation (IMV) can be viewed as two parallel ventilator circuits, one for spontaneous and the other for mechanical ventilation. Patient work of breathing is related to the amount of spontaneous ventilation.

Pressure support, or pressure assist ventilation, is a fairly recent ventilator mode. With initiation of each inspiratory effort, the patient receives a pressure assist to a set level, which reduces inspiratory work of breathing. The greater the work of breathing, the more pressure support is necessary. The interplay between the patient's inspiratory capability, work of breathing, and level of pressure support determines the respiratory rate and tidal volume. This mode is not suitable for patients who lack satisfactory initiation of inspiratory effort.

Mechanical ventilation results in a greater impairment in cardiac output than spontaneous ventilation in most circumstances. Patients with a reduced cardiac output as a result of hypovolemia may benefit from the IMV mode, in which a portion of the ventilation is spontaneous. This mode assumes, of course, that the patient is capable of supplying part of the minute ventilation. The degree of ventilatory support is therefore balanced with cardiovascular status in selecting a ventilator mode.

VENTILATOR-IMPOSED WORK

The amount of inspiratory and expiratory work imposed by the ventilator is frequently overlooked. Most volume ventilators contain a demand valve that must be "opened" by patient inspiratory effort to obtain gas flow. The resistance of these valves can impose a considerable work burden to patients [16]. If inspiratory flow is delayed or insufficient to meet the patient's peak flow, then work of breathing is further increased. Decreasing the sensitivity of the sensitivity control valve in the assist/control mode will also increase patient work. Work is also necessary to overcome the resistance of the expiratory valves of the ventilator [17, 18].

I : E RATIO

The relationship of inspiratory (I) to expiratory (E) time as a function of the total respiratory cycle is the I : E ratio. During mechanical ventilation, the I : E ratio is primarily a function of respiratory rate, peak flow rate, tidal volume, and flow generation pattern. Attention to the ratio is important but is commonly ignored. A COPD patient would benefit from a prolonged expiratory time, which would allow time for alveolar emptying, which in turn is usually prolonged by the loss of elastic recoil and increased resistance. In adult respiratory distress syndrome (ARDS), oxygenation may be improved by increasing the inspiratory time, presumably by allowing the alveolus to spend more time above the closing capacity, resulting in an increase in ventilation.

TRANSPORT VENTILATORS

Mechanically ventilated patients frequently require intrahospital transport and are often manually ventilated during transport, resulting in significant variation in minute ventilation and consequently $PaCO_2$. A reduction in ventilation in a patient with intracranial hypertension may have disastrous consequences.

Patients requiring high airway pressures, PEEP, and high FiO_2 to maintain oxygenation cannot be effectively ventilated manually. The risk of a disturbance in ventilation or oxygenation in such patients is great. Dysrhythmias and blood pressure fluctuations have been demonstrated during transport in which manual ventilation is employed [19]. Patients requiring close control of $PaCO_2$ and those with a significant abnormality in oxygenation should be transported using a portable transport ventilator.

PEEP AND CPAP

PEEP and CPAP produce alveolar splinting and recruitment, thereby increasing FRC and explaining the beneficial effect of these modalities in acute restrictive (low FRC) lung disease. The effect is directly proportional to compliance and presents a potential problem in situations with nonhomogeneous pathology. Consider the patient with unilateral aspiration pneumonia. Increasing PEEP levels will preferentially increase the FRC and possibly the pulmonary vascular resistance (PVR) of the normally compliant lung. The increased PVR may shift pulmonary blood flow to the diseased lung. Rarely, differential ventilation and PEEP via a double-lumen tube and two ventilators is required to overcome this problem.

Numerous approaches for adjusting PEEP exist. PEEP has been titrated to (1) a reduction in FiO_2 to a "nontoxic" range (e.g., FiO_2 of less than 0.5), (2) a $\dot{Q}s/\dot{Q}T$ of less than 20 percent, (3) the optimal point of oxygen delivery, (4) optimum compliance, and (5) a narrowing of the $P(a-et)CO_2$. The most commonly utilized approach is probably a combination of choices (1) and (3). PEEP is increased, usually leading to a reduction in FiO_2, and if oxygen delivery is reduced secondary to a diminished cardiac output, volume loading and/or inotropic therapy is instituted.

Knowledge of the effect of PEEP and CPAP on FRC should prevent it being used in pathologic conditions characterized by an elevated FRC. The FRC of COPD or asthmatic patients is frequently elevated, occasionally to 80 percent of the total lung capacity. Inappropriate use of PEEP or CPAP in these situations may cause oxygenation to become worse, decrease cardiac output, and increase work of breathing.

The effect of PEEP or CPAP on the inspiratory work of breathing is primarily a function of its effect on pulmonary compliance. The lung is least compliant at both low and high lung volumes. Therefore, if PEEP or CPAP increases FRC to a more normal level, the elastic work of breathing is lessened (Fig. 3-10). Resistance is also reduced by increasing the FRC. Weaning from mechanical ventilation is enhanced with the use of optimum CPAP (best compliance) in patients recovering from ARDS [20]. On the other hand, PEEP, either mechanical or intrinsic, can produce overdistention in conditions characterized by elevated FRC, thereby decreasing compliance.

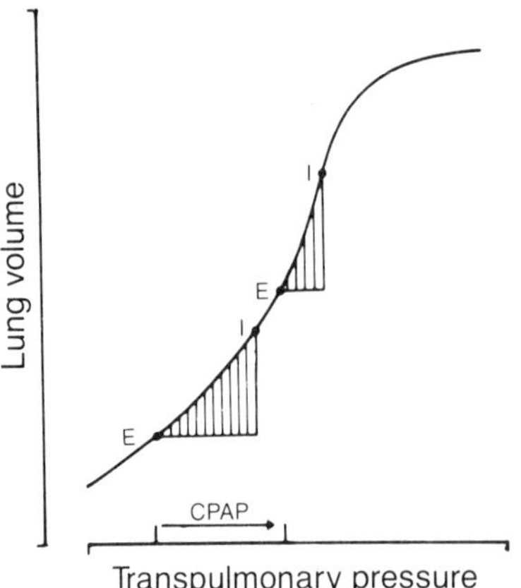

Fig. 3-10. Application of CPAP (continuous positive airway pressure) increases FRC (E) to a more normal level, with resultant improved compliance and reduced work of breathing. (From J. B. Downs. Airway Pressure Support. In J. M. Civetta, R. W. Taylor, and R. R. Kirby [eds.], *Critical Care.* Philadelphia: Lippincott, 1988. With permission.)

HEMODYNAMIC EFFECTS

The potential hemodynamic effects of PEEP and CPAP include (1) a reduction in venous return, (2) an increase in pulmonary vascular resistance, (3) a decrease in left ventricular compliance secondary to a possible shift of the interventricular septum into the left ventricle and an increase in juxtacardiac pressure, and (4) a reduction in left ventricular afterload. Positive pressure ventilation (PPV) is associated with the same effects, although in a phasic manner [21]. The importance of these various possibilities depends on many cardiopulmonary factors such as the homogeneity of pulmonary pathology, FRC, intravascular volume, and pulmonary, chest wall, and cardiac compliance.

Positive airway pressure will impair venous return by increasing intrathoracic pressure, which is directly proportional to pulmonary compliance and inversely proportional to thoracoabdominal (extrapulmonary) compliance. Thus, it is the transmission of the airway pressure to the pleural space, tempered by thoracoabdominal compliance, that determines the intrathoracic pressure. High compliance states (e.g., COPD) involve a greater increase in intrathoracic pressure than low compliance situations (e.g., ARDS) for the same airway pressure and extrapulmonary compliance.

The effect of mechanical ventilation on systemic blood pressure can be used as a rough assessment of intravascular volume [22]. The blood pressure will rise initially as the tidal volume is delivered, reflecting an increase in preload to the left ventricle as blood is "squeezed" from the lungs to the left ventricle. Decreased afterload may also augment the stroke volume. After a short period (e.g., three heart beats), the systolic pressure will decrease as a result of diminished venous return and other factors. The systolic pressure variation (SPV) derived from comparing the expiratory phase blood pressure with the peak inspiratory pressure will be a reflection of intravascular volume tempered by intrathoracic pressure [23]. For the same intrathoracic pressure, the SPV will generally be greater in hypovolemic patients.

Hypotension is not infrequently observed after commencing mechanical ventilation. Besides impaired venous return, other factors must be considered. Air trapping will increase FRC and intrathoracic pressure and impair cardiac output by a number of mechanisms.

In a patient struggling to perform the work of breathing, catecholamine levels and arteriolar tone are increased. With institution of mechanical ventilation, the stress of impending respiratory failure is removed, and catecholamine levels may drop, with a corresponding fall in blood pressure. In addition, narcotics or sedatives may be administered at the time of intubation and mechanical ventilation, which may decrease arterial and venous tone and may also cause myocardial depression. It is important to be cognizant of these factors, particularly in the patient with a tenuous cardiovascular status secondary to hypovolemia or diminished cardiac function.

SPECIFIC EXAMPLES

CHRONIC OBSTRUCTIVE PULMONARY DISEASE

Patients with severe COPD are prone to air trapping under certain circumstances, particularly when they are on mechanic ventilation [24]. Since elastic recoil of the lungs is diminished and resistance to air flow (obstruction) is present, the expiratory time necessary to prevent air trapping is prolonged. Hyperinflation will have many effects. Gas exchange will be worsened by increasing $\dot{V}/\dot{Q}$ mismatch. Barotrauma risk is heightened, which in patients prone to this problem is of considerable concern. Cardiac output will be impaired by decreased venous return secondary to increased intrathoracic pressure, which is inordinately increased because of the high pulmonary compliance. An increase in PVR or juxtacardiac pressure from the hyperexpanded lungs may decrease preload and thus cardiac output. Ventilatory muscle function will be impaired because understretching will result in a reduction in tension or strength. Compliance will be decreased, thereby increasing the work of breathing.

Intrinsic or auto-PEEP is a fairly common cause of hyperinflation and must be considered in COPD patients, particularly those with hypotension [25]. Auto-PEEP is defined as the pressure difference between the true alveolar end expiratory pressures and the end-expiratory pressure measured proximally. It arises when insufficient time is allowed for alveolar emptying.

Auto-PEEP can be detected by occluding the expiratory limb of the ventilatory circuit at end expiration while preventing the next inspiration. Any rise in the proximal pressure above the initial end-expiratory pressure is the amount of auto-PEEP.

ASTHMA

In patients with asthma a reduction in the work of breathing before the ventilatory pump fatigues under the load is the primary therapeutic objective. Resistance is the main component of the work; however, compliance is reduced if significant air trapping is present. Many of the points concerning hyperexpansion covered in the section on COPD also pertain to bronchoconstriction. During spontaneous ventilation, prolongation of exhalation will limit inspiratory time, necessitating an increase in inspiratory flow rate through narrowed airways, thus increasing resistance and consequently the work of breathing. This degree of work requires a great transpulmonary pressure gradient and results in a large negative pleural pressure, which partially explains pulsus paradox in asthma.

ADULT RESPIRATORY DISTRESS SYNDROME

Representing an acute severe reduction in pulmonary compliance and FRC, ARDS is on the opposite end of the spectrum from COPD with respect to lung volumes and compliance. Required ventilator settings will be quite different. PEEP is a mainstay in ventilator management. Expiratory time is typically shortened, allowing a greater inspiratory time and thus improved oxygen transfer to the alveolus. In fact, inverse I : E ratio ventilation (e.g., 3 : 1) can improve oxygenation in certain patients [26]. Mean airway pressures typically increase as inspiratory time is lengthened; therefore a reduction in cardiac output is possible. This effect is lessened by the low pulmonary compliance, which results in decreased transmission of pressure to the pleural space and a diminished rise in intrathoracic pressure.

PATIENT-VENTILATOR DYSCOORDINATION

Patient agitation and "fighting the ventilator" may have profound effects on gas exchange. Coughing, "bucking," or any inappropriate contraction of the ventilatory muscles will increase airway pressure by reducing extrapulmonary compliance as the inspired volume is delivered. Barotrauma risk is increased, and insufficient tidal volume delivery may result if the ventilator is pressure limited and the remaining volume is "popped off." Forceful coughing will also tend to reduce the FRC and oxygenation transiently. Agitation will also increase oxygen consumption, possibly reducing $P\bar{v}O_2$ and thus PaO_2 in a patient with a significant shunt. Hyperventilation may occur in agitated patients during assist/control ventilation, and frequent inspiratory efforts may produce air trapping in patients in whom exhalation is impaired.

Agitation during mechanical ventilation should be considered an indicator of a potentially serious problem. Fighting the ventilator has been the first clue to hypoxemia, pneumothorax, main stem intubation, pulmonary embolus, endotracheal tube obstruction, and many other serious events. As such, it should prompt an investigation for the cause and not lead to the reflex administration of sedation.

Muscle relaxants are rarely necessary to treat patient-ventilator dyscoordination if adequate doses of sedatives and/or analgesics are utilized. The use of muscle relaxants to "quiet" the patient without adequate sedation and analgesia should be avoided to prevent the disturbing experience of "paralysis while awake." A minority of patients will require muscle relaxants to reduce airway pressures. In this situation, analgesic and sedative requirements can be somewhat guided by monitoring the "sympathetic responses" (e.g., tachycardia, hypertension) to pain and agitation and by evaluating the response to treatment. Alternatively, periodic withholding of muscle relaxants may allow assessment of the adequacy of sedation and analgesia.

HEAD TRAUMA

In the great majority of patients with severe brain injury, oxygenation abnormalities will occur at some point during hospitalization. Severe hypoxemia may be present on admission as a result of aspiration pneumonitis or neurogenic pulmonary edema. Ventilator therapy for an acute severe restrictive pulmonary process is diametrically opposed to that typically utilized for intracranial hypertension. Since raising the intrathoracic pressure may increase intracranial pressure (ICP) by impairing intracranial and cerebral venous return, mean airway pressure should be kept low by shortening inspiratory time and avoiding PEEP. Management of ARDS, however, would dictate application of PEEP and frequently a lengthening of the inspiratory time. Increasing inspiratory time and PEEP must be done judiciously in patients with intracranial hypertension. However, if PEEP is necessary to achieve adequate arterial oxygen saturation, it should obviously be utilized. PEEP-induced hypotension must be aggressively addressed because this will worsen the neurologic injury.

The impact of airway pressure on ICP is a function of three compliances. Pulmonary and thoracoabdominal compliance and the interaction of the two in determining intrathoracic pressure has been previously discussed. Fortunately, the low compliance characteristics of ARDS will decrease airway pressure transmission, and the rise in intrathoracic pressure will thus be decreased, thereby producing less impairment of cerebral venous return. The volume position on the intracranial compliance curve will determine the effect of an increase in volume on ICP (see Chapter 13, Fig. 13-4). Measurement of ICP is indicated when airway pressures are significantly elevated in a patient with a serious brain injury.

FLAIL CHEST

Flail chest often produces an acute reduction in ventilatory pump function. Work of breathing is frequently increased by atelectasis, pneumonia, chest wall edema, or pulmonary contusion. It is the interplay between the reduced ventilatory capability and the increased work of breathing that determines the need for mechanical ventilation. Shallowing breathing secondary to pain and decreased ventilatory capability promote atelectasis and a further reduction in compliance, thus increasing the work of breathing. Therapy is directed at aggressive control of pain and reducing the work of breathing. Clearing bronchial secretions and treatment of any bronchoconstriction will aid in reducing the work needed to overcome resistance. Elastic work is decreased by treatment of the underlying pulmonary pathology and possibly CPAP to increase FRC and thus compliance.

CARDIOGENIC PULMONARY EDEMA

Many aspects of cardiopulmonary interaction are illustrated by pulmonary edema secondary to inadequate cardiac function (Fig. 3-11). Pulmonary edema decreases pulmonary compliance, thereby increasing the oxygen cost (work) of breathing. This increased oxygen delivery to the ventilatory muscles is required of a heart that is already producing an inadequate output and of lungs that may be incapable of complete oxygen saturation of the blood. Therefore, the cardiopulmonary system may be unable to maintain adequate oxygen delivery. The markedly desaturated mixed venous blood will also contribute to hypoxemia. As oxygen delivery fails, the oxygen supply to the ventilatory muscles will decrease, resulting in acute ventilatory failure.

Patient attempts to overcome the low pulmonary compliance will cause pleural pressures to become more negative. This reduction in intrathoracic pressure will enhance venous return and worsen pulmonary congestion. Greater negative intrathoracic pressure will also increase the afterload on the left ventricle, potentially reducing cardiac output even further and increasing pulmonary edema. In contrast, positive intrathoracic pressure has been demonstrated to augment cardiac performance in this situation [27].

Mechanical ventilation, particularly with PEEP, will attenuate many of these factors. Patient work is diminished as a result of increased FRC. Work of breathing is performed by the ventilator, thereby allowing delivery of more oxygen to other organs. Cardiac work is reduced, a fact that is significant in many situations but particularly in patients with coronary artery disease. Mixed venous oxygen content may improve, thereby increasing the

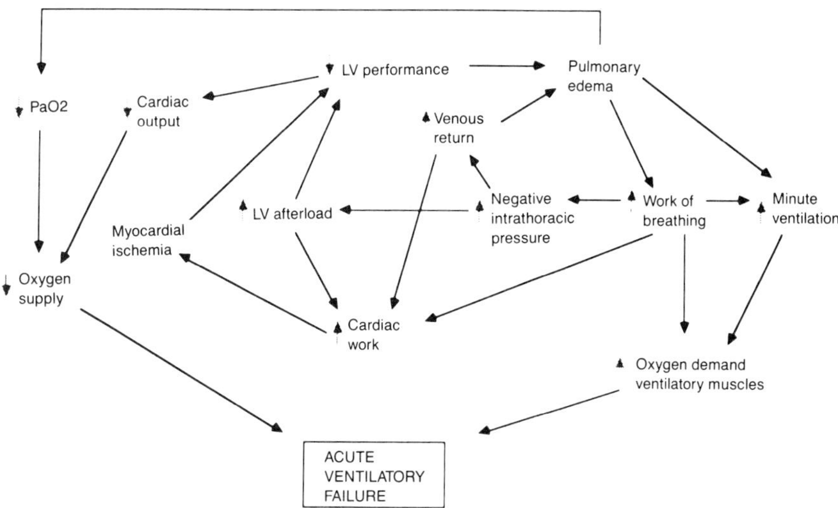

Fig. 3-11. Possible interplay of factors resulting in acute ventilatory failure in patients with cardiogenic pulmonary edema.

arterial content. Pulmonary congestion is decreased as the positive intrathoracic pressure reduces venous return and left ventricular afterload. CPAP has been demonstrated to produce many of the same salutary effects [28].

CONCLUSION

This chapter has attempted to bridge the gap that frequently exists between an understanding of normal and pathologic physiology and common clinical situations encountered in the treatment of pulmonary disorders. The artificial separation between "basic" physiology and "clinical" medicine results in suboptimal management. An attempt has been made to weave or blend the physiologic factors with clinical examples to obscure the separation and provide the physiologic basis for management tactics. It is hoped that a better understanding of the clinical management of disordered pulmonary physiology has been imparted.

REFERENCES

1. Gilbert, R., and Keighley, J. F. The arterial/alveolar oxygen tension ratio. An index of gas exchange applicable to varying inspired oxygen concentrations. *Am. Rev. Resp. Dis.* 109:142–145, 1974.
2. Covelli, H. D., Nessan, V. J., and Tuttle, W. K., III. Oxygen derived variables in acute respiratory failure. *Crit. Care Med.* 1:646–649, 1983.

3. Gilbert, R., Auchincloss, J. H., Kuppinger, M., et al. Stability of the arterial/alveolar oxygen partial pressure ratio. *Crit. Care Med.* 7:267–272, 1979.
4. Roussos, C. Function and fatigue of respiratory muscles. *Chest* 885:1245–1325, 1985.
5. Morganroth, M. L. Morganroth, J. L., Nett, L. M., et al. Criteria for weaning from prolonged mechanical ventilation. *Arch. Intern. Med.* 144:1012–1016, 1984.
6. Fiastro, J. F., Habib, M. P., Shon, B. T., et al. Comparison of standard weaning parameters and the mechanical work of breathing in mechanically ventilated patients. *Chest* 94:232–238, 1988.
7. Dehaven, C. B., Hurst, J. M., and Branson, R. D. Evaluation of two different extubation criteria: Attributes contributing to success. *Crit. Care Med.* 14:92–94, 1986.
8. Dantzker, D. R., and Tobin, M. J. Monitoring respiratory muscle function. *Respir. Care* 30:422–431, 1985.
9. Tobin, M. J., Chadha, T. S., Jenouri, G., et al. Breathing patterns 2. Diseased subjects. *Chest* 84:286–294, 1983.
10. Field, S., Kelly, S. M., and Macklem, P. T. The oxygen cost of breathing in patients with cardiorespiratory disease. *Am. Rev. Respir. Dis.* 126:9–13, 1982.
11. Viires, N., Sillye, G., Aubier, M., et al. Regional blood flow distribution in dog during induced hypotension and low cardiac output. *J. Clin. Invest.* 72:935–947, 1983.
12. Räsänen, J., Nikki, P., and Heikkilä, J. Acute myocardial infarction complicated by respiratory failure. *Chest* 85:21–28, 1984.
13. Yamanaka, M. K., and Sue, D. Y. Comparison of arterial-end-tidal PCO_2 difference and dead space/tidal volume ratio in respiratory failure. *Chest* 92:832–835, 1987.
14. Dark, D. S., Pingleton, S. K., and Kerby, G. R. Hypercapnia during weaning: A complication of nutritional support. *Chest* 88:141–143, 1985.
15. Marini, J. J., Capps, J. S., and Culver, B. H. The inspiratory work of breathing during assisted mechanical ventilation. *Chest* 87:612–618, 1985.
16. Christopher, K. L., Neff, T. A., Bowman, J. L., et al. Demand and continuous flow intermittent mandatory ventilation systems. *Chest* 87:625–630, 1985.
17. Marini, J. J., Culver, B. H., and Kirk, W. Flow resistance of exhalation valves and positive end-expiratory pressure devices used in mechanical ventilation. *Am. Rev. Respir. Dis.* 131:850–854, 1985.
18. Banner, M. J., Lampotang, S., Boysen, P. G., et al. Flow resistance of expiratory positive-pressure valve systems. *Chest* 90:212–217, 1986.
19. Braman, S. S., Dunn, S. M., Amico, C. A., et al. Complications of intrahospital transport in critically ill patients. *Ann. Intern. Med.* 107:469–473, 1987.
20. Katz, J. A., and Marks, J. D. Inspiratory work with and without continuous positive airway pressure in patients with acute respiratory failure. *Anesthesiology* 63:598–607, 1985.
21. Luce, J. M. The cardiovascular effects of mechanical ventilation and positive end-expiratory pressure. *J.A.M.A.* 252:807–811, 1984.
22. Coyle, J. P., Teplick, R. S., Long, M. C., et al. Respiratory variation in systemic arterial pressure as an indicator of volume status (abstract). *Anesthesiology* 59:A53, 1983.
23. Perel, A., Pizov, R., and Cotev, S. Systolic blood pressure variation is a sensitive indicator of hypovolemia in ventilated dogs subjected to graded hemorrhage. *Anesthesiology* 67:498–502, 1987.
24. Tuxen, D. V., and Lane, S. The effects of ventilatory pattern on hyperinflation, airway pressures, and circulation in mechanical ventilation of patients with severe air-flow obstruction. *Am. Rev. Respir. Dis.* 136:872–879, 1987.
25. Pepe, P. E., and Marini, J. J. Occult positive end-expiratory pressure in mechani-

cally ventilated patients with airflow obstruction. *Am. Rev. Respir. Dis.* 126:166–170, 1982.
26. Gurevitch, M. J., VanDyke, J., Young, E. S., et al. Improved oxygenation and lower peak airway pressure in severe adult respiratory distress syndrome. Treatment with inverse ratio ventilation. *Chest* 89:211–213, 1986.
27. Pinsky, M. R., and Summer, W. R. Cardiac augmentation by phasic high intrathoracic pressure support in man. *Chest* 84:370–375, 1983.
28. Räsänen, J., Heikkilä, J., Downs, J., et al. Continuous positive airway pressure by face mask in acute cardiogenic pulmonary edema. *Am. J. Cardiol.* 55:296–300, 1985.

4. Cardiac Perspectives

Glenn S. Vanstrum

In this chapter, we will consider the special problems of the cardiac patient. For an organ that has such a simple function, i.e., a blood pump, the heart never ceases to amaze scientists and clinicians as secret after secret of anatomy and physiology is revealed, leading to constant improvements in pharmacology and therapy. Cardiac care draws the interest of many because proper function of the heart is an indisputable, final determinant of life— with it, one has at least a chance of living. Without it, or without a mechanical or transplant substitute, one is dead. In this chapter, we will begin to examine this organ system from the perspective of anesthesia and emergency medicine by studying airway management, coronary supply and demand, and cardiac monitoring. We will then discuss various life-saving treatment modalities and conclude with condensed discussions of some cardiac clinical entities.

AIRWAY MANAGEMENT AND CORONARY SUPPLY AND DEMAND

OXYGENATION AND CARDIAC PERFORMANCE

The desired result of cardiac function, in simplistic terms, is to transport essential oxygen to the peripheral tissues and to carry waste carbon dioxide back from tissues to the lungs. The heart itself, of course, utilizes respiration to maintain its own cellular integrity and function. Hence, optimizing oxygenation and ventilation cannot be neglected as one is distracted by cardiac considerations such as the monitoring of filling pressures and titration of nitroglycerin drips. Hypoxia, caused by shunt, $\dot{V}/\dot{Q}$ mismatch, hypoventilation, or decreased FIO_2, can quickly exacerbate an ongoing cardiac catastrophe. As cardiac output drops and oxygen extraction increases, mixed venous PO_2 falls. When this blood passes through lungs rendered inefficient by $\dot{V}/\dot{Q}$ mismatch and shunt, it becomes poorly oxygenated arterial blood [1], and a downward spiraling vicious circle is formed. Hence the considerations presented in Chapters 2 and 3 must be kept in mind as one becomes immersed in the complexities of cardiotonic drips, bypass equipment, and left ventricular stroke work indices.

The literature is not replete with data on the exact energy price paid for the work of breathing by a patient with cardiac compromise. Once interstitial and alveolar filling from left ventricular failure occurs, however, a much greater percentage of the cardiac output is needed to supply the bellows mechanism of the now stiff and poorly compliant lungs (see Chapter 3). Not only do intubation and positive pressure ventilation relieve the heart of this energy expenditure but also they often improve oxygenation by recruitment of collapsed alveoli. Hypoxic vasoconstriction and similar vascular effects of hypercarbia lead to increased afterload for the right ventricle and can be relieved by positive pressure high FIO_2 ventilation. Positive end-expiratory pressure (PEEP), a mainstay of treatment for $\dot{V}/\dot{Q}$ mismatch, can best be applied after intubation.

Recent work by Lemaire and associates has shown that fluid-loaded patients on mechanical ventilation had marked increases (relative to the same patients after diuresis) in pulmonary artery occlusion presssures, preload, and afterload, during a trial of spontaneous respiration [2]. Permutt, in analyzing their data, has hypothesized that the transdiaphragmatic pressure differential may be an explanation of their findings [3]. Thus, during spontaneous ventilation, when the diaphragm contracts, intra-abdominal pressure increases and encourages diversion of abdominal splanchnic blood into the relatively low pressure thorax. The institution of mechanical ventilation suppresses this effect and improves hemodynamics in the volume-congested emergency patient in pulmonary edema.

Obviously, it is not common practice to put all patients in pulmonary edema or those having a myocardial infarction on the ventilator. A major downside of such treatment, in addition to the more chronic sequelae of pulmonary infectious disease and barotrauma, is the extreme stimulus of the intubating procedure itself. Intubation in healthy patients, whether oral or nasal, is well known by anesthesiologists to require as much or more anesthetic to prevent unwanted tachycardia and hypertension as surgical interventions such as skin incision or sternal splitting. The epinephrine discharge caused by intubation in a patient who is teetering on the edge of a positive balance between oxygen supply and demand, and disaster, can cause fatal dysrhythmias.

Epinephrine, on the other hand, is one of the few drugs that has maintained a place in the cardiac arrest pharmacopeia. Thus, a patient who is near cardiac extremis may benefit from the endogenous sympathomimetic discharge that results from intubation, and a patient in full cardiac arrest may need several milligrams of the drug in addition to intubation (see below under Critical Treatment Options for a discussion of the epinephrine dosing controversy). Deciding whether to ameliorate or to augment the hyperdynamic response to intubation requires a thorough understanding of the physiology and drugs involved and a good feel for the location of the patient in the spectrum of cardiac disease. This is where the art of medicine comes into play.

Once a patient is intubated, great care must be taken to monitor the effect of positive pressure ventilation on cardiac function. Large tidal volumes and PEEP, while beneficial for recruitment of collapsed alveoli and hence oxygenation, do diminish venous return to the left ventricle and increase functional afterload to the right ventricle. Often one is forced to use high (60 to 100% O_2) FiO_2s with relatively small tidal volumes (10 ml/kg) and higher rates initially until cardiac performance is optimal. When PEEP is introduced, it is often necessary to monitor its depressant effect on cardiac output via a pulmonary artery (PA) catheter. Thus, the clinician must juggle inotropic drips and PEEP to optimize cardiac output and PO_2.

CORONARY SUPPLY AND DEMAND— CLINICAL CORRELATES

Coronary Supply

Optimization of cardiac function requires an understanding of coronary artery supply and demand. Supply is determined by coronary resistance, diastolic time intervals, and the gradient between diastolic blood pressure and left ventricular end-diastolic pressure (LVEDP). Coronary resistance may be modified by nitrates or calcium channel blockers. The author prefers to use the intravenous nitroglycerin infusion, mixed as 50 mg in 250 ml of diluent and titrated at 3 to 30 ml/hr to give an infusion rate of 0.1 to 1.5 μg/kg/min in a 70-kg patient. In the emergency department (ED), one may also use 10 mg of sublingual nifedipine, sublingual nitroglycerin, nitroglycerin gels or slow-release patches. Sodium nitroprusside, which indiscriminately dilates epicardial and small coronary collateral vessels, may well cause a "coronary steal" phenomenon, in which ischemic areas of myocardium, normally favored by local collateral dilatation, are "robbed" by the widespread and nonselective dilatation caused by the drug [4]. Nitroglycerin, on the other hand, seems to dilate only the large epicardial vessels and does not cause this problem. Another advantage of nitroglycerin is its venous dilatory property, which relaxes an overstretched ventricle and reduces preload in an overly volume replete patient, moving end-diastolic volume to a more favorable position on the Starling curve.

The second determinant of coronary artery supply, diastolic time interval, is explained by the fact that blood cannot flow well in the contracting, systolic heart. Diastole is the red cell's chance to "sneak" into the ischemic wall of muscle and deliver oxygen. Unfortunately, tachycardia occurs at the expense of diastole, not systole. It has been shown by Slogoff and Keats that perioperative myocardial ischemia is significantly related to tachycardia [5–7]. Surprisingly, they also showed [5] that the manner in which the individual physician treats such patients is more closely related to eventual infarction than the initial severity of the patient's disease. In Slogoff and Keats' well-designed study, there was one physician whose patients (probably receiving less preinduction medication) had consistently higher heart rates. These patients, no different from the other anesthesiologists' patients, had a higher rate of perioperative myocardial infarction. The implications of this fact for the emergency physician treating acute myocardial infarction should be obvious. In the setting of critical myocardial ischemia, tachycardia must be treated, whether by volume loading, narcotic pain management (bradycardia is a welcome vagomimetic side effect of narcotics such as morphine or fentanyl), or, more directly, by the use of beta blockers or calcium channel blockers that are negative dromotropes (e.g., verapamil) (Fig. 4-1).

Often inotropic support in the form of dopamine or dobutamine will be

DECREASED MYOCARDIAL OXYGEN SUPPLY

1. Decreased coronary blood flow
   a. Tachycardia
   b. Diastolic hypotension
   c. Increased preload
   d. Hypocapnia
   e. Coronary spasm
2. Decreased oxygen delivery
   a. Anemia
   b. Hypoxia
   c. Decreased 2,3 DPG

INCREASED MYOCARDIAL OXYGEN DEMAND

1. Tachycardia
2. Increased wall tension
   a. Increased preload
   b. Increased afterload
3. Increased contractility

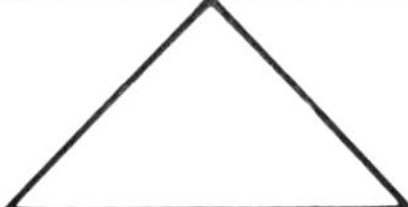

Fig. 4-1. Detrimental changes that can occur in the myocardial oxygen balance are demonstrated. Tachycardia and increased preload are marked to stand out, since they appear on both sides of the balance. (From R. D. Miller [ed.]. *Anesthesia* [2nd ed.]. New York: Churchill Livingstone, 1986. With permission.)

required after use of beta blockade in critically ischemic cardiac patients requiring treatment for tachycardia. Because of the obvious dangers of giving beta blockers with durations of action measured in hours, such as propranolol, some now recommend the initial use of the new, ultra-short-acting drug esmolol [8]. With its half-life of 9 minutes and a duration of action of about 5 minutes, not only is it efficatious for acute situations such as intubation, but also one can gauge the effect of such therapy for more long-term treatment and, ideally, abandon it quickly if necessary. A loading dose of 0.5 mg/kg esmolol is followed by a drip of 50 to 100 µg/kg/min. Because of wide individual variations in adrenergic receptor populations, all beta blockade dosing schedules must be considered approximate. Careful titration is no exception in this instance, and an arterial line is recommended for second-to-second blood pressure monitoring.

The third determinant of coronary supply, the pressure gradient between diastolic blood pressure and LVEDP, requires the optimization of systemic blood pressure, whether by volume or inotropic support, and the maintenance of the lowest LVEDP that still can generate a good cardiac output. Obviously, arterial line and pulmonary artery catheter monitoring is needed to best manipulate these variables. Still, one can do a great deal without invasive monitoring if the basic principles are understood and a thorough physical examination is performed. One does not need a PA catheter to know that a trial of volume is needed for a cardiac patient with flat neck veins who is having chest pain and hypotension after trauma or bowel surgery. Although some clinicians in emergency medicine have recommended inflation of the MAST suit as a reversible alternative to a fluid infusion in such a case, simple head-down bed positioning is faster and even more physiologic (see Chapter 12 for a discussion of the MAST suit). Either strategem, however, decreases ventilation efficiency, the former by abdominal restriction, the latter by the effect of positioning. In a similar vein, one does not need a PA catheter to know that a patient with rales two-thirds of the way up the lung fields and bulging neck veins needs nitrates, diuretics, opiates, and, possibly, inotropic support to decrease LVEDP.

Coronary Demand

The determinants of coronary perfusion demand are the state of contractility, preload and afterload, and cardiac rate and rhythm. Cardiac contractility, or inotropy, can be reduced, when appropriate, by the use of beta blockade, calcium channel blockade, or intravenous and volatile anesthetics. The special need to ameliorate the hyperdynamic response to intubation in the cardiac patient requires careful consideration. If a patient has serious pump failure, it is best to avoid strong myocardial depressants such as IV sodium thiopental for intubation. Even benzodiazepines have enough myocardial depressant qualities [9, 10] that they should be avoided in patients with fulminant cardiac failure. In such situations 50 to 100 μg of IV fentanyl (1 to 2 ml), or 5 to 10 μg of IV sufentanil, is probably the best regimen, in addition to muscle relaxation and possibly some IV lidocaine. Ketamine may also be considered as a useful drug in this situation, although the indirect increase in blood pressure and heart rate due to it may not be seen in a catechol-depleted patient (see Chapters 5 and 15).

Preload and afterload are directly reduced by vasodilators. *Afterload* is defined, strictly speaking, as myocardial wall tension, but clinically it is approximated by the systemic vascular resistance (SVR). SVR is calculated in dynes/cm/sec^{-5} by the formula:

$$\frac{(\text{Mean arterial pressure}) - (\text{central venous pressure})}{\text{cardiac output}} \times 80$$

Hydralazine is a relatively pure afterload reduction agent and may be used to good effect to treat elevated SVR (normal is 800 to 1600) in a dose of 5 to 20 mg every 4 hours. It takes 10 to 20 minutes to gauge the effect of an IV bolus of 5 mg of hydralazine, and the effects last for 3 to 4 hours. Over-titration of the drug can usually be reversed with volume loading. Nitroprusside dilates both arterial and venous beds and has the coronary steal effect mentioned above; however, it is commonly used for recalcitrant hypertension in a drip preparation (50 mg in 250 ml of diluent) that can be rapidly titrated. Nitroglycerin is predominantly a preload or venous dilator, but it does have some arterial dilatory effects and should be used in hypertensive patients with ischemic cardiac disease in a dose up to 100 μg/min before adding nitroprusside.

If diastolic blood pressure is low, it may be raised by volume, inotropic support (dopamine, dobutamine, digoxin), or alpha-agonist drugs such as phenylephrine (Neo-synephrine) or norepinephrine (Levophed). It is important to remember that the failing heart's performance will be adversely affected by alpha-agonist use [11] and that such drugs should probably be reserved for situations involving lowered SVR (e.g., sepsis, postcardiopulmonary bypass rewarming). There is some recent evidence, however, that alpha-agonist drugs may be underused in the setting of cardiac arrest (see Alpha- vs Beta-Adrenergic Drugs in Cardiac Arrest). Deciding which modality to use and how to use it is greatly facilitated by PA catheter data, but, prior to obtaining such data, one must use the physical examination and clinical situation to make a best educated guess. A more thorough discussion of intotropic drips will follow below.

Heart rate and rhythm are fundamental to coronary demand as well as to supply. New onset of atrial fibrillation or atrial tachycardia can be catastrophic to a patient teetering on the edge of disaster (especially a patient with stenotic valvular disease, see below). Dramatic and dangerous as it may seem, electric cardioversion is often the indicated therapy in such cases. The author has induced ventricular fibrillation in the ED after attempted cardioversion in a confused, hypotensive patient with atrial tachycardia. Although prompt defibrillation resulted in normal sinus rhythm, it was not without considerable stress to both the physician's and the patient's coronaries—still, even in retrospect, the treatment was proper. Although some might use IV verapamil in this situation, it is important to make sure that it is considered only for narrow complex atrial tachycardias. Use of verapamil in a patient with ventricular tachycardia who has a blood pressure that has been misdiagnosed as atrial tachycardia with aberrancy can lead to irretrievable asystole. Asystole can also occur if the drug is used in patients who have already been treated with digoxin and beta-blocking drugs [4].

MONITORING IN THE CARDIAC PATIENT

ELECTROCARDIOGRAM

The subject of 12-lead electrocardiography (ECG) has been well covered in other volumes. Such devices are too cumbersome for monitoring in the second-to-second sense of the word, and three- to five-lead monitors are used for that purpose in the ED and the operating suite. The ongoing knowledge of cardiac electrical activity provided by these ubiquitous devices has great clinical utility in detecting dysrhythmias and myocardial ischemia.

Dysrhythmias can be precipitated by ischemic cardiac disease, catheter insertions, hypokalemia, anesthetic agents such as halothane, intracranial pathology, and vagal or other reflexes [12]. Bipolar leads such as the three-electrode monitoring systems used in most EDs and ORs can be modified from their usual left arm, left leg, right arm positions to improve detection of atrial dysrhythmias, conduction defects, and bundle branch blocks. For example, the MCL_1 (modified central lead) is obtained by placing the left arm electrode under the outer third of the left clavicle and the left leg electrode in the fourth intercostal space to the right of the sternum, with lead III selected [12].

Ischemia, shown by ST-segment depression, and myocardial injury or coronary spasm, shown by ST-segment elevation, can be best detected by a unipolar system such as the modified precordial lead placement used in the 12-lead ECG. Unlike bipolar leads, which measure electric current between two distinct points, a unipolar system measures electric potential between a single point and a common central terminal created by three or four standard leads connected through resistances of 5000 ohms each. Five-electrode systems are currently marketed in which a lead is attached to each limb and a fifth lead is attached to the V_5 position. Blackburn has recommended use of this lead because he demonstrated that 89 percent of ST-segment information can be found in V_5 [13]. This system produces all six bipolar limb leads and a true, ischemia-sensitive V_5 lead, and is used in many cardiac surgical centers.

One may still use a three-lead bipolar system to monitor ischemia with some confidence. To approximate the V_5 unipolar lead, one may attach the right arm lead under the right clavicle, and the left arm lead in the V_5 position, with lead I selected. The left leg electrode is then placed as usual, providing a lead II configuration for detection of dysrhythmia when lead II is selected (Fig. 4-2).

In monitoring ST segments during a period of time, it is important to realize that many ECG monitors have two modes, a sensitive "diagnostic" mode and a heavily filtered "monitoring" mode. The latter is relatively unaffected by movement, nearby electric currents, wandering baselines, and the like but may create spurious ST-segment changes [12]. The former can give an accurate ST tracing but is extremely sensitive.

PULMONARY ARTERY CATHETERS

We have mentioned the importance of pulmonary artery pressure monitoring above. Although such PA or Swan-Ganz catheters are not often used in most emergency departments [11], they are frequently used in anesthesia

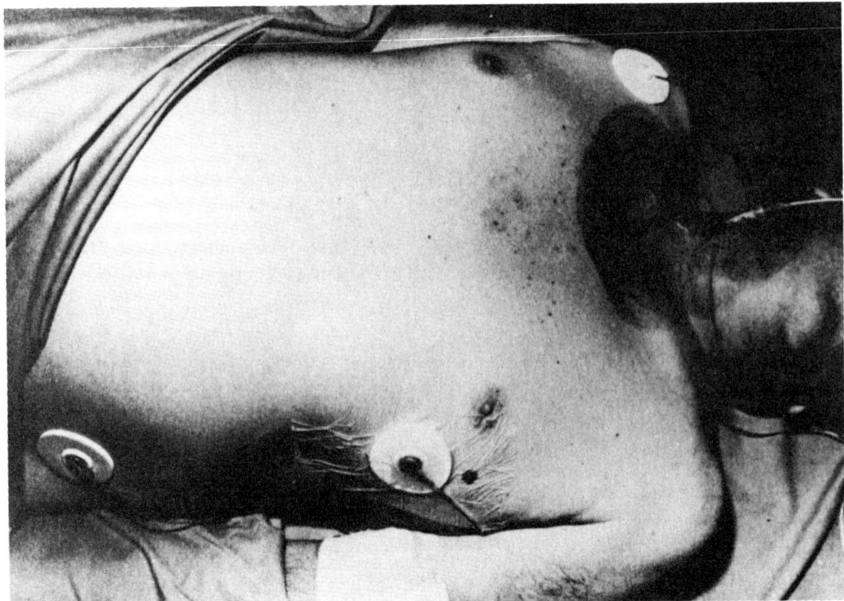

Fig. 4-2. A modified CS5 lead is demonstrated in which the left arm lead has been moved down to the V_5 position. Lead I can then be turned on to measure from the right arm to the V_5 position (CS5), which is a common lead on which to detect ischemia. Lead II can be used to detect inferior wall ischemia and dysrhythmias. (From R. D. Miller [ed.], *Anesthesia* [2nd ed.]. New York: Churchill Livingstone, 1986. With permission.)

and in intensive care units. There is controversy about the possible underuse or overuse of such devices. They do represent a considerable added expense, they require considerable training on the part of both physicians and nursing personnel, and, most important, there is a small but significant amount of potential morbidity and mortality related to their use.

Proponents of the devices point out the well-known disparity betwen PA catheter data and right-sided pressure data from the central venous pressure (CVP) catheter, which is used frequently in emergency medicine. Knowing cardiac output enables one to calculate SVR (see above), which, in conjunction with wedge pressure data, is invaluable in treating hypotension. A vast amount of additional data, from interpreting cardiac rhythms to diagnosing valvular disease or pulmonary embolus, is also available to the sophisticated user of the PA catheter [14]. PA catheters are now manufactured that deliver constant mixed venous oxygen saturation data [15]. Such data are invaluable as an early warning system for decreased cardiac output (the usual cause of lowered mixed venous saturation).

Should the PA catheter be used more often in emergency medicine? This author's opinion, obtained after having worked on both sides of the fence, is a qualified yes. If a sufficient number of critical cardiac patients spend an hour or more in the emergency department, if an emergency physician is adequately trained to place the catheter and interpret the data, and if pressure monitoring equipment is maintained in the ED, it is not unreasonable to use a PA catheter. Certainly if an ED physician feels compelled to place a central line in either a cardiac patient or an elderly trauma patient with probable cardiac disease, at the very least he or she should consider placing that hospital's introducer sheath for a later PA catheter. Most PA catheter complications, such as pneumothorax or hematoma, are related to central line placement. The three remaining complication categories include infection, which mandates careful sterile technique (see Chapter 11), dysrhythmia, which usually occurs as the catheter is passed through the right ventricle and can be treated by rapid insertion into the pulmonary artery or withdrawal, and, finally, pulmonary hemorrhage. Failure to recognize the wedge position in patients with pulmonary hypertension and mitral regurgitation, in which a large V wave can resemble the PA tracing, is a prime contributor to such hemorrhage [16].

If one is contemplating placing a PA catheter, the following points are best considered.

1. Make sure the patient is returned to a level position from the head-down position after central line insertion. Insert the catheter to the 20-cm mark before expanding the balloon.
2. Never use more than the recommended amount of air in the balloon (1.5 cc), and never withdraw the catheter with the balloon expanded.
3. Active deflation of the balloon predisposes to balloon rupture. Hence, let the balloon deflate passively.
4. Always watch the pressure trace while inserting the catheter, and if possible, pass the catheter relatively rapidly through the right ventricle. Not only will this diminish the chance of ventricular dysrhythmias, but it also seems to diminish intraventricular coiling. If the right ventricle is extremely irritable, premature ventricular contractions (PVCs) that are noncontractile may inhibit blood flow (Fig. 4-3). In this case, slow passage of the catheter may be successful in allowing placement of the distal tip in the pulmonary artery.
5. On reaching the pulmonary artery (noted by the increase in diastolic pressure and the disappearance of the characteristic right ventricular wave form), it is best to slow the insertion of the catheter. Usually the PA trace is noted at 40 cm if the right internal jugular approach is used, 35 cm with the subclavian approach. Be aware that, if the patient has mitral regurgitation, the wedge wave form will be very similar to the PA wave form. Extreme caution is mandated here. Often the PA diastolic pressure can substitute for

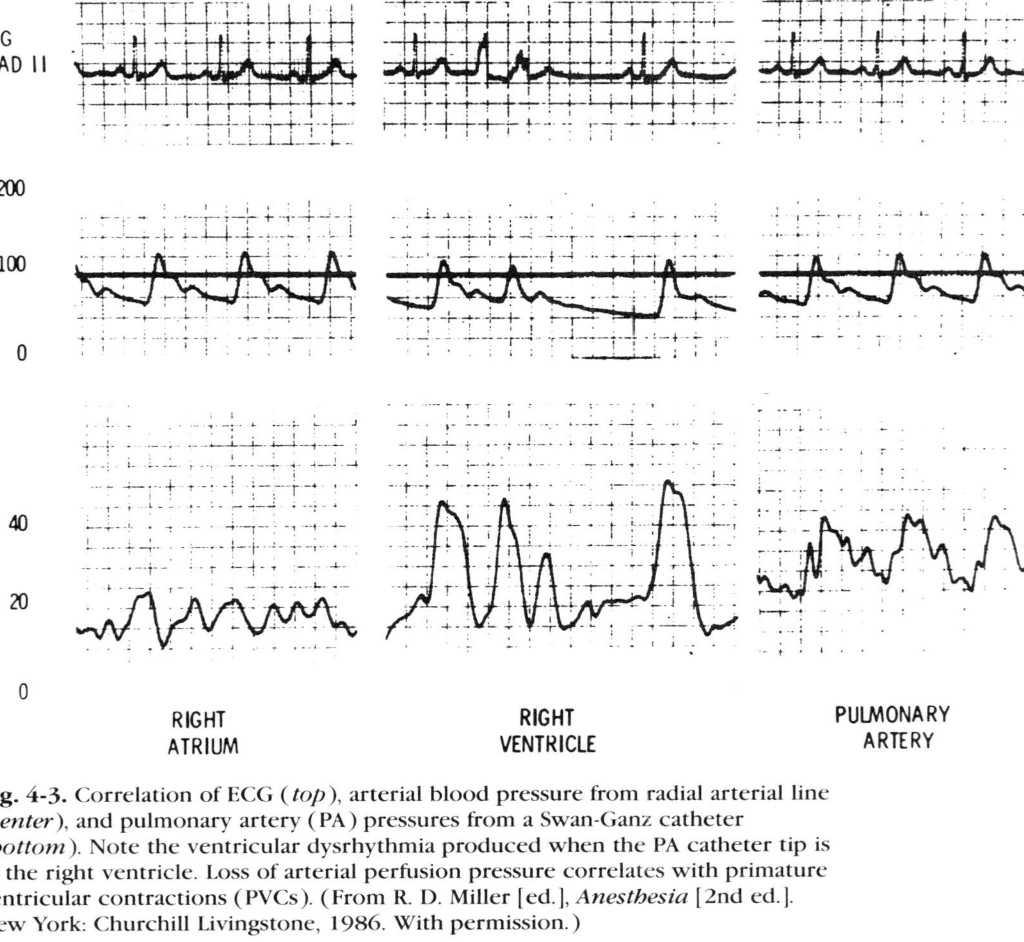

Fig. 4-3. Correlation of ECG (*top*), arterial blood pressure from radial arterial line (*center*), and pulmonary artery (PA) pressures from a Swan-Ganz catheter (*bottom*). Note the ventricular dysrhythmia produced when the PA catheter tip is in the right ventricle. Loss of arterial perfusion pressure correlates with primature ventricular contractions (PVCs). (From R. D. Miller [ed.], *Anesthesia* [2nd ed.]. New York: Churchill Livingstone, 1986. With permission.)

the wedge pressure, and the risk of causing pulmonary hemorrhage by persistent wedging or "wedge-searching" is real, especially in patients with pulmonary hypertension or coagulopathies.
6. If one has difficulty in passing the catheter, try positioning the patient differently (head-up, head-down, tilt), or consider using fluo-
roscopy or waiting for help from a more experienced colleague.
7. *Never become so engrossed with the procedure that the clinical
condition (especially the airway) of the patient is ignored.*

Whether or not an emergency physician places the catheter, often knowledge of wave forms and the data generated will be useful should he or she
be required to resuscitate a patient who already has a PA line in a non-
emergency department location, such as in a late night ICU cardiac arrest.
Although cardiac anesthesiologists place such lines routinely, other anesthesiologists may either be unfamiliar with them or use them rarely. Generally
speaking, if a clinical situation such as major bowel surgery or major trauma
mandates a CVP anyway, and if a patient has a history of significant cardiac
disease, it is usually worth the risk and expense to place a PA catheter. (For
a discussion of arterial line monitoring, see Chapter 12.)

NONINVASIVE ESOPHAGEAL MONITORING

A number of noninvasive monitoring techniques are revolutionizing the
practice of anesthesiology. In Chapter 2, oxygen saturation and end-tidal
CO_2 monitors were discussed in detail as adjuncts for monitoring the function of respiration. In this author's opinion, it is only a matter of time before
these monitors are not only used routinely in emergency medicine but become the "standard of practice." The importance of respiratory function for
optimal cardiac response is discussed above. However, in the patient with
adequate respiratory function and a failing heart, a reduction in peripheral
oxygen saturation may only be a terminal sign of poor cardiac output, as
will a reduction in end-tidal CO_2 production. Thus, additional monitors
have been developed to assist in the noninvasive monitoring of the cardiac
system, in addition to the ECG, which is now indispensable but some 30
years ago was still considered experimental.

Transesophageal two-dimensional echocardiography has been evaluated
for use in cardiac anesthesiology [17]. Not strictly noninvasive, because it
requires the esophageal placement of a fairly large tube, it does give valuable information to trained observers about regional wall motion abnormalities that are noted with ischemia. Such abnormalities have been shown
to occur before electrocardiographic evidence of ischemia appears [18].
The use of this device, unfortunately, requires a general anesthetic or a comatose patient, and hence it will probably find limited applicability in the
emergency department.

An enhancement of this apparatus is the esophageal Doppler ultrasonography cardiac output device [19]. Although it also requires a comatose or anesthetized patient, it may still be useful in the ED because it can supply repeated and reproducible cardiac output data. The value of such data without the filling pressure data supplied by the PA catheter is, however, yet to be determined. The ultrasound device is fashioned into a standard-sized esophageal stethoscope tube and hence is easily placed in an atraumatic manner.

A final esophageal technique that bears mentioning is esophageal electrode electrocardiography. This device can be helpful in the accurate characterization of atrial tachycardias [12, 20].

ACID-BASE CONSIDERATIONS IN CARDIAC ARREST

Recently, the excessive use of sodium bicarbonate therapy, engendered in part by ACLS algorithms in the early 1980s, has been called into question [21, 22]. A study by Weil and others of acid-base conditions in 105 patients during and after cardiopulmonary resuscitation (CPR), demonstrated sharp decreases in survival when arterial pH exceeded 7.55 [23]. The cardiac depression that supposedly was treated with bicarbonate is most probably due to the severe respiratory acidosis found in cardiac arrests [24]. Although acidotic hypoxic heart muscle has slightly depressed contractility compared with alkalotic hypoxic heart muscle, once reoxygenation occurs the acidotic muscle has nearly twice the contractility [25], presumably due to preservation of energy stores.

The factor determining contractility is intracellular pH [26], which drops slowly with metabolic acidosis but much more rapidly with either hypoventilation (respiratory acidosis) or the administration of sodium bicarbonate, which rapidly increased blood PCO_2 as well as pH [27]. Bicarbonate "fizzes" when it is added to blood. This CO_2 then diffuses intracellularly and exacerbates intracellular acidosis. In addition, the pH change causes leftward shifting of the oxyhemoglobin saturation curve, with resultant decreased unloading of tissue oxygen. All these effects of sodium bicarbonate are deleterious and indicate very careful use of the substance, if it is to be used at all, in conjunction with ongoing acid-base monitoring by means of arterial blood gas tension analysis.

Many rationalize the use of bicarbonate therapy to increase the efficacy of catecholamine infusion. Although the blunting effect of acidosis on catechols in cardiac arrest has yet to be studied, other studies suggest that this effect is moderate (30 percent in animals) and can most probably be erased with hyperventilation and increased dosing of catechols [24, 28, 29]. There is still a place for bicarbonate, but it should be used solely for severe metabolic acidosis and with careful monitoring of blood gases to avoid alkalinization.

CRITICAL TREATMENT OPTIONS

CARDIOTONIC DRIPS

Epinephrine

The prototype of all sympathomimetic drugs, epinephrine has a combined alpha and beta effect. After cardiopulmonary bypass or cardiac arrest, for example, Kaplan speaks of a "stunned myocardium," which needs a "kick" [30], and epinephrine is clearly the drug of choice for such treatment. At low doses (1 to 2 μg/min or 0.01 to 0.03 μg/kg/min), the beta effects (increased inotropy and vasodilatation) predominate; at moderate doses (2 to 10 μg/min), alpha-adrenergic effects appear; and at high doses, alpha effects, i.e., intense vasoconstriction, predominate [30]. One can also give a bolus dose for acute hypotensive reactions varying along a wide spectrum. Thus one might inject 2 to 8 μg for, say, marked hypotension following a dose of a drug such as sodium thiopental or morphine. Should such a dose prove ineffective in 30 to 60 seconds, one can increase the bolus dose to 10 μg, then 50 μg, then 100 μg, and so on, until the desired result is achieved. Initiation of a drip at this point will maintain therapeutic levels in an optimal fashion (see Chapter 5). The use of the drug in this manner is not often appreciated by many emergency physicians, who are more accustomed to giving 1 mg or 1000 μg doses in the cardiac arrest situation. Over-reaction and overdosage of epinephrine, not uncommon in a drug with dosages that vary over several orders of magnitude, result in prompt marked hypertension and tachycardia as well as possible ventricular ectopy and fibrillation. Nevertheless, when the clinical situation is deteriorating rapidly, it is a reliably efficacious drug.

Recently, controversy has emerged concerning the proper dose of epinephrine in cardiac arrest situations [24]. The current ACLS recommendation for this clinical situation is 1 mg IV q5min [31]. If averaged out as a drip, this dose approximates a 3 μg/min drip for a 70-kg adult, which, as we have seen above, is a relatively low dose, considered by Callahan to be homeopathic for this situation [24]. Recent studies involving CPR in swine [32, 33] and dogs [34] indicate that much larger doses, i.e., 100 to 200 μg/ kg (7 to 14 mg in a 70-kg adult) have much greater efficacy in raising and prolonging diastolic blood pressure and in promoting cerebral and myocardial cellular survival.

It has also been claimed that epinephrine can convert the more ominous "fine" ventricular fibrillation into the more convertible "coarse" variety. Weaver and colleagues have demonstrated that although fine ventricular fibrillation is indeed a good predictor of increased mortality, epinephrine does little to alter this [35].

Alpha- versus Beta-Adrenergic Drugs in Cardiac Arrest

As the above discussion indicates, there is considerable clinical evidence that only alpha-range epinephrine is efficacious in the cardiac arrest situation. Otto and associates demonstrated in a convincing study that alpha blockade was uniformly fatal in a dog CPR model [36]. Redding and colleagues have demonstrated the efficacy of methoxamine, a pure long-acting alpha-adrenergic drug [37] and have gone on to postulate the superiority of such a drug in cardiac arrest to epinephrine, which still has some myocardial oxygen consumption–increasing beta effect. Holmes and associates [38] demonstrated that isoproterenol, a pure beta-1 and beta-2 agonist, decreases coronary perfusion in a dog arrest model, probably at the expense of increased blood flow to nonessential organ systems such as muscle. Thus, there may be a place in the treatment of cardiac arrest for alpha-agonist agents such as norepinephrine and phenylephrine because both are easily titratable alpha agonists. The former drug is a very strong alpha-adrenergic agent with a short duration of action and may be used in a drip in a fashion similar to epinephrine. Lindner and associates recently compared the use of epinephrine and norepinephrine in a porcine arrest model [39]. They showed that norepinephrine increased myocardial blood flow almost as much as epinephrine but caused significantly less myocardial oxygen consumption and increased coronary sinus oxygen values. They attributed this effect to the diminished beta-2 effect of the norepinephrine.

To further confuse the issue, Brown and colleagues showed improved myocardial extraction ratios and blood flow with epinephrine as opposed to phenylephrine in a swine arrest model [33]. Obviously, more research is needed in this area.

Although pharmacologic scholars may argue about what drug to use in patients with cardiac arrest, it seems clear that rapid defibrillation is the most important factor leading to survival [31, 40]. Defibrillation was the only beneficial treatment performed by paramedics in a Salt Lake City study by Dean and colleagues on the effect of mobile prehospital care of myocardial infarction patients [41]. There is also recent evidence that patients undergoing arrest who do not respond to paramedic interventions such as defibrillation and airway management have a dismal chance of responding to in-hospital therapy [42]. The implications of such a study on when to desist from a Code Blue resuscitation attempt for in-house patients should be considered.

Drip Combinations

In less severe cardiac disease treatment trends have changed from use of alpha drugs to beta-adrenergic drugs. For example, vasodilators such as nitroglycerin or nitroprusside are added to epinephrine drips to reduce afterload and related myocardial oxygen demand as well as to increase perfusion to the kidneys and gut [30]. In patients with pulmonary hypertension and right heart failure, one may infuse pressors such as epinephrine through a surgically placed left atrial line and simultaneously give, through a PA catheter line, a vasodilator such as nitroprusside or prostaglandin E_1 [43].

Dopamine hydrochloride is a popular drug for moderate hypotension and myocardial inotropic boost, although most agree that it has no place in treating cardiac arrest. Its unique low dose (0.5 to 3 μg/kg/min) dopaminergic effects increase renal blood flow. At moderate doses, 1 to 10 μg/kg/min, beta effects predominate, and at still higher doses alpha effects take over. Unfortunately, tachycardia is a common deleterious side effect, Dobutamine, on the other hand, a predominant beta-agonist drug, causes mild vascular dilatation and increased inotropy at normal clinical doses (2.5 to 10 μg/kg/min) with less tachycardia. Although these effects have shown dobutamine to be superior to dopamine in cardiac failure [44], more recent work shows that a combination of both yields a synergistic improvement compared with either alone [45].

PACEMAKERS

The usual setting in the ED in which a pacemaker is required is the presentation of a patient with a right coronary artery occlusion, inferior myocardial infarction, and severe bradycardia refractory to pharmacologic intervention [46]. Overdose of beta blockade drugs may also produce bradyasystolic arrest requiring prompt intervention [47]. Although in the past a transvenous pacing catheter may have been applied in these settings, such a catheter requires central venous access, demands considerable skill and time for electrode insertion, and has a high complication rate [48]. Although balloon-tipped, flow-directed venous catheters can assist nonfluoroscopic placement in the right ventricle, failure to capture can still occur. Recently, external cardiac pacing, in which a pacing stimulus is rapidly, reliably, and safely delivered through two large electrodes placed anteriorly and posteriorly, has become an important modality in emergency departments, ICUs, and operating rooms [49, 50]. Its use in prehospital care has also been demonstrated [51]. Although some muscle contraction invariably occurs and may concern the patient, this is a minor problem and does not stand in the way of making these devices the standard of care in any well-equipped facility.

Should a patient with a permanent pacemaker present to the ED, it is useful to know that when the battery power is low, the rate will be programmed to drop slightly as a warning, e.g., from 72 to 65. Hence, it is important to investigate prior program settings. If a patient is undergoing surgery, electrocautery will interfere with the sensing mode, preventing many permanently implanted transvenous pacemakers from firing. By placing an appropriate magnet over the implanted unit, one can convert the system to the fixed rate mode and alleviate this problem [52].

CARDIOPULMONARY BYPASS

Although initially developed for surgical procedures such as coronary artery bypass grafting and valve replacement, cardiopulmonary bypass (CPB) has been adapted for novel uses and locations in past years. In a nutshell, sterile cannulae are placed in large veins (femoral, internal jugular, or, most commonly, venae cavae) and in the arterial tree (femoral, aorta). Anticoagulation is achieved with heparin. Blood is drained into a venous reservoir below the cannulation site, pumped by a roller or vortex pump head through a membrane or bubble oxygenator, then through a heat exchanger, and back to the patient. A variety of gauges report oxygen saturation, pressures, and flow rates [53].

New uses for CPB include treatment of profound hypothermia and treatment of selected cases of acute myocardial infarction. Patients with profound hypothermia may be rewarmed most successfully by a variety of internal rewarming techniques, including peritoneal dialysis, hemodialysis, and inhalation of warmed oxygen. In the asystolic, hypothermic patient the most efficient warming method available should be used, and that is extracorporeal circulation [54]. Seuffert recently described just such a successful resuscitation in an Alaskan woman [55]. Drawbacks to this technique include the obvious need for sophisticated equipment and personnel as well as the need for total systemic anticoagulation. Heparinization can lead to massive hemorrhage in a hypothermic patient with undiagnosed traumatic injuries; hence, CPB should probably be instituted only for isolated hypothermic insults.

Development of portable pump oxygenators that contain only the most essential items to provide a cardiac output of from 2 to 2.5 liters/min have made institution of CPB possible outside of the operating room [56]. Bypass is initiated via a percutaneous Seldinger technique in which dilators enable a skilled physician to place large femoral arterial and venous cannulae. Although CPB has been reported to be useful in selected, moribund patients with acute myocardial infarction [57] and in a dog cardiac arrest model [58], the impact of the new portable technology in such situations has yet to be determined.

ICU use of left and right ventricular assist devices (LVADs and RVADs), which provide cardiac output only without oxygenation, has allowed patients with refractory pump failure to "rest" for prolonged periods [59]. Because the lungs must be included in the circuit, an open chest is required for insertion. Unfortunately, these devices also require anticoagulation, and prolonged use is harmful to platelet function.

A final device that may be encountered by an emergency physician or anesthesiologist is the intra-aortic balloon pump (IABP), in which a CO_2 or helium gas–powered balloon is placed through a femoral artery to a location just distal to the aortic arch. The balloon is expanded during diastole to increase coronary blood flow and deflated just as systole begins to augment ejection. These devices are also placed percutaneously and are (compared to CPB) safe, simple, and predictable. They do not produce a cardiac output, they only augment an existing output. Although they may be safer than prolonged CPB, they have been associated with life- and, especially, limb-threatening complications [60]. Sometimes, however, the IABP can tip the balance between myocardial oxygen consumption and supply favorably enough to be life saving.

As a final aside, most clinical decisions made during the use of CPB and other assist devices revolve around the patient's blood pressure, data that are usually recorded as radial arterial line pressure (see Chapter 12 for a more complete discussion of arterial lines). A number of reports have appeared that suggest that from 17 to 72 percent of postbypass radial line blood pressures are falsely low [61, 62]. This phenomenon is due to peripheral resistance and volume factors and not to compromised cardiac function, as shown by simultaneously recorded normal or elevated central aortic root pressures. Thus, measuring femoral or aortic root pressures (via the intra-aortic balloon pump) can dispel doubts about the veracity of radial line pressures in immediate postbypass situations and prevent unwarranted and dangerous therapy.

OPEN CHEST CARDIAC MASSAGE

Although abandoned with the onset of closed chest cardiac massage, the role of open chest massage in cardiac arrest is being reexamined. Sanders and colleagues [63] compared closed chest massage controls with open chest cardiac massage in a dog model and found that coronary perfusion pressure was increased tenfold (from 5 to 51 mm Hg) with direct cardiac compression. Survival was improved, however, only when the thoracotomy was initiated within 15 minutes after initiation of ventricular fibrillation. Other studies support these findings [64, 65].

Geehr and Lewis reported a randomized trial of open heart massage versus conventional CPR [66] in prehospital treatment of nontraumatic cardiac arrest. Of 23 patients in the former group and 26 patients in the latter, only three from each group survived to be admitted, and all eventually died. They concluded that the technique should be used only when cardiac tamponade is suspected. The obvious disadvantages of open massage include all the problems of nonoperating room thoracotomy (see Chapter 3), not the least of which is infection risk for the operator as well as danger of ventricular damage from overzealous manual manipulation.

Less mechanistic objections to the widespread use of open chest massage for cardiac arrest revolve around the perception that few patients are allowed to die in hospital without a Code Blue attempt, perhaps due to medicolegal fears. The concept of "death with dignity" is thought by many to be a valid one, and ritual thoracotomy on patients as a last act does seem to violate this idea. Open cardiac massage may well be underused in certain clinical situations; however, it is not clear at present exactly how to define such exigencies.

SPECIFIC CARDIAC EMERGENCY SETTINGS

THE STATUS POST CORONARY BYPASS GRAFT PATIENT

As coronary artery bypass grafting (CABG) becomes more commonly performed, both anesthesiologists and emergency physicians will see more and more patients who have had the procedure. For example, patients may present to the ED with nonrelated problems such as gastrointestinal hemorrhage or related problems such as new onset of ischemia. This history should trigger several considerations. If the patient is being prepared for emergent "re-do" heart surgery, increased blood loss is to be expected, extra large-bore (14-gauge) IV lines should be prepared, and blood and blood products should be readied in the blood bank. As a rule, should a patient who is status post-CABG deteriorate suddenly, emergent operation and cannulation will depend on femoral access because rapid dissection through the mass of sternal adhesions may be formidable. Hence, it is best to use great caution in placing femoral lines and to avoid hematoma formation in that region either by placing lines elsewhere or by skillful technique with adequate manual tamponade if needed.

The natural history and prognosis of patients who have had CABG surgery is variable. Often these patients have marked diminution of anginal symptoms or are totally pain free and have good exercise tolerance. Other patients may have initial relief of symptoms, but, due either to irretrievably damaged myocardium from prior infarcts or to progression of atherosclerosis, they continue to have increased symptoms and decreased exercise tolerance. A multifactorial study of 82 patients followed for 10 years after CABG surgery revealed that, of 132 total grafts patent 1 year following surgery, 50 grafts were unaffected after 10 years, 43 grafts were narrowed, and 39 grafts were occluded [67]. Thus, whatever clinical problem a post-CABG patient may have, it should be recognized that coronary artery disease is progressive and that the longer the time elapsed since surgery the greater the chance for renewed myocardial compromise.

VALVULAR DISEASE

It is not within the scope of this chapter to discuss the many characteristics of valvular heart disease. There are, however, some general principles regarding these patients that bear mentioning. First, any valvular lesion, whether stenotic or regurgitative, predisposes to turbulent blood flow (hence the murmer), and such flow predisposes to the formation of bacterial endocarditis. Hence, extreme care in avoiding bacteremia should be maintained during any procedure. Second, one should not always assume that a murmur is due to valvular blood flow because it may be due to a patent ventricular or atrial septal defect. Although during most of the cardiac cycle shunting is left-to-right, it is now accepted from Doppler echocardiographic studies that there are moments during the cardiac cycle when right-to-left flow occurs. When one also considers that a sizable minority of patients have a potentially patent foramen ovale, it becomes clear that *any* patient has the potential for right-to-left blood flow. Thus extreme care should always be taken to clear air out of intravenous apparati and to avoid injecting even tiny bubbles when administering IV medication.

Finally, it is useful to consider stenotic and regurgitant valvular lesions as groups. Aortic stenosis (AS) and mitral stenosis (MS) have a generally poorer prognosis than aortic regurgitation (AR) and mitral regurgitation (MR) [68]. Hemodynamically, it is best to keep in mind that for stenotic lesions, maintaining preload is the best defense against hypotension, especially with AS. A second goal is avoidance of dysrhythmia, especially new atrial fibrillation or marked tachycardia in MS or extreme bradycardia or tachycardia in AS. Thus, if confronted with a patient with AS who is hypotensive, one should refrain from use of pressors and inotropes and instead make sure that adequate volume and cardiac rhythm are maintained. CPR in an arrested AS patient is rarely successful in the best of circumstances but absolutely futile in a patient with inadequate volume loading. MS patients may already be volume overloaded with pulmonary congestion; hence, should they deteriorate one might try gentle inotropic support or, if MR/MS or extreme pulmonary hypertension exists, gentle vasodilatation.

Regurgitant lesions respond favorably to vasodilatation and mild tachycardia. Unlike stenotic lesions, there is no fixed orifice to limit stroke volume; instead, the problem is that blood may flow either forward or backward. Vasodilation and avoidance of bradycardia favor forward flow and are key foundations for treating compromised patients with AR or MR. For a more complete discussion of valvular heart disease and associated hemodynamic management, the interested reader is referred to an excellent discussion by Jackson and Thomas [69].

THROMBOLYTIC AND ANGIOPLASTY THERAPY

The use of thrombolytic therapy has logically followed the realization that thrombotic occlusion is the most common cause of a transmural myocardial infarction [70]. The therapeutic goal is increased plasmin, which is formed from the inactive proenzyme plasminogen by "activators." Plasmin then lyses the offending fresh fibrin clot. It is now clear that there are two types of plasmin activators—exogenous activators, such as urokinase or streptokinase, which activate plasmin more or less indiscriminately, and extrinsic activators, such as tissue-type plasminogen activator (TPA), which binds to fibrin clot. Only then, in the fibrin matrix, does plasminogen become bound and subsequently converted to plasmin [71]. The former activators have a higher propensity for hemorrhagic complications, and, based on a preliminary study, the latter activator, prototype TPA, is not only safer but almost twice as effective [72]. Now that TPA has been introduced clinically, the former drugs will no doubt be used less. Nevertheless, they have been efficacious in selected patients. Both intracoronary "cath lab" use and emergency medicine intravenous use (500,000 to 1.7 million IV units of streptokinase) have been studied [73]. It is not clear how best to treat persistent hemorrhage after streptokinase- or urokinase-induced hemorrhage other than by resupplying exogenous clotting factors, administration of epsilonaminocaproic acid [74] and allowing the drug to be metabolized. Unfortunately, there is no analogue to the use of protamine in heparin-treated patients. Hence, it is best to prevent complications by careful patient selection. Thus, exogenous plasminogen activator therapy should be considered only in patients with elevated ST segments and typical chest pain who do not have Q waves or recent surgery, a recent history of CPR, CVA, or other predisposition to hemorrhagic complications.

As TPA becomes more commonly used, emergency physicians may be recruited to administer the drug as they were for administering intravenous streptokinase. A controlled study from the National Heart Foundation of Australia examined the use of TPA within 4 hours from onset of symptoms [75]. Because of proved efficacy of thrombolytic therapy in patients with symptoms less than 2 hours old [76], they excluded such patients from randomization and possible placebo administration. Thus, because earlier therapy works better, emergency treatment may be warranted. Thorough preparation for reperfusion dysrhythmias, concomitant heparin therapy, and proper patient selection should precede such use of the drug. Interestingly, the National Institutes of Health (NIH) is currently performing a prehospital clinical trial on the use of TPA by paramedics in patients with classic MI symptoms and 12 lead-ECG telephone diagnosis by base station physician (personal communication, Joseph Gifford, M.D., Seattle, Washington). Preliminary results indicate that therapy is rendered 60 to 90 minutes earlier with such a program than by ED therapy.

RUPTURED AORTIC ANEURYSM

Definitive diagnosis for acute rupture of the aorta, whether thoracic or abdominal, rests on angiography, although on occasion a patient in shock may undergo exploratory surgery. Once the diagnosis is made, large-bore intravenous catheterization, CVP or PA catheterization, and arterial line placement should proceed as preparations for surgery. These patients require a great deal of volume replacement, as a rule, and this should be initiated in the ED with appropriate warming. It may be necessary to give noncrossmatched blood in the ED as well. In spite of the best efforts, this diagnosis carries a high mortality.

Medical treatment, which may be more precisely defined as drug therapy prior to proximal surgical control of the aneurysm, depends on controlling the blood pressure and limiting cardiac inotropy. Thus, administration of IV sodium nitroprusside alone may result in a reflex tachycardia with no diminution of inotropy and resultant increased stress on the aortic wall. One must therefore give adequate IV beta blocker drugs, e.g., propranolol or esmolol, concomitantly with the vasodilator. A heart rate of less than 70 bpm is a reasonable goal, and this may require up to 4 mg of IV propranolol per hour. An alternate medical regimen utilizes IV titration of the ganglionic blocker, trimethophan camsylate (Arfonad, 500 mg in 500 ml diluent, drip-titrated to blood pressure). This drug has a vagotonic action to accompany its vasodilatory effects and does not require beta blockade. Drawbacks include rapid tachyphylaxis, dilatation of the pupils (which can confuse neurologic examination), and the unfamiliarity of many physicians with its use.

CARDIAC TRANSPLANTS

The once heroic and experimental cardiac transplant is becoming a more and more accepted procedure at selected cardiac surgery centers around the United States, mostly due to the success of the immunosuppressant agent cyclosporin. In fact, over 50 percent of the 2577 transplants registered in 1986 were performed during the period from 1984 to 1986 [77]. Any emergency physician or anesthesiologist in a noncardiac transplant hospital may still be called on to give resuscitative care for a potential donor, usually a trauma victim with an isolated head injury. General management should include airway management, adequate volume replacement as measured by CVP, and preservation of adequate coronary perfusion pressures, usually measured indirectly by an arterial line. Some patients may require low to mid-dose dopamine in the face of hypotension with adequate volume replacement. Often these donor patients will develop diabetes insipidus secondary to their cranial injuries. This is primarily a water loss by the kidneys and should be replaced with crystalloid on a milliliter for milliliter basis in conjunction with intramuscular vasopressin. During anesthesia for removal of the heart, spinal reflexes can cause hypertension even in patients with no documented cerebral blood flow. Although IV narcotic can smooth anesthetic management, many prefer treatment with a strict vasodilator such as nitroprusside.

Criteria for brain death are discussed in Chapters 13 and 14 and may include cerebral blood flow studies. In California, two physicians must sign an affidavit prior to any transplant procedure. Anesthetic management for the recipient [78] is of interest to the emergency physician because an increased number of patients with denervated hearts may seek emergency care. Although their cardiac accelerators do not function, these patients can mount a tachycardia over time, if needed, by serum catecholamines. Nevertheless, if bradycardia is a clinical problem, anticholinergics such as atropine are not efficacious, and one should use a drug such as isoproterenol. These patients are immunosuppressed, and corresponding care should be taken to prevent infection. Symptoms of graft rejection, which usually mandate admission and cardiology consult, are secondary to decreased cardiac output and poor ventricular compliance. They include complaints of weakness, fatigue, or malaise [79].

TRAUMA

For discussion involving cardiac trauma, see Chapter 12.

CONCLUSION

To ensure a smooth transition for a cardiac patient from life outside the hospital, through the ED, to the catheter laboratory or operating room, to the ICU and the ward, and back to life on the outside, it is important for practitioners in all areas to have an understanding of the physiology, pharmacology, and various medical equipment options that may be utilized. Both anesthesiologists and emergency physicians may be required to intervene at any time and in many places to assist in airway management, cardiac arrest, or other immediate cardiac emergencies. We have endeavored in this chapter to discuss these problems from such a perspective.

REFERENCES

1. Cheney, F. W., and Colley, P. S. The effect of cardiac output on arterial blood oxygenation. *Anesthesiology* 52:496–503, 1980.
2. Lemaire, F., Teboul, J. L., Cinotti, L., et al. Acute left ventricular dysfunction during unsuccessful weaning from mechanical ventilation. *Anesthesiology* 69:171–179, 1988.
3. Permutt, S. Circulatory effects of weaning from mechanical ventilation: The importance of transdiaphragmatic pressure. *Anesthesiology* 69:157–160, 1988.
4. Kates, R. A. Antianginal Drug Therapy. In J. A. Kaplan (ed.), *Cardiac Anesthesia* (2nd ed.). New York: Grune & Stratton, 1987. Pp. 451–517.
5. Slogoff, S., and Keats, A. S. Does perioperative myocardial ischemia lead to postoperative myocardial infarction? *Anesthesiology* 62:107–114, 1985.
6. Lowenstein, E. Perianesthetic ischemic episodes cause myocardial infarction in humans—a hypothesis confirmed. *Anesthesiology* 62:103–106, 1985.
7. Slogoff, S., and Keats, A. S. *Anesthesiology* 65:539–542, 1986.
8. Harrison, L., Ralley, F. E., Wynands, J. E., et al. The role of an ultra short-acting adrenergic blocker (esmolol) in patients undergoing coronary bypass surgery. *Anesthesiology* 66:413–418, 1987.
9. Reves, J. G., Kissin, I., Fournier, S. E., et al. Additive negative inotropic effect of a combination of diazepam and fentanyl. *Anesth. Analg.* 63:97–100, 1984.
10. Stanley, T. H., and Webster, L. R. Anesthetic requirements and cardiovascular effects of fentanyl-oxygen and fentanyl-diazepam-oxygen anesthesia in man. *Anesth. Analg.* 57:411–416, 1978.
11. Franaszek, J. B. Congestive Heart Failure. In P. Rosen, et al. (ed.), *Emergency Medicine.* St. Louis: Mosby, 1988. Pp. 1303–1314.
12. Thys, D. M., and Kaplan, J. A. Recent Advances in Electrocardiographic Techniques. In J. A. Kaplan (ed.), *Cardiac Anesthesia* (2nd ed.). New York: Grune & Stratton, 1987. Pp. 227–253.

13. Blackburn, H., and Katigbak, R. What electrocardiographic leads to take after exercise? *Am. Heart J.* 67:184, 1964.
14. Sharkey, S. W. Beyond the wedge: Clinical physiology and the Swan-Ganz catheter. *Am. J. Med.* 83:111–122, 1987.
15. Reinhart, K., Moser, N., Rudolph, T., et al. Comparison of two mixed-venous saturation catheters in critically ill patients. *Anesthesiology* 67:A182, 1987.
16. Foote, G. A., Schabel, S. I., and Hodges, M. Pulmonary complications of the flow-directed balloon-tipped catheter. *N. Engl. J. Med.* 290:927–931, 1974.
17. Abel, M. D., Nishimura, R. A., Callahan, M. J., et al. Evaluation of intraoperative transesophageal two-dimensional echocardiography. *Anesthesiology* 66:64–68, 1987.
18. Smith, J. S., Cahalan, M. K., Benefiel, D. J., et al. Intraoperative detection of myocardial ischemia in high risk patients: Electrocardiography vs. two-dimensional echocardiography. *Circulation* 72:1015–1021, 1985.
19. Mark, J. B., Steinbrook, R. A., Gugino, L. D., et al. Continuous noninvasive monitoring of cardiac output with esophageal Doppler ultrasound during cardiac surgery. *Anesth. Analg.* 65:1013–1020, 1986.
20. Greeley, W. J., Kates, R. A., Bushman, G. A., et al. Intraoperative esophageal electrocardiography for dysrhythmia analysis and therapy in pediatric cardiac surgical patients. *Anesthesiology* 65:669–672, 1986.
21. Stacpoole, P. W. Lactic acidosis: The case against bicarbonate therapy. *Ann. Intern. Med.* 105:276–278, 1986.
22. Marinez, R. Sodium bicarbonate therapy in cardiac arrest. *West. J. Med.* 146:603–604, 1987.
23. Weil, M. H., Ruiz, C. E., Michaels, S., et al. Acid-base determinants of survival after cardiopulmonary resuscitation. *Crit. Care Med.* 13:888–892, 1985.
24. Callahan, M. Advances in the management of cardiac arrest. *West. J. Med.* 145:670–675, 1986.
25. Bing, O.H.L., Brooks, W. W., and Messer, J. V. Heart muscle viability following hypoxia: Protective effect of acidosis. *Science* 180:1297–1298, 1973.
26. Kagiyama, Y., Hill, J. L., and Gettes, L. S. Interaction of acidosis and increased extracellular potassium on action potential characteristics and conduction in guinea pig ventricular muscle. *Circ. Res.* 51:614–623, 1982.
27. Surawicz, B. Ventricular fibrillation. *J. Am. Coll. Cardiol.* 5:43B–45B, 1985.
28. Houle, D. B., Weil, M. H., Brown, E. B., et al. Influence of respiratory acidosis on ECG and pressor responses to epinephrine, norepinephrine, and metaraminol. *Proc. Soc. Exp. Biol. Med.* 94:561–564, 1957.
29. Zwanger, M. L., Domeier, R. M., Bock, B. F. Effect of epinephrine on cardiovascular hemodynamics during metabolic acidosis. *Ann. Emerg. Med.* 15:638, 1986.
30. Kaplan, J. A. Treatment of perioperative left heart failure. In J. A. Kaplan (ed.), *Cardiac Anesthesia* (2nd ed.). New York: Grune & Stratton, 1987.
31. Standards and guidelines for cardiopulmonary resuscitation (CPR) and emergency cardiac care (ECC). *J.A.M.A.* 255:2905–2973, 1986.
32. Brown, C. G., Werman, H. A., Davis, E. A., et al. Comparative effect of graded doses of epinephrine on regional brain blood flow during CPR in a swine model. *Ann. Emerg. Med.* 15:1138–1144, 1986.
33. Brown, C. G., Taylor, R. B., Werman, H. A., et al. Myocardial oxygen delivery/consumption during cardiopulmonary resuscitation: A comparison of epinephrine and phenylephrine. *Ann. Emerg. Med.* 17:302–308, 1988.
34. Kosnik, J. W., Jackson, R. E., Keats, S., et al. Dose-related response of centrally administered epinephrine on the change in aortic diastolic pressure during closed-chest massage in dogs. *Ann. Emerg. Med.* 14:204–208, 1985.
35. Weaver, W. D., Cobb, L. A., Dennis, D., et al. Amplitude of ventricular fibrillation waveform and outcome after cardiac arrest. *Ann. Intern. Med.* 102:53–55, 1985.

36. Otto, C. W., Yakaitis, R. W., and Blitt, C. D. Mechanism of action of epinephrine in resuscitation from asphyxial arrest. *Crit. Care Med.* 9:365–365, 1981.
37. Redding, J. S., Haynes, R. R., and Thomas, J. D. Drug therapy in resuscitation from electromechanical dissociation. *Crit. Care Med.* 11:681–684, 1983.
38. Holmes, H. R., Babbs, C. F., Voorhees, W. D., et al. Influence of adrenergic drugs upon vital organ perfusion during CPR. *Crit. Care Med.* 8:137–140, 1980.
39. Lindner, K. H., Ahnefield, F. W., Schurmann, W., et al. A comparison of epinephrine and norepinephrine on myocardial oxygen delivery and consumption during cardiopulmonary resuscitation. *Anesthesiology* 69:3A(S):A96, 1988.
40. Eisenberg, M. S., Bergner, L., Hallstrom, A. P., et al. Sudden cardiac death. *Sci. Am.* 245:37–43, 1986.
41. Dean, N. C., Haug, P. J., and Hawker, P. J. Effect of mobile paramedic units on outcome in patients with myocardial infarction. *Ann. Emerg. Med.* 17:1034–1041.
42. Kellerman, A. L., Staves, D. R., and Hackman, B. B. In-hospital resuscitation following unsuccessful prehospital advanced cardiac life support: "Heroic efforts" or an exercise in futility? *Ann. Emerg. Med.* 17:589–594, 1988.
43. D'Ambra, M. N., LaRaia, P. J., Philbin, D. M., et al. Prostaglandin E_1. *J. Thorac. Cardiovasc. Surg.* 89:567–572, 1985.
44. Leier, C. V., Heban, P.T., Huss, P., et al. Comparative systemic and regional hemodynamic effects of dopamine and dobutamine in patients with cardiomyopathic heart failure. *Circulation* 58:446–475, 1978.
45. Richard, C., Ricome, J. L., Rimailho, A., et al. Combined effects of dopamine and dobutamine in cardiogenic shock. *Circulation* 67:620–626, 1983.
46. Little, T. External cardiac pacing in right ventricular infarction. *Ann. Emerg. Med.* 17:640–643, 1988.
47. Kenyon, C. J., Aldinger, G. E., Joshipura, P., et al. Successful resuscitation using external cardiac pacing in beta adrenergic antagonist-induced bradyasystolic arrest. *Ann. Emerg. Med.* 17:711–713, 1988.
48. Austin, J. L., Preis, L. K., Crampton, R. S., et al. Analysis of pacemaker malfunction and complications of temporary pacing in the coronary care unit. *Am. J. Cardiol.* 49:301–306, 1982.
49. Falk, R. H., Zoll, P. M., and Zoll, R. H. Safety and efficacy of noninvasive cardiac pacing. *N. Engl. J. Med.* 309:1166–1168, 1983.
50. Rhee, K. J. Transcutaneous cardiac pacing. *West. J. Med.* 146:605, 1987.
51. Paris, P. M., Stewart, R. D., and Kaplan, R. M. Transcutaneous pacing for bradyasystolic cardiac arrests in prehospital care. *Ann. Emerg. Med.* 14:320–323, 1985.
52. Ludmer, P. I., and Goldschlager, N. Cardiac pacing in the 80's. *N. Engl. J. Med.* 311:1671–1680, 1984.
53. Tinker, J. H., and Roberts, S. L. Management of Cardiopulmonary Bypass. In J. A. Kaplan (ed.), *Cardiac Anesthesia* (2nd ed.). New York: Grune & Stratton, 1987. Pp. 895–926.
54. Paton, B. C. Accidental hypothermia. *Pharmacol. Ther.* 22:331–377, 1983.
55. Seuffert, G. An Alaskan experience with cardiopulmonary bypass in resuscitating patients with profound hypothermia and cardiac arrest. *Alaska Med.* 26:31–33, 1984.
56. Phillips, S. J., Ballentine, B., Slonine, D., et al. Percutaneous initiation of cardiopulmonary bypass. *Ann. Thorac. Surg.* 36:223–225, 1983.
57. Stuckey, J. H., Newman, M. M., Dennis, C., et al. The use of the heart-lung machine in selected cases of acute myocardial infarction. *Surg. Forum* 8:342–344, 1985.
58. Levine, R., Gorayeb, M., Safar, P., et al. Cardiopulmonary bypass after cardiac arrest and prolonged closed chest CPR in dogs. *Ann. Emerg. Med.* 16:620–627, 1987.

59. Dembitsky, W. P., Daily, P. O., Raney, A. A., et al. Temporary extracorporeal support of the right ventricle. *J. Thorac. Cardiovasc. Surg.* 91:518–525, 1986.

60. Silvay, G., Litwak, R. S., and Griepp, R. B. Circulatory Assist Devices. In J. A. Kaplan (ed.), *Cardiac Anesthesia* (2nd ed.). New York: Grune & Stratton, 1987. Pp. 1021–1038.

61. Mohr, R., Lavee, J., and Goor, D. A. Inaccuracy of radial artery pressure measurements after cardiac operations. *J. Thorac. Cardiovasc. Surg.* 94:286–290, 1987.

62. Stern, D. H., Gerson, J. I., Allen, F. B., et al. Can we trust the direct radial artery pressure immediately following cardiopulmonary bypass? *Anesthesiology* 62:557–561, 1985.

63. Sanders, A. B., Kern, K. B., Atlas, M., et al. Importance of the duration of inadequate coronary perfusion pressure on resuscitation from cardiac arrest. *J. Am. Coll. Cardiol.* 6:113–118, 1985.

64. Bircher, N., and Safar, P. Manual open chest cardiopulmonary resuscitation. *Ann. Emerg. Med.* 13:770–773, 1984.

65. Sanders, A. B., Kern, K. B., Ewy, G. A., et al. Improved resuscitation from cardiac arrest with open chest massage. *Ann. Emerg. Med.* 13:672–675, 1984.

66. Geehr, E. C., Lewis, F. R., and Auerbach, P. S. Failure of open-heart massage to improve survival after prehospital nontraumatic cardiac arrest. *N. Engl. J. Med.* 314:1189–1190, 1986.

67. Campeau, L., Enjalbert, M., Lesperance, J., et al. The relation of risk factors to the development of atherosclerosis in saphenous-vein bypass grafts and the progression of disease in the native circulation. *N. Engl. J. Med.* 311:1329–1339, 1984.

68. Rapaport, E. Natural history of aortic and mitral valve disease. *Am. J. Cardiol.* 35:221–227, 1975.

69. Jackson, J. M., and Thomas, S. J. Valvular Heart Disease. In J. A. Kaplan (ed.), *Cardiac Anesthesia* (2nd ed.). New York: Grune & Stratton, 1987. Pp. 589–633.

70. DeWood, M. A., Spores, J., Hensley, G. R., et al. Coronary arteriographic findings in acute transmural infarction. *Circulation* 68 (Suppl. I):39–49, 1983.

71. Estafanous, F. G. Management of Emergency Revascularization or Cardiac Reoperation. In J. A. Kaplan (ed.), *Cardiac Anesthesia* (2nd ed.). New York: Grune & Stratton, 1987. Pp. 833–854.

72. TIMI Study Group. The thrombolysis in myocardial infarction (TIMI) trial, Phase I findings. *N. Engl. J. Med.* 312:932–936, 1985.

73. Alderman, E. L., Jutzy, K. R., Berti, L. E., et al. Randomized comparison of intravenous versus intracoronary streptokinase for myocardial infarction. *Am. J. Cardiol.* 54:14–19, 1984.

74. Fabian, J. A., and Stewart, L. Fibrinolytic Therapy. In Ellison, N., and Jobes, D. R. (ed.), *Effective Hemostasis in Cardiac Surgery.* Philadelphia: Saunders, 1988. Pp. 57–68.

75. National Heart Foundation of Australia Coronary Thrombolysis Group. Coronary thrombolysis and myocardial salvage by tissue plasminogen activator given up to 4 hours after onset of myocardial infarction. *Lancet* 1:203–208, 1988.

76. Gruppo Italiano per lo Studio della Strepochinasi nell' Infarto Miocardico (GISSO). Effectiveness of intravenous thrombolytic treatment in acute myocardial infarction. *Lancet* 397–401, 1986.

77. Copeland, J. G., Emery, R. W., Levinson, M. M., et al. Selection of patients for cardiac transplantation. *Circulation* 75:2–9, 1987.

78. Hensley, F. A., Martin, D. E., Larach, D. R., et al. Anesthetic management for cardiac transplant in North America—1986. *J. Cardiothorac. Anesth.* 1:429–437, 1987.

79. Trento, A., Hardsty, R. L., and Griffith, B. P. Heart Transplantation. In Shoemaker, W. C., Ayres, S., Grenvik, A., et al. (ed.), *Textbook of Critical Care* (2nd ed.). Philadelphia: Saunders, 1989.

5. Pharmacology

Christopher A. Mills

Case 1

A frail elderly woman is brought by her husband to the emergency department. The woman is so tachypneic that she cannot talk and indeed appears only barely able to cooperate; her husband relates a long-standing history of chronic obstructive pulmonary disease (COPD), characterized by emphysema and periodic attacks of asthma. The woman had been complaining for 6 months or more of increasing dyspnea on exertion, which abruptly worsened the morning of admission; the dyspnea was accompanied by nausea and palpitations. During the last 3 hours the shortness of breath progressed to the point where she could only sit bolt upright; her usual antiasthma drugs were completely ineffective. On admission her blood pressure is 90/50 mm Hg, the pulse is regular at 120 beats/min (bpm), and respirations are 44/min. On 4 liters of oxygen by nonrebreathing mask, arterial blood gases are reported as follows: pH 7.19, PCO_2 74, PO_2 48, and hemoglobin 16.3. What should be done next?

Case 2

An 18-year-old male was riding his Moped home from school without benefit of a helmet. While traveling at about 30 miles an hour, he hit an automobile broadside, was catapulted over the car, and landed on the sidewalk. The paramedics report that on their arrival about 5 minutes after the accident the patient was breathing, not moving any extremity, and was unresponsive. After protecting the cervical spine, they brought the patient to the emergency department, where he began to scream and move his arms and legs vigorously; he was still not coherent. Aside from the mental status changes, a brief neurologic examination was negative. Although the patient is becoming combative, the vital signs are stable, and consultation is sought with a neurosurgeon and a trauma surgeon, who order CT scans of the head and abdomen, respectively. What should be done next?

Case 3

A 78-year-old male was scheduled for colonic endoscopy to evaluate occult rectal bleeding. The patient had had coronary artery bypass grafting 8 years previously, and during the past 3 years his angina has returned. In addition to "mild" type II diabetes that is responsive to oral agents and chronic hypertension that is fairly well controlled by calcium channel blockers and a diuretic, the patient has a known abdominal aortic aneurysm that has grown slightly by echocardiography during the past 6 months. The patient was very uncomfortable during the colonoscopy and received intravenous sedation consisting of 7 mg of midazolam (Versed) and 14 mg of morphine sulfate. His blood pressure was relatively stable in the range of 160/100 during the procedure, which was terminated after 45 minutes. Five minutes afterward he was difficult to rouse and was brought downstairs to the emergency department. Oxygen is administered by nasal cannulae; his vital signs include a blood pressure of 108/76, pulse of 46 bpm, and respirations between

8 and 10 per minute. Transcutaneous pulse oximetry shows an arterial saturation of 98 percent. This outpatient is barely responsive; the endoscopist and the patient's wife anxiously await the emergency physician's report on how to arouse him so he can go home. What should be done next?

Each of the preceding case reports is hypothetical yet represents a plausible situation that might occur in the emergency department. This chapter will make periodic reference to these cases as important points concerning phamracologic principles of anesthesia and emergency medicine are developed. The first part of this chapter consists of a brief and very basic overview of pharmacokinetics—how the drugs given to patients get to the site of their action, and how their actions are later terminated. Specific drug categories—namely, hypnotics/cerebral depressants, narcotics and antagonists, muscle relaxants, and the anesthetic vapors—will be discussed. The pharmacology of local anesthetics is discussed in Chapter 6 of this book.

PHARMACOKINETICS

The movement of drugs into and out of the various body fluids and tissues and the interaction of drugs with receptors to bring about specific actions is referred to as pharmacokinetics. A much more complete treatment of this complex subject can be found elsewhere [1–5]; the intent of this section is to introduce the reader to basic concepts such as volume of distribution, distribution and elimination half-life, and the differences between intravenous bolus and infusion drug administration.

VOLUME OF DISTRIBUTION

The fluids and tissues into which a drug disperses are called its volume of distribution. This is the apparent volume needed to reach the serum concentration that is found after a known amount of drug is administered. For example, if a bucket contained 1 liter of fluid and 1 gram of a drug—say penicillin—was put into the bucket and then measured, 1 gram of penicillin per liter of fluid would be found, which is the volume into which the penicillin is distributed. But if a different 1-liter bucket were used that was lined with a membrane that absorbed half the penicillin it came in contact with, then only one-half gram of penicillin per liter of fluid would be found. To get the same concentration as that found in the first bucket, you would need twice the penicillin. The volume of distribution in the second bucket, the one that sequesters the penicillin, is twice that of the normal bucket; the second bucket appears to be twice as big as the first. Thus a drug that leaves the plasma (which is our bucket in the previous example) and preferentially binds to the tissue will have a relatively large volume of distribution. This

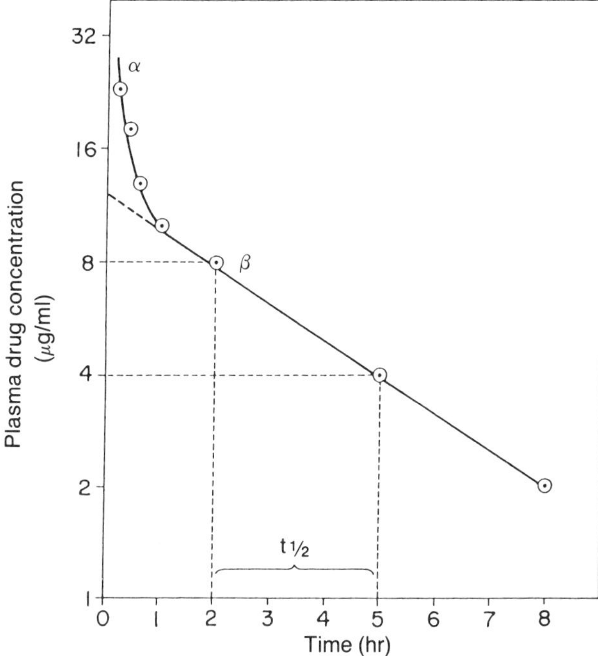

Fig. 5-1. Pharmacokinetics of a single IV bolus. The plasma concentration following administration of a single dose of a drug is shown. The rapid alpha elimination and slower beta elimination (3 hours in this case) are illustrated. (From A. G. Gilman and L. Goodman [eds.], *The Pharmacologic Basis of Therapeutics.* New York: Macmillan, 1980. With permission.)

class of drugs tends to be highly lipophilic. The volume of distribution varies with the drug and with the disease process: it tends to be larger in patients with renal failure, for instance. In healthy patients, of course, the volume of distribution is most closely related to patient weight. Heavier patients are bigger "buckets," and so the initial dose of drug needs to be higher to reach the same serum level and, presumably, drug effect.

THE SINGLE BOLUS; DISTRIBUTION AND ELIMINATION HALF-LIVES

As detailed in Figure 5-1, when a drug is administered intravenously as a "push" or "bolus," it reaches peak blood concentration very rapidly—in seconds. This drug-rich volume of blood is itself rapidly redistributed, first into the vessel-rich group of body organs that includes the heart and brain. Simply put, after an IV push, drug concentrations will reach extraordinarily high concentrations in a matter of seconds; these high concentrations will be delivered to the heart and brain in one "arm-to-brain" circulation time.

If you read the following sentence aloud, not quickly, but not slowly, you will have an idea of what that circulation time is:

> The drug has just entered the arm through the IV tubing. It travels up the arm, over to the heart, around the heart, and out to the lungs. It travels through the lungs, back to the heart, around the heart, and up the carotid arteries to the brain.

From that point on, the concentration of the drug, particularly in the *vessel-rich group,* will fall. At first this diminution of drug level will be very rapid; this decrease is referred to as the *alpha* or *distribution half-life* and reflects (1) the dilution of the initial high concentration by successive "tides" of blood that had not been exposed to the drug during its bolus administration, and (2) the blood circulating to and depositing drug at other, more slowly perfused tissues in the body. These tissues are referred to as the *vessel-poor* group.

Again, as seen in Figure 5-1, following the redistribution the drug is then slowly eliminated from the body via some combination of metabolism and excretion. This *beta* or *elimination half-life* follows first-order kinetics. Such kinetics dictate that a constant fraction is reduced per unit of time; if the elimination half-life is 1 hour, then half of the drug is eliminated in the first hour, half of what remains (i.e., one-quarter of the initial dose) is eliminated during the second hour, and so on. After four elimination half-lives, only one-sixteenth of the drug remains, and for all intents and purposes, the drug has been eliminated.

For most drugs administered in the emergency department, the alpha half-life is on the order of 5 to 10 minutes, and the beta half-life is on the order of 1 to 3 hours. One glaring exception is succinylcholine: its beta elimination half-life is so fast that it interferes with the redistribution of the drug.

Drugs may be eliminated by a variety of methods; they may be metabolized in the liver, transported back to the gut through the enterohepatic circulation and excreted through the feces, or metabolized to compounds excreted in the urine. Drugs may be excreted directly in the urine; compounds, particularly inhaled agents, may be eliminated through the lungs.

Repeated doses of a drug will cause cumulative effects. Boluses given at fixed doses and intervals reach plateau concentrations at about four half-lives, as shown in Figure 5-2.

Note, however, that there are still relatively wide changes in serum drug concentration about this "plateau" level; for some drugs, the peak concentration may be too high or the trough too low to be of benefit to the patient.

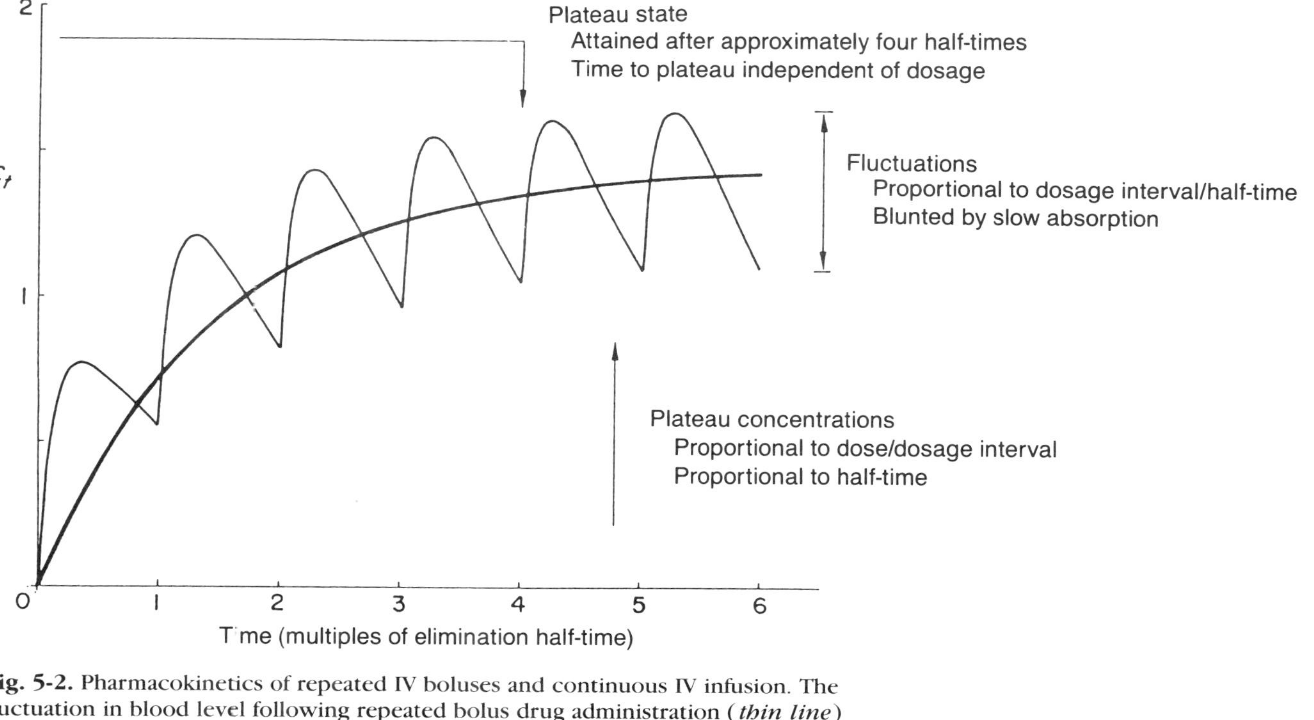

Fig. 5-2. Pharmacokinetics of repeated IV boluses and continuous IV infusion. The fluctuation in blood level following repeated bolus drug administration (*thin line*) is illustrated. The more smooth curve (*thick line*) represents a constant intravenous infusion of the drug. A plateau is reached after about 4 beta half-lives of drug administration. (From A. G. Gilman and L. Goodman [eds.], *The Pharmacologic Basis of Therapeutics.* New York: Macmillan, 1980. With permission.)

THE CONSTANT INFUSION

The desired serum drug level can be reached quickly, and this level maintained smoothly, if a loading dose is followed by a constant intravenous infusion (Fig. 5-3). This technique is particularly valuable in administering drugs with fast beta-elimination half-lives that would otherwise require very frequent repeated bolus doses, such as lidocaine. The bolus of drug is calculated by the volume of distribution into which the drug is dispersing; the rate of infusion is calculated by knowing the half-life, or beta elimination. (Common vasoactive drugs that are given by constant infusion are listed in Table 5-1.)

Of concern are drugs metabolized into compounds that are themselves active. Vecuronium, a nondepolarizing skeletal muscle relaxant, for example, is metabolized into compounds that have no action of their own. A similar compound, pancuronium bromide, is metabolized into a compound that is itself half as potent as its parent. If the correct amount of drug is given exactly every half-life, and the drug is metabolized into inactive compounds, a steady-state will be reached as outlined previously (see Fig. 5-2). However, if active metabolites remain, the action of the drug appears to increase; the beta elimination of the effect of the drug increases, and the intervals between drug doses need to be lengthened.

Although the drug is physically eliminated from the body during the beta, or elimination, half-life, the majority of offsets of action of most drugs administered in the acute setting of the emergency department or the operating room are based on the alpha, or redistribution half-life. Many of the drugs, including sodium thiopental, vecuronium, fentanyl, and even morphine, undergo a curtailing of effect not because they are being eliminated through the liver or kidneys but because they are being redistributed from organ systems sensitive to their actions, such as the brain, to organ systems that are relatively unaffected by them, such as the fat and skin. As can be seen from Figure 5-1, the decrease in concentration during the 30 minutes of redistribution (from 32 to 8, or 24 μg/ml) is about three times the decrease (from 8 to 2, or 6 μg/ml) that takes place during the next 7 hours of metabolism. It is apparent that if no drug effect is seen at or below a plasma drug concentration of 15 μg/ml, for example, metabolism per se of this single bolus is of virtually no effect in terms of offset of action. By contrast, for a drug given by repeated boluses, or constant infusion, metabolism plays a very large role in determining drug effect.

Exceptionally large doses of narcotics are often used in cardiac anesthesia; such doses may be two orders of magnitude higher than doses encountered for pain relief in the emergency department. At such high doses, the usual offset of action of the narcotic becomes much more dependent on drug elimination (rather than redistribution). Remember that in reversing the action of narcotics in such high doses (which may also be encountered in drug addicts), the action of naloxone, for example, will be depen-

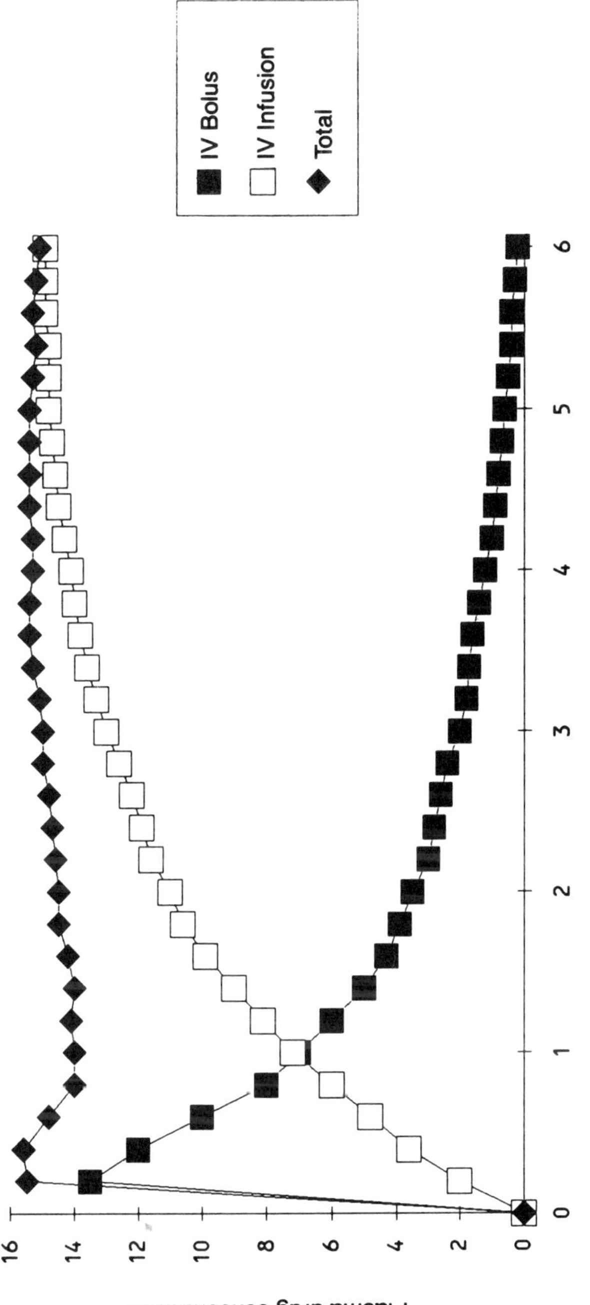

Fig. 5-3. Pharmacokinetics of IV bolus followed by constant infusion. An initial (or loading) dose followed by an infusion results in a more constant blood level, which is reached very quickly. This technique is particularly useful for drugs with short beta-elimination half-lives, such as epinephrine or lidocaine.

Table 5-1. Vasoactive drug delivery chart

Drug	Mix in 250 ml 5% D/W except as noted	Strength	Dose (usual or moderate)	IV rate (ml/hr) according to body weight (kg/lb)					
				50 kg/ 110 lb	60 kg/ 132 lb	70 kg/ 154 lb	80 kg/ 176 lb	90 kg/ 198 lb	100 kg/ 220 lb
Aminophylline[a]	500 mg	2 mg/ml	0.5 mg/kg/hr	12.5	15	17.5	20	22.5	25
Amrinone[b]	100 mg + 20 ml NS	2.5 mg/ml	5 µg/kg/min	6	7.2	8.4	9.6	10.8	12
Dobutamine	500 mg	2 mg/ml	5 µg/kg/min	7.5	9	10.5	12	13.5	15
Dopamine	400 mg	1600 µg/ml	5 µg/kg/min	9.4	11.25	13.1	15	16.9	18.8
Epinephrine	2 mg	8 µg/ml	2 µg/min			2 µ/min	=	15 ml/hr	
Esmolol[f]	2.5 gm	10 mg/ml	5 µg/kg/min	15	18	21	24	27	30
Hydralazine	250 mg (100 mg/ 100 ml)	1 mg/ml	5 µg/kg/min	15	18	21	24	26	30
Insulin	25 u/100 ml NS	0.25 u/ml	1 u/hr (1-4)			1 u/hr = 4 ml/hr			
Isoproterenol	1 mg	4 µg/ml	1 µg/min			1 µg/min	=	15 ml/hr	
Metaraminol	100 mg	400 µg/ml	50 µg/min			50 µg/min	=	7.5 ml/hr	
Naloxone	10 mg (4 mg/ 100 ml)	40 µg/ml			10 µg/min	=	0.6 mg/hr	=	15 ml/hr

Phenylephrine	33.3 (20 mg/ 150 ml)	133 µg/ml	0.5 µg/kg/min	11.25	13.5	15.75	18	20.25	22.5
Nitroglycerin	50 mg	200 µg/ml	0.5 µg/kg/min (µg/min)	7.5 (25)	9 (30)	10.5 (35)	12 (40)	13.5 (45)	15 (50)
Nitroprusside	50 mg	200 µg/ml	0.5 µg/kg/min	7.5	9	10.5	12	13.5	15
Norepinephrine	4 mg	16 µg/ml	4 µg/min			4 µg/min	=	15 ml/hr	
Prostaglandin E_1	2000 µg/100 ml	20 µg/ml	20–100 ng/kg/ min	3–15	3.6–18	4.2–21	4.8–24	5.4–26	6–30
Trimethaphan	500 mg	2 mg/ml	250 µg/kg/min	6.25	7.5	8.75	10	11.25	12.5
Lidocaine[c]	2 gm	8 mg/ml	1–4 mg/min			2 mg/min	=	15 ml/hr	
Procainamide[d]	2 gm	8 mg/ml	1–4 mg/min			2 mg/min	=	15 ml/hr	
Bretylium[c]	2 gm	8 mg/ml	1–4 mg/min			2 mg/min	=	15 ml/hr	

The commonly used vasoactive drugs, and dilutions that are common to our operating room and intensive care units are shown. A "usual" or moderate dose is shown, and the intravenous delivery rate in ml/hr for various body weights is charted. Example: Dopamine is needed in a 60 kg patient at 5 µg/ kg/min. Look across *Dopamine*: dilute 400 mg in 250 ml of 5% D/W, and for a 60-kg patient, infuse at 11.25 ml/hr to deliver 5 µg/kg/hr. *Example*: A standard nitroglycerine drip is running at 35 ml/hr in a 75-kg patient. What dose is being delivered? Interpolate rates between 70 and 80 kg to arrive at 11.2 ml/hr: this patient is on about triple that, or 0.5 × 3 = 1.5 µg/kg/min (or 112.5 µg/min).

NS = normal saline

[a]Aminophylline: Load 6 mg/kg.

[b]Amrinone: Load 0.75 mg/kg and may repeat once.

[c]Lidocaine: Load 1-1.5 mg/kg.

[d]Procainamide: Load 100 mg q 5 min to 1 gm total.

[e]Bretylium: Load 5 mg/kg and may repeat to a total of 30 mg/kg.

[f]Esmolol: Load 0.5 mg/kg.

dent on redistribution and will be of shorter duration than that of the narcotic. This concept is discussed in further detail later in this chapter.

OTHER ROUTES OF ADMINISTRATION

The physician is not limited to getting drugs into a patient directly by vein, although venous administration is certainly the fastest and surest method of delivery. Venous access may be impossible in a patient who habitually self-administers intravenous drugs or in a patient in cardiovascular collapse. Alternatives include intramuscular, subcutaneous, oral, sublingual, rectal, intratracheal, inhalational, and peridural administration; these routes should be kept in mind for a patient who is without immediate venous access.

Intramuscular (IM) and subcutaneous (subQ) administration depends on local blood flow; anything that diminishes that flow will delay the onset of the drug. Indeed, drugs that themselves have a deleterious effect on local blood flow, such as epinephrine, may slow their own appearance in the blood stream. Thus the toxic dose of local anesthetics used for infiltration is about 50 percent higher when combined with epinephrine because the absorption into the vasculature is delayed by the vasoconstrictive effect of the epinephrine.

In general, whereas the appearance of drug effect after intravenous administration is on the order of 2 to 10 minutes, the onset after IM or subQ administration is delayed to between 30 and 90 minutes, and the immediacy of effect is blunted because serum drug levels rise gradually. Concomitantly, drug offset is also slower, so the serum drug level after intramuscular or subcutaneous administration rises more slowly and to a lower peak level, and diminishes more slowly than after an intravenous dose. If regional blood flow is low enough, as in severe hypothermia or cardiovascular collapse, the drug may never be adequately mobilized from the muscle to the blood stream, so adequate serum drug levels will never be reached. Some medications, including diazepam, are very unreliably absorbed after intramuscular injections.

Oral and rectal dosing also rely on local blood flow; in addition, for sublingual drugs to be effective, they must be dissolved in the saliva. In general, these routes are intermediate in efficacy between the IV and IM/subQ routes. Drugs absorbed from the rectum differ from those absorbed higher in the gastrointestinal system: Rectal drugs miss the liver in their first pass through the body. This may result in higher peak levels because even during one pass, the liver can be a very efficient site for metabolism of medication.

Intrathecal and peridural drug administration can result in complex and variable effects. It must be remembered that these routes of administration, although involving very small quantities of medication (0.4 mg of morphine, for example) can deliver levels of drug at the brain that are much higher than might otherwise be expected because the blood-brain barrier has been bypassed.

Intratracheal drug administration is a convenient method of administering drugs to an intubated patient who has no venous access. Epinephrine is the most commonly used drug given by intratracheal administration; the usual adult dose is 1 mg, or 10 ml of a 1:1000 solution [6]. Atropine, isoproterenol, and nitroglycerin should also be effective by this route. Lidocaine and naloxone are also effective when given through an endotracheal tube; calcium chloride, sodium bicarbonate, and diazepam are contraindicated by this route because of potential toxicity to the pulmonary parenchyma from either the drug itself (the former drugs) or the diluent (diazepam).

The inhalation of bronchoactive drugs such as beta-2-specific agonists has been an accepted method of administration for many years; remember that in patients suffering from extreme bronchospasm, such medications may not reach the distal reactive airways and thus may not be efficacious. Generally, systemic absorption via the tracheobronchial tree is as fast as direct intravenous administration. Inhalational administration of other medications is essentially limited to the anesthetic vapors, which will be discussed near the end of this chapter.

THE INTRAVENOUS AGENTS

For the purposes of discussion in the following sections, some terms need to be defined. Remember that many of the agents in the pharmacopeia are very specific in their actions, although this may be difficult to discern by simple observation. For example, an adequately ventilated patient who has been given 70 mg of morphine will superficially appear identical to one given 7 mg of pancuronium, but their underlying states of consciousness, central adrenergic tones, and responses to pain will be very different.

In the following sections, terms will be used according to the following definitions. *Analgesia* is insensitivity to pain; note that this definition is without comment on consciousness. Given enough pure analgesia, a patient may be quite aware of his surroundings but may not experience the sensation or physiologic sequelae of noxious stimuli. *Amnesia* is loss of memory for an event, likewise without comment on physiologic response to pain. *Hypnosis* is a state resembling sleep (i.e., unarousable, eyes closed), whereas *sedation* (according to *Webster's New Collegiate Dictionary*) is a "relaxed easy state" (i.e., arousable, eyes often open); a sedated patient or one under the effect of pure hypnotics may have intact responses to pain. *Tranquilize* means to reduce mental tension and anxiety (*ibid.*), specifically through two classes of drugs called *neuroleptics* and *minor tranquilizers*. *Dissociate* means to disrupt normal mental processes, inhibiting cognition. A patient who is *anesthetized* has been rendered insensitive to the surroundings, no matter what the surroundings are doing to him; anesthesia may involve a patient generally, affecting the total body, or locally, affecting a region of the body. *Relaxed* and *relaxation* are two terms specific to anesthesia, referring to muscle tone; enough "relaxation" will result in complete muscle paralysis. Unless adequately sedated or tranquilized, or anesthetized, a muscularly "relaxed" patient will be mentally quite "tense."

BARBITURATES

There are four barbiturates in common use: sodium thiopental (STP, Pentothal), thiamylal sodium (Surital), methohexital (Brevital), and pentobarbital (Nembutal). Etomidate (Amidate), although not a barbiturate will also be discussed in this section. The eugonols, for example, propanidid, and the steroids, for example, althesin and minaxolone, are not used in this country, partly because of an unacceptably high rate of sensitivity and side effects with higher doses. They will not be mentioned further in this chapter.

Sodium Thiopental

Sodium thiopental is the most commonly used agent for the induction of general anesthesia. Barbiturates, because of their quick onset and offset of action, are often used to induce a brief state of "general anesthesia" during which other treatments can be accomplished, such as tracheal intubation, cardioversion, or beginning other forms of anesthesia such as infiltration of local anesthetics or induction of inhalational anesthesia. All barbiturates including thiopental have a distinct lack of analgesia and, in fact, induce mild hyperesthesia; they are not often used for the maintenance of anesthesia in this country. Their pharmacokinetics are presented in Figs. 5-4 and 5-5.

Thiopental is lipophilic and un-ionized, and has rapid brain uptake—one circulation time—in spite of high protein binding. The fast offset of action derives from its redistribution back out of brain tissue rather than from metabolism. The properties of thiopental will be presented as a generic representation of the entire class of barbiturates; differences in the individual agents will be described later.

The metabolism of thiopental is hepatic, at about 20 percent per hour, with a beta elimination of about 2½ hours. The metabolism is depressed in patients with liver disease; this, of course, would not significantly affect the kinetics of a single IV bolus, which depends on redistribution.

The barbiturates are all direct myocardial depressants in a dose-related fashion. Venodilation, arterial dilation, increased myocardial oxygen consumption, arrhythmias, and decreased cardiac output are commonly seen with barbiturates, especially with rapid (IV bolus) administration [7]. These effects can be spectacular, and in patients susceptible to cardiovascular collapse, the barbiturates may not be the agents of choice for rendering the patient unconscious.

In our Case 1, described earlier, concerning the elderly COPD woman with a blood pressure of 90/50 and pulse of 120, if the object is to intubate

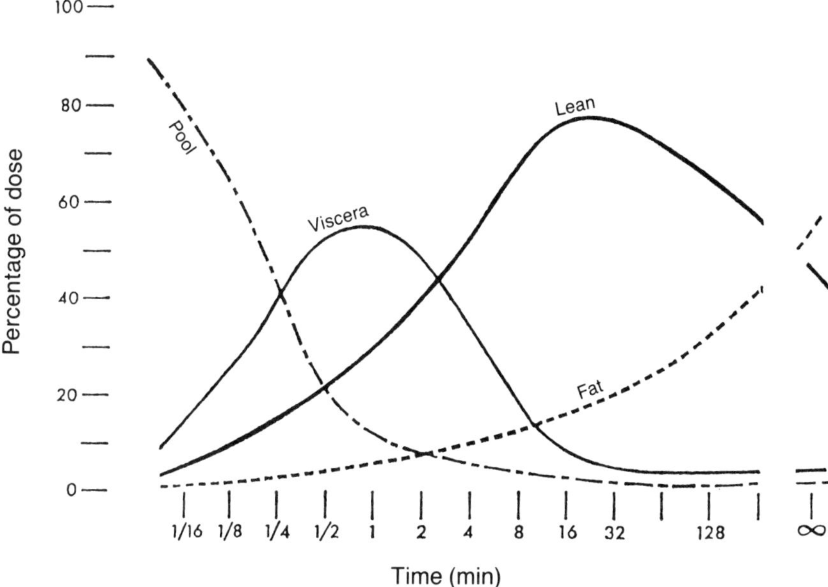

Fig. 5-4. Distribution of pentothal following an IV bolus. As the "pool" (or mixed venous) concentration decreases, the rise in concentration in the vessel-rich (visceral, including brain) group precedes that of the more poorly perfused tissues. Note that the peak in drug concentration in the visceral group has been reached in less than 2 minutes and by 8 minutes is nearly zero. (From J. W. Dundee and G. Wyant. *Intravenous Anesthesia.* London: Churchill Livingstone, 1974. With permission.)

the patient, a barbiturate would almost certainly *not* be the drug of choice for rendering the patient unconscious or amnestic. Her demise from complete cardiovascular collapse might follow a dose of pentothal as low as 2 mg/kg.

The barbiturates depress both the rate and depth of respirations, and they reduce the sensitivity of the central respiratory drive to carbon dioxide. They are all cerebral depressants; in fact, in high enough doses, on the order of 30 mg/kg, they can completely abolish cerebral electrical activity. In such circumstances, cerebral metabolism is also severely diminished; the brain is "protected," and high-dose barbiturates are often looked on as a form of "cerebroplegia." Intracranial pressure is reduced by barbiturates, making them ideal for use in patients with closed head injuries or other intracranial mass lesions. In the second case report, above, our otherwise healthy, cardiovascularly strong, combative ex-motorcycle rider would be a perfect patient in whom to use a barbiturate to induce unconsciousness and unresponsiveness for a brief time during intubation; the intracranial pressure would also be lowered.

True allergy to barbiturates in general is said to be rare, and anaphylaxis

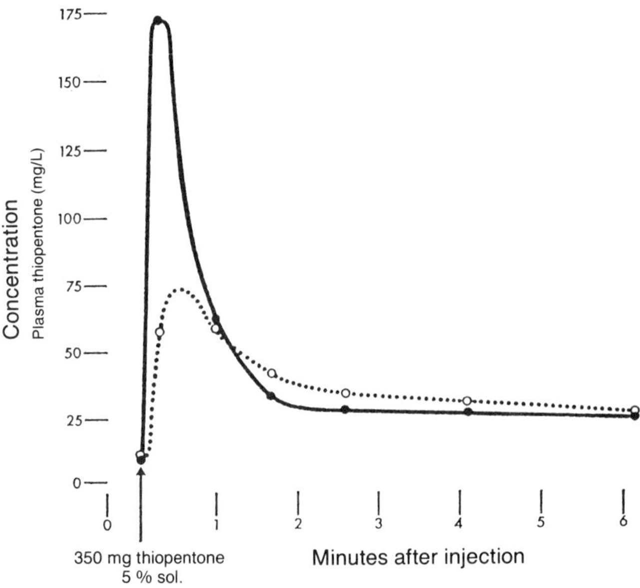

Fig. 5-5. Pharmacokinetics of an IV bolus of thiopental. The arterial (*solid line*) and jugular venous (*dashed line*) concentrations of pentothal following a 350-mg intravenous bolus are illustrated. (From J. W. Dundee and G. Wyant. *Intravenous Anesthesia.* London: Churchill Livingstone, 1974. With permission.)

is even more uncommon. A demyelinating exacerbation of *acute intermittent* and *variegated porphyria* may follow barbiturate but not etomidate administration; these diseases constitute an absolute contraindication to barbiturate use.

The usual intravenous dose of thiopental is 3 to 5 mg/kg. The larger and faster the bolus, the higher the initial blood concentration, and the deeper the cardiovascular-respiratory-cerebral depression. Judicious timing of the excitement of the medical intervention, for example intubation, with the depression of the induction by thiopental may act to smooth out hemodynamics.

Thiamylal

Thiamylal (Surital) substitutes an allyl group for the R_{5a} ethyl of thiopental. Thiamylal is, for all intents and purposes, merely a different and often less expensive version of pentothal; the two are equipotent and have virtually identical effects and toxicities.

Methohexital

Methohexital (Brevital) is an oxybarbiturate about three times as potent as pentothal. Compared to thiopental, methohexital has greater CNS stimulatory effects that result more commonly in hiccups and limit its usefulness in epileptics; it reduces peripheral vascular resistance more, resulting in more tachycardia and often in a lower blood pressure. It has a slightly faster offset of action and incites allergic reactions even less than thiopental. A standard induction dose is 1 mg/kg, although for fast procedures requiring only amnesia, such as cardioversions, half the usual induction dose or less may be adequate. Because of its rapid redistribution time, a very fast IV bolus is recommended; if it is "dribbled in," it may redistribute so fast that adequate cerebral drug levels will not be reached.

Pentobarbital

Pentobarbital (Nembutal) can be administered rectally, in a dose of about 4 mg/kg, 2 hours prior to a procedure that requires sedation; 2 to 4 mg/kg given intramusuclarly, 1 hour prior to the procedure would accomplish the same result. This medicine is used primarily in the pediatric population, as a preoperative medication, or as a sedative prior to a nonpainful procedure such as computed tomography (CT) or magnetic resonance imaging (MRI) scan. Not surprisingly, because of its route of administration, both onset and offset of action are prolonged. In these doses, mild cardiovascular and respiratory depression can be expected to accompany the sedation.

Etomidate

Etomidate (Amidate) is an imidazole that can be used as an intravenous induction agent, particularly in patients with limited cardiovascular reserve. Like thiopental, it is a poor analgesic, and it decreases cerebral oxygen consumption and blood flow. At a dose of 0.3 mg/kg it induces anesthesia somewhat more slowly than thiopental, but recovery is slightly faster. Two distinct disadvantages include pain on injection into a peripheral vein and myoclonia/dystonia. Its main advantage is less cardiovascular depression: Cardiac rate, output, stroke volume, and oxygen consumption are essentially unchanged after etomidate given to healthy patients. Respiratory depression, however, may occur. Allergy is rare, and the porphyrias are not exacerbated by its administration. Recent literature [8, 9] attributes to etomidate the suppression of adrenocortical steroid secretion, especially during prolonged sedation in an intensive care unit (ICU); the implication is that the normal stress response is adversely affected. The usual IV induction dose is 0.3 mg/kg.

NARCOTICS

There are five narcotics in common use: meperidine, morphine, fentanyl, sufentanil, and alfentanil. The pure narcotic antagonists will be presented in the following section, and the agonist-antagonists will be described afterward. In this section, morphine sulfate will be presented as a parent compound, to which the others will be compared. The sites of action, or receptors, of the opioids are specific: See the section on narcotic agonist-antagonists.

Whereas barbiturates are much better hypnotics than analgesics, the narcotics offer profound analgesia and usually produce moderate hypnosis. Amnesia from narcotics is unreliable, and some supplementation is usually given to obviate patient awareness.

Morphine

Morphine sulfate is an inexpensive and naturally occurring opioid derived from the poppy. Intravenous morphine is rapidly redistributed following an IV bolus, and it has a long beta half-life—over 2 hours (Fig. 5-6). It is apparently retained in the central nervous system out of proportion to its blood levels, so redistribution has a lesser effect on its duration of action. Morphine is metabolized and conjugated in the liver and excreted by the kidneys. Narcotic metabolism is highly dependent on hepatic function and blood flow; any factor that decreases hepatic function will prolong the beta elimination of any of the narcotics. Aging also appears to inhibit morphine metabolism.

Morphine sulfate per se is not a cardiac depressant, although hypotension, hypertension, and dysrhythmias may occur with its use [10]. Morphine is associated with histamine-induced vascular dilation; venous dilation is more profound and lasts longer than arterial dilation. Possibly as a central nervous system reflex against such vasodilation, scrum catecholamines such as epinephrine and norepinephrine may actually increase following morphine administration, particularly in lower doses. More often, however, vagotonia, histamine release, and decreased sympathetic tone are the sequelae of morphine administration. In hypovolemic patients, the vascular atonia may lead to a profound drop in blood pressure; before giving morphine, especially in high doses, one must be prepared to "fill up the tank" to maintain cardiac filling pressure and cardiac output. On the other hand, in a patient suffering from cardiovascular overload, as in congestive heart failure or pulmonary edema, administration of morphine may open the vasculature and promote rather than diminish cardiac output (see Chapter 4).

Respiratory depression is a well-known side effect of narcotics, occurring in a dose-related fashion, probably at the level of the brain stem. It is hard to overemphasize the following: If narcotics are given, ventilatory minute-volume will decrease, as will sensitivity to carbon dioxide. The higher the dose of narcotic, the greater the ventilatory depression. Generally, the respiratory rate is lowered relatively more than the tidal volume. The respiratory effects of the anesthetic adjuncts, which will be discussed below, are additive to those of the narcotics.

Hand-in-hand with respiratory depression is analgesia: The higher the dose of opioid, the deeper the analgesia. Stimulation of the central nervous

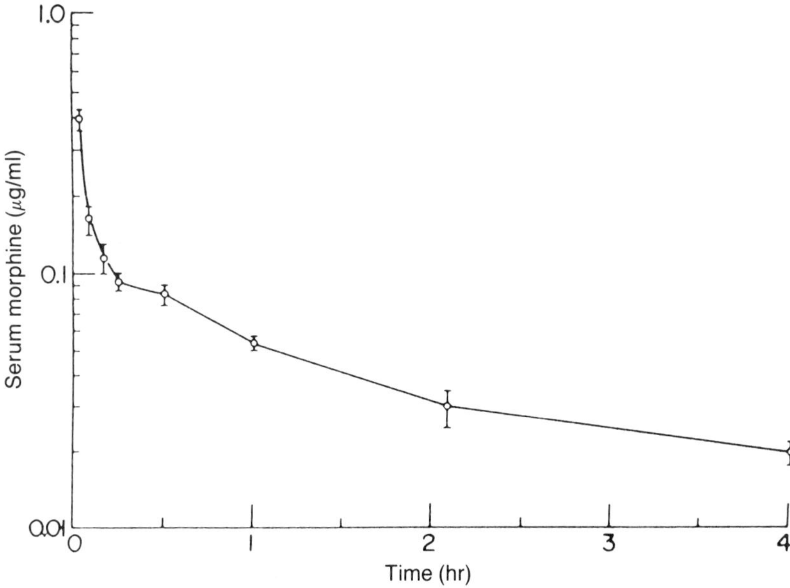

Fig. 5-6. Pharmacokinetics of an IV bolus of morphine sulfate. The average serum morphine concentration following a single IV administration of 10 mg of morphine in a 70-kg patient is shown. Note that during the initial 15-minute alpha elimination phase the concentration falls by about a factor of four; during the beta elimination phase more than 4 hours are required to reduce the concentration by the same factor. (From R. G. Miller [ed.]. *Anesthesia.* New York: Churchill Livingstone, 1981. With permission.)

system from whatever cause—trauma, surgery, cardiac failure—will activate the adrenergic nervous system; catecholamine secretion, hyperventilation, blood pressure elevation, tachycardia, mydriasis, and even hyperthermia may result. Each of these effects is counteracted by narcotic administration; thus a balance must be struck. Too little narcotic, and the adverse physiologic sequelae of pain will occur; too much narcotic, and respiratory depression will predominate. This balance is made more difficult because whereas the amount of narcotic given can be controlled, the amount of pain often cannot.

In Case 3, concerning the man who had had colonoscopy, the amount of narcotic he had received was "just right" during this painful procedure, during which he was as comfortable as possible given the circumstances. Once the colonoscope was withdrawn, however, he was left with a relative narcotic overdose; the balance had tipped in favor of respiratory depression. We will return to this patient in a later section, when we figure out how to tip the scales back toward a more physiologic position.

Narcotics are emetics and cause some degree of spasm of the smooth muscle of the gut—specifically the sphincter of Oddi. The corollaries are biliary spasm and constipation. Narcotic antagonists will also antagonize these side effects (see the following two sections, Narcotic Antagonists, and Narcotic Agonist-Antagonists). Narcotics do not produce muscle relaxation; in fact, rigidity, particularly of the trunk muscles, can occur, especially with rapid administration of the more potent narcotics.

Dosages of morphine are variable, reflecting the variability not only of patient response (addicts may be virtually "unnarcotizable") but also of the stimulation at hand. For mild to moderate pain, morphine in incremental intravenous doses, on the order of 0.05 mg/kg every 5 to 10 minutes, may be a good place to start. Intramuscular and subcutaneous doses are well absorbed from adequately perfused tissue. Slow administration accompanied by fluid replacement for the inevitable vasodilation are the mainstays of morphine administration, particularly in the high doses used during general anesthesia.

Meperidine

Meperidine (Demerol) is a little more than one-tenth as potent as morphine, so it should be given in eight- to tenfold higher doses. Unlike morphine, however, it is a direct cardiac depressant in clinical doses [11]. Its pharmacokinetics are similar to those of morphine, and in aging patients its metabolism is delayed significantly. In equipotent doses, meperidine is more likely than morphine to release histamine [12]; this characteristic, coupled with its direct cardiovascular depression, make hypotension and tachycardia more likely to occur after meperidine than after morphine [13].

Fentanyl

Fentanyl (Sublimaze) is a newer synthetic narcotic related to meperidine. Fentanyl is about 100 times more potent than morphine and has a faster time of onset and a shorter duration of action. It is highly lipophilic and appears in the CNS more rapidly than morphine. Fentanyl is about 70 percent protein bound (morphine is about 30 percent); the shorter duration of action of fentanyl is related to its rapid redistribution out of the CNS. Unlike morphine, fentanyl is not "trapped" in the CNS tissue, and blood-brain fentanyl levels are correlated closely. The beta half-life of fentanyl is longer than that of morphine, so fentanyl is more highly cumulative in repeated doses. Fentanyl is metabolized in the liver with a beta elimination half-life on the order of 2 to 4 hours.

Fentanyl is without direct cardiovascular effects, and it almost never incites histamine release [11, 12]. After the administration of fentanyl (or enough of any narcotic, for that matter), the central sympathetic outflow, with its attendant catecholamine secretion, may be markedly diminished. In addition, fentanyl is vagotonic. These factors would be expected to result in diminished heart rate, blood pressure, stroke volume, cardiac output, and oxygen metabolism. Please note that these effects are not directly related to fentanyl; rather, they result from a diminished central sympathetic outflow. In fact, the fentanyl family of drugs was developed largely because they are devoid of direct cardiovascular effects. In combination with other agents, most notably nitrous oxide and the benzodiazepines, fentanyl will result in some degree of direct cardiovascular compromise [14, 15].

Dosages of fentanyl are characterized as low (less than 10 μg/kg), mid-level (10 to 50 μg/kg), and the so-called high-dose range (50 μg/kg to 150 μg/kg or more). Fairly rapid IV administration is associated with loss of consciousness at drug levels of about 10 μg/kg. Fentanyl is supplied for IV administration at 50 μg/ml; 50 to 100 μg, or 1 to 2 ml, will accomplish the same result as that achieved with 1 to 2 mg of morphine, and sooner, but it will *not* result in histamine release or vasodilation; the duration of effect from these lower doses of fentanyl will be less than that from morphine.

Sufentanil

Sufentanil (Sufenta) is a newer and more potent narcotic, about seven times as potent as fentanyl. It differs from fentanyl most in potency; its onset of action and half-life may be slightly shorter, and it is more lipophilic. Sufentanil is more highly protein bound and has a smaller volume of distribution than fentanyl; it, too, is devoid of any direct cardiovascular side effects, and its potency bespeaks an incredibly high margin of safety (see DeCastro [11] for a very well-written commentary on narcotic safety.)

Alfentanil

Alfentanil (Alfenta) is the newest of the synthetic opioids. It has a relatively fast beta elimination, about 90 minutes, which is about half that of all other narcotics, and it is touted as particularly effective in outpatient anesthesia. Alfentanil is about one-third as potent as fentanyl; an initial dose on the order of 5 to 10 μg/kg should provide adequate analgesia without undue respiratory depression and should last 30 minutes or less. It, too, is virtually without direct cardiovascular effect.

In case 3 above (the colonoscopy patient given morphine sulfate), perhaps a large part of the analgesic and sedative effects could be expected to be waning had alfentanil been chosen instead of morphine.

NARCOTIC ANTAGONISTS

To fully understand the action of narcotic agonists and antagonists, it is necessary to present a brief synopsis of narcotic receptor theory as it is currently understood. The science of opioid receptors is relatively new and is hampered in large part by a lack of pure agonists or antagonists to any given narcotic receptor. The location, mechanisms of action, pharmacokinetics and physiologic effects of the different receptors have not yet been completely worked out [16–21]; indeed, there is probably a large overlap among the various receptors.

Opioid Receptors

The mu receptor (standing for morphine) was probably discovered first and has since been subdivided into two receptors—the mu_1 and the mu_2. Of these, the mu_1 is the more ubiquitous and has the property of "common" binding, meaning that both exogenous opioids such as morphine and endogenous opioids such as enkephalin can interact with high affinity to stimulate the receptor. The mu_1 receptor is found throughout the brain, especially in the periaqueductal gray and other midline structures. This receptor is not associated with respiratory depression, gastrointestinal dysmotility, or sedation; it seems to be a more "pure" analgesic receptor. Naloxazone and naloxonazine appear to block this receptor.

The mu_2 receptor is more morphine-specific, although it binds morphine with less affinity than the mu_1 receptor. The mu_2 receptor is found in the central, or "supraspinal" nervous system, and is responsible for the sedation, respiratory depression, and gastrointestinal side effects common to opioids.

The delta receptor (for D-Ala2-D-Leu5-enkephalin) appears to be enkephalin-specific, although it is of lower affinity than the mu_1 receptor. It, too, exists in a central location in the nervous system.

The kappa receptor (for ethylKetocyclazocine) appears to exist in a more peripheral or "spinal" location; it is naloxone-resistant and seems not to produce respiratory depression. Most of the mixed agonist-antagonist analgesics seem to bind to the kappa receptor.

The sigma receptor (for SKF 10047) appears to be associated with many of the less desirable aspects of the opiates. The phencyclidine (PCP) receptor may be a sigma site. Respiratory stimulation and dysphoria are characteristics of sigma stimulation.

In summary, there appear to be four classes of opiate receptors: (1) the mu, divided into mu_1 (common to exogenous and endogenous opioids, of high affinity, and central) and mu_2 (morphine, low affinity, central, respiratory depression, and sedation), (2) the delta (enkephalin, central), (3) kappa (spinal, agonist-antagonist, no respiratory depression), and (4) sigma (PCP-like, respiratory stimulation). These receptors are presented in Table 5-2.

Currently two pure opioid antagonists are available: naloxone (Narcan) and naltrexone. The latter is a newly arrived drug with physiologic effects identical to those of naloxone. Naltrexone is more potent, much more efficacious orally, and has a much longer half-life (about 10 hours) than naloxone.

Table 5-2. Opioid receptors

Receptor name	Location in nervous system	Binding	Respiratory effect	Central effect
Mu$_1$	Central	EO, O, A, A-A	?None	?Pure analgesia
Mu$_2$	Central	O, A, A-A	Depression	Sedation
Delta	Central	EO	?	?
Kappa	Spinal	A-A	None	None
Sigma	Central	PCP, A-A	Stimulation	PCP

EO = Endogenous opioids (enkephalins); O = opioids; A = antagonists; A-A = agonist-antagonists; PCP = phencyclidine-like.

Naloxone

Naloxone is virtually devoid of agonist properties. It is a prompt, pure, and complete narcotic antagonist and works at all receptors but is less effective at the kappa receptor. It is most effective at the mu receptor and may be less effective at antagonising effects of the agonist-antagonists (which work at the kappa receptor) than of the pure opioid agonists.

Naloxone is metabolized and conjugated in the liver. Because of this rapid hepatic clearance it is only one-fiftieth as effective orally as intravenously. Its beta-elimination half-life of between 20 minutes [22] and 1.5 hours [1] is considerably shorter than that of any of the other commonly used narcotics except alfentanil; its effectiveness should be expected to dissipate after about an hour or less. This waning of effect is termed *renarcatization*; it may be attenuated by repeating the dose of naloxone at intervals or by giving the drug by continuous infusion, or by giving additional drug in a fashion that would prolong its duration of action, such as intramuscularly.

In persons not addicted to opioids, naloxone in small doses completely reverses all effects seen after narcotic administration: morphine's vasodilation, sedation, and biliary colic; fentanyl's vagotonia, and anesthesia. This reversal occurs in one circulation time.

In narcotic addicts naloxone may rarely be responsible for a virtual explosion of the central sympathetic nervous system. This "overshoot" phenomenon has been ascribed to acute narcotic withdrawal; it includes nausea, vomiting, tachycardia, arrhythmias, hypertension, restlessness, sweating, hyperventilation, and pulmonary edema [23]. In the majority of cases, however, naloxone treatment of an acute narcotic overdose in an addict will not result in physiologic calamity and indeed may be life saving.

Unfortunately, virtually identical physiologic misadventure has been described following even low-dose naloxone administration to otherwise normal patients given narcotics in the course of general anesthesia [24–35]. Similar hyperdynamic sequelae after naloxone treatment have also been reported in the emergency medicine literature [23]. Some have attributed these effects to the unmasking of acute addiction, or tolerance, following even one-time narcotic administration.

One adult ampule (0.4 mg) of naloxone has a large amount of "narcotic-reducing" power; the author is personally unaware of studies titrating naloxone reversal against narcotic dosage. Based on personal experience in the laboratory, a guess would be that 0.4 mg of naloxone would completely, although temporarily, reverse a dose of at least 50 μg/kg of fentanyl or 1 mg/kg of morphine. Lower doses of naloxone would carry lower "reversing power"; just as the "right dose" of narcotic is arrived at by a combination of pharmacologic savvy, patient response, and experience, the amount of naloxone that will reverse just enough of the excess opioid to leave the patient breathing and comfortable cannot be foretold. Titration, purposefully aiming low, is probably the safest procedure in reversing narcosis.

Of interest is the role played by hypercarbia, which will accompany narcosis in the absence of ventilatory support, in narcotic antagonism. It appears from experimental work that the sympathetic stimulation following narcotic reversal by a pure antagonist is more profound—that is, that the hypertension, tachycardia, and catecholamine release are worse—when naloxone is given during a period of hypoventilation and hypercarbia than when given during hypo- or even normocarbia [36].

Naloxone has been used in very high doses to treat acute spinal cord injury and septic shock [37–40]. For spinal cord injury, the theory is that the spinal cord microcirculation is somehow aided by the narcotic antagonism. The doses needed are very high: 5 mg/kg—which is to say, about 10 adult ampules per kilogram—as a loading dose, and about three-fourths of that per hour as an infusion. These "megadoses" are needed, it is claimed, to antagonize the kappa receptors; a kappa-specific antagonist seems to provide the same protection at much lower doses.

In septic shock, endogenous opioids, particularly the beta-endorphins, are secreted, along with adrenocorticotropin hormone (ACTH), to cause vasodilation. Blocking the endorphins, in theory, would help to reverse the vasodilation and improve hemodynamics. There are ample data in animals [40] to support this claim; unfortunately, the results for humans are much more controversial [39].

Briefly review case 3, above. Now for a word of caution: In an otherwise normal patient who has been given enough narcotics to slow breathing to a worrisome point—like our patient in case 3 after his colonic endoscopy, naloxone almost certainly will nearly instantly reverse the effects of the opioids. Overshoot, the return of physiologic parameters to levels higher and possibly more detrimental than baseline, has been described as a frequent companion of naloxone use. Recall that there were enough accompanying circumstances in that patient, such as failing cardiac bypass grafts, aortic aneurysm, and coexisting hypertension, to make sudden narcotic reversal potentially hazardous. As that patient was wheeled into the emergency department, he was probably not hypoxic, yet he almost certainly was hypercarbic. Although an ampule of naloxone might wake him up, the hemodynamic and physiologic consequences could be devastating.

This brings us to the conclusion of this section on pure narcotic reversal: It is presumed that the administration of narcotics, except by addicts to themselves, is chosen for a specific expected benefit—blunted central sympathetic outflow, patient analgesia, and sedation. If the given dose is in excess of the requirements, resulting in hypoventilation, two choices need to be made; first, is narcotic reversal really needed, and second, if it is, should it be accomplished by a pure antagonist or a partial agonist-antagonist? Recall that all of the benefits of narcotic use will be erased, perhaps resulting in physiologic parameters far more pathologic than the prenarcotic baseline. This calamity may occur nearly instantly on administration of naloxone. Remember that beyond the initial histamine release and vasodilation (which do not accompany the fentanyl family of opioids), the only side effect of narcosis is hypoventilation, and breathing for patients is usually relatively straightforward.

NARCOTIC AGONIST-ANTAGONISTS

The "antagonism" of narcotic action may represent interference of opioid action at one type of receptor, stimulation of narcotic action at another opposing receptor, or a combination of both. A drug may block certain receptors (antagonism) and stimulate others (agonism) at the same time, with additive *or* conflicting results; such drugs are classified as agonist-antagonists. A concise summary of receptor theory is presented by Flacke [19].

Nalbuphine (Nubain) will be presented as the prototype compound. It does seem to offer advantages over the other agonist-antagonists, listed in Table 5-3, including absence of abuse potential and a ceiling on respiratory depression (see below) [41, 42].

Recall that stimulation of the mu receptor results in pain relief, respiratory depression, euphoria, and physical dependence. Nalbuphine is a mu-receptor antagonist, which is to say that it competitively inhibits the action of opioids at that receptor. As such, it would be surprising if nalbuphine itself caused physical addiction, and it does not; indeed, it is not scheduled under the Controlled Substances Act. Nalbuphine is a kappa receptor agonist and results in respiratory depression, sedation, and analgesia, probably at the spinal cord level. In very high doses, nalbuphine might stimulate the sigma receptor, leading to dysphoric reactions, although nalbuphine's sigma activity is very limited.

It is apparent that two of the actions of nalbuphine are mutually competitive: It causes respiratory depression by stimulating the kappa receptor but antagonizes the respiratory depression caused by opioid action through its mu receptor antagonism. Nalbuphine is said to have a ceiling effect on re-

Table 5-3. Receptor pharmacology for agonist, partial agonist-antagonist, and antagonist drugs

| Drug | Brand name | Receptor-stimulated | | | Respiratory depression (approx. CO ceiling) | Abuse potential |
		mu	kappa	sigma		
Buprenorphine	Buprenex	Partial +[a]	Antag	None	Mild (?45 torr)	Low
Butorphanol	Stadol	Weak +[b]	+	+	Mod (50-55 torr)	Yes
Nalbuphine	Nubain	Antag	+	Little	Mild (45-48 torr)	No
Nalorphine	Nalline	Weak +	+−	+	Mild	? (Not avail)
Pentazocine	Talwin	Antag	+++	+	Mod (50-55 torr)	Yes
Morphine		+++	+−+	? None	High (no limit)	Yes
Naloxone	Narcan	Antag	Antag	Antag	No	No
Naltrexone	Trexan	Antag	Antag	Antag	No	No

The drugs, brand names, and receptor interactions are shown. See text for details on physiological effects of receptor stimulation.
[a]Buprenorphine avidly binds to the mu receptor, causing partial agonistic effects. Its onset of action is slow, reducing its abuse potential. Because of its tenacious receptor binding, an antagonist such as naloxone has reduced efficacy since the antagonist cannot easily displace buprenorphine from the receptor.
[b]Butorphanol is an antagonist at the mu receptor in the animal (*Physician's Desk Reference*), but data for binding at the mu receptor in man are lacking.
The superb contribution of Craig Moldenhauer, M.D., is gratefully acknowledged.

spiratory depression: at low doses, in the absence of other opioid action, nalbuphine will diminish the sensitivity of the central nervous system to carbon dioxide, and mild hypoventilation will ensue. However, at higher doses, or if respiratory depression has already been established by the prior administration of an opioid, the mu-antagonistic activity of nalbuphine will result in the sensitivity of the respiratory center returning toward, but probably not quite to, normal [43].

In summary, when nalbuphine is given to a patient, the first actions seen result from kappa stimulation: mild analgesia and respiratory depression up to a ceiling, beyond which further doses of the drug will not result in further analgesia or respiratory depression. The dose at which this ceiling effect occurs is on the order of 10 mg in an adult patient. Indeed, at very high doses, above 50 mg, the sigma stimulation may result in dysphoria. On the other hand, if the patient has first been given an opioid and has a baseline of analgesia and respiratory depression, the administration of even low-dose nalbuphine (1 to 5 mg) will result in antagonism of the opioid action: sensitivity to carbon dioxide will be returned toward normal, and at least some of the analgesia will be undone.

Investigation of the comparison of nalbuphine reversal with naloxone reversal of opioid action has centered on two areas: first, the hormonal differences between the two drugs, i.e., catecholamine secretion in response to the reversal, and second, the differences in reversal between patients with hypercapnia and those with hypocapnia. It turns out that nalbuphine results in a "gentler" reversal of narcotic action; the increases in blood pressure, heart rate, and epinephrine and norepinephrine secretion are significantly less after nalbuphine reversal than after naloxone administration [35]. Further, even in periods of hypercapnia during which naloxone reversal caused abrupt and sustained increases in blood pressure, heart rate, and catecholamine levels, nalbuphine resulted in a lesser increase in heart rate and blood pressure, and no significant increase in epinephrine or norepinephrine [19]. The implication is that narcotic reversal by an agonist-antagonist is of a completely different quality than that by a pure antagonist.

The pharmacokinetics of nalbuphine also differ from those of naloxone: Although both have a fast onset of action, about 2 minutes, the beta-elimination half life of naloxone (between ½ and 1½ hours) is significantly less than that of nalbuphine (3 to 5 hours). Recall that the half-life of all opioids except alfentanil is at least twice that of naloxone; renarcotization is certainly possible, if not probable, following a single IV bolus of naloxone.

The two other commonly used partial agonists, or agonist-antagonists, are butorphanol (Stadol) and pentazocine (Talwin). They differ from each other and from nalbuphine in a number of ways. The activity of pentazocine is almost entirely due to kappa-receptor agonism; the drug is probably a mu-receptor antagonist. There are two consequences: Because of its mu-antagonism, pentazocine can precipitate withdrawal symptoms if it is administered to narcotic addicts; and because of its strong kappa activity it can lead to psychomimetic dependence—addiction. Euphoria, nausea, vomiting, and respiratory depression are the most frequent side effects.

Butorphanol is a partial mu agonist and a weak kappa agonist. It, too, probably causes tolerance and addiction. Sedation, and, more infrequently, nausea, vertigo, and confusion are its side effects.

The agonist-antagonists and their mechanisms of action are listed in Table 5-3.

TRANQUILIZERS

The benzodiazepines (diazepam, lorazepam, and midazolam) and a butyrophenone (droperidol) will be described. These agents are used to promote tranquility, mental detachment, and amnesia. They are not analgesics and are poor hypnotics even in relatively high doses.

Benzodiazepines

The benzodiazepines produce a feeling of sedated tranquility, with drowsiness a prominent feature. In high doses unconsciousness may occur. Particularly with lorazepam, the patient may seem to be awake and making appropriate responses, although later he is found to have been completely amnestic for conversation and other events.

Diazepam. Diazepam (Valium) is a water-insoluble compound dissolved in propylene glycol, ethyl alcohol, and sodium benzoate in benzoic acid to a pH of about 6.7. It is very painful on intravenous administration and is painful and poorly absorbed when given intramuscularly. The pain of IV administration can be lessened by preceding the diazepam with a narcotic, with a small dose of lidocaine (20 mg or so), by giving the drug through a central venous cannula, or by preparing an emulsification of diazepam in lidocaine. Venous sequelae such as thrombosis and phlebitis are a significant problem with diazepam administration, increasing in frequency with the age of the patient. Oral absorption produces higher and more consistent blood levels than intramuscular administration.

Among patients, serum concentrations may vary by a factor of three following a standard IV dose of diazepam. This, coupled with the variability of patient effect, the long time needed for onset, active metabolites, and long beta half-life (30 to 90 hours in some patients) limit the usefulness of diazepam as an induction agent [44]. In the emergency department, diazepam should be expected to have a prolonged duration of action.

Metabolism is primarily hepatic, and cirrhosis may increase the terminal half-life fivefold. Diazepam has an unfortunate propensity to cross the placenta readily; the acute effects on a baby born to a mother given diazepam include depression and impaired temperature control.

A "second peak" of diazepam effect has been found about 6 to 8 hours following a single oral or intravenous administration, possibly due to enterohepatic recirculation. Patients may become more drowsy then and certainly should be warned to abstain from activity requiring mental or physical acuity for at least 24 hours following diazepam administration.

Despite occasional reports of cardiovascular collapse following diazepam use, it is said to be virtually free from direct cardiac effects, although in combination with high-dose narcotics there is a diminution of cardiovascular function [14, 15]. Alone, it is a "mild" respiratory depressant, mostly at the expense of tidal volume, which is generally of no harmful effect in a normal patient. In combination with narcotics or in debilitated patients, even low-dose diazepam may exert severe and/or prolonged respiratory depression.

Diazepam raises the seizure threshold and is a commonly used anticonvulsant. Amnesia from the benzodiazepines is well known, although as Figures 5-7 and 5-8 show, perhaps too much reliance is placed on the ability of diazepam in particular to render the patient amnestic.

There are reports of the ability of physostigmine and aminophylline to reverse the effects of benzodiazepines [45–48], although many, including this author, have not had such success [49–51]. A diazepam-specific antagonist is currently undergoing clinical trials and will probably be available in the near future.

The dose of diazepam varies: 0.1 to 0.15 mg/kg will produce some sedation if given orally; the same dose given intravenously will produce moderate and medium-lasting sedation.

Lorazepam. Lorazepam (Ativan) is more potent than diazepam and is well absorbed intramuscularly. Compared with diazepam, lorazepam is of slower onset and has even more prolonged action. Particularly following intravenous use it is a very powerful amnestic agent, even at doses that may not cause deep sedation. Like diazepam, it will raise the seizure threshold and act as an anticonvulsant. The incidence of pain on injection and venous sequelae are much reduced with lorazepam, which must be given after diluting it in normal saline because of its high viscosity.

Lorazepam is a good sedative-hypnotic for sleep; 2 to 4 mg orally will be a powerful soporific. The same dose given intramuscularly will result about an hour later in rather profound sedation and probably nearly complete amnesia. A dose of 1 or 2 mg given intravenously prior to an unpleasant procedure may allay anxiety, blur memory, and not unduly suppress respirations. The price, however, is prolonged sedation, and lorazepam is inappropriate for many outpatient or emergency department procedures. It has no analgesic properties; sedation and amnesia are characteristics of its use, and if relief from pain is needed, an opioid needs to be administered.

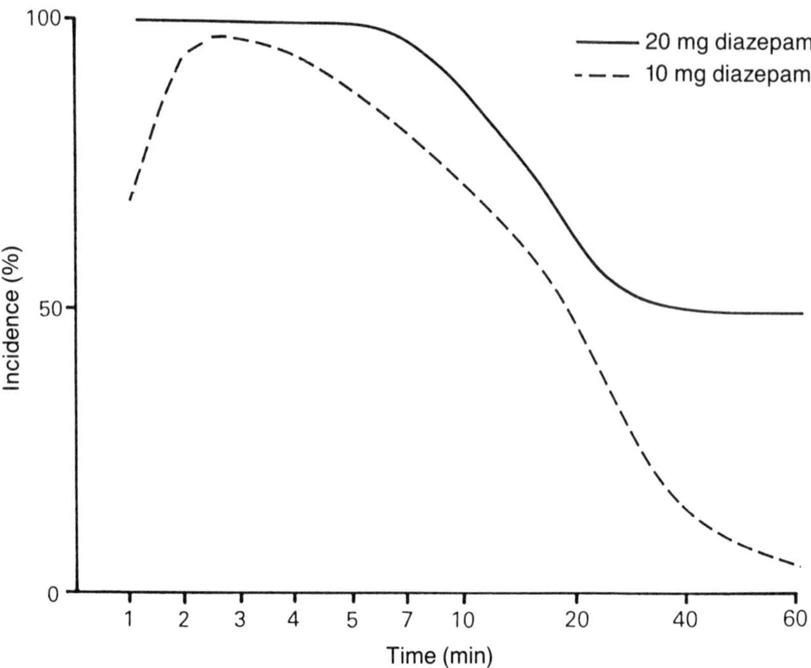

Fig. 5-7. The amnestic effects of diazepam. The percentage of patients who were amnestic for conversation following the IV administration of diazepam 10 mg (*dashed line*) or 20 mg (*solid line*) is shown. The sedative effects can be expected to far outlast the amnestic effects. (From J. W. Dundee and G. Wyant. *Intravenous Anesthesia.* London: Churchill Livingstone, 1974. With permission.)

Midazolam. Midazolam (Versed) is a new benzodiazepine that is two to three times as potent as diazepam but water soluble; it greatly diminishes the venous sequelae and enhances IM absorption. Its beta elimination is about twice as fast as that of diazepam. Midazolam is transported across the placenta less easily than diazepam. In combination with narcotics, it too has been shown to produce cardiovascular depression. Incremental doses of 1 or 2 mg can be titrated to promote sedation and lessen anxiety; the usual dose is in the range of 3 to 6 mg. The sedative effect will begin to wane after about an hour; this dose, as expected, is about half that required for diazepam, and the duration of action is also about half.

Neuroleptics

Of the phenothiazines and butyrophenones, only droperidol (Inapsine), an example of the latter, is used as an intravenous adjunctive anesthetic agent. Because of extrapyramidal side effects (dystonia, parkinsonism, akathisia, dyskinesia, and tremor), cardiovascular effects (alpha blockade, vasodilation, and hypotension), and other problems associated more with long-term

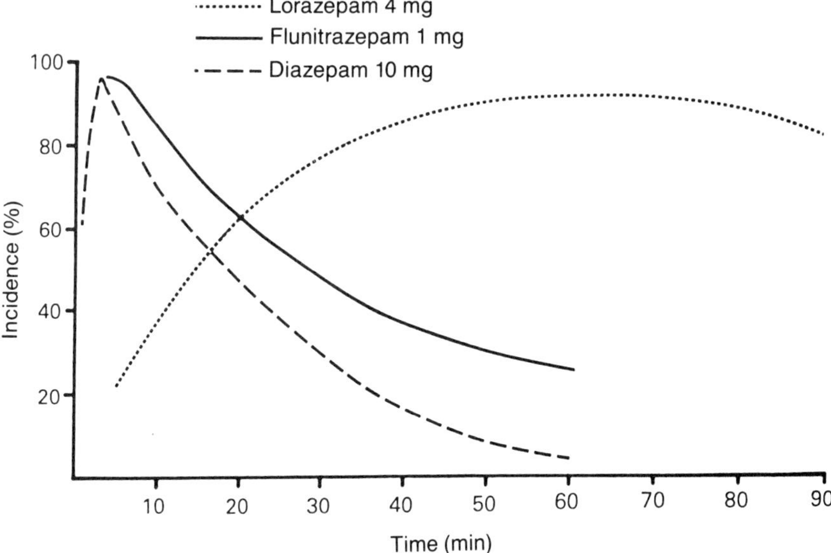

Fig. 5-8. Amnestic effects of lorazepam and diazepam. Note the far-superior and much longer lasting amnesia afforded by a single intravenous dose of 4 mg of lorazepam; again, very prolonged sedation would accompany such a dose. (From J. W. Dundee and G. Wyant. *Intravenous Anesthesia.* London: Churchill Livingstone, 1974. With permission.)

use (obstructive jaundice, skin pigmentation, hypercholesterolemia, and blood dyscrasias), the neuroleptic agents in general and phenothiazines in particular are only infrequently used as intravenous anesthetic agents. The exception is prochlorperazine (Compazine), which is a fairly potent anti-emetic; it is most frequently administered rectally or intramuscularly; side effects including sedation and dystonias limit its usefulness.

Droperidol. Droperidol produces an affect of indifference, apathy, or mental detachment that may belie a psyche that is far from calm. Particularly when used alone, droperidol as a sedative may actually induce apprehension; it has fallen out of favor as a preoperative premedication because of an unacceptably high incidence of patients cancelling surgery or complaining of heightened anxiety after its use, despite reports of impartial observers that the patients appeared outwardly calm and composed. After its effects have retreated, patients are unable to pinpoint why they cancelled surgery; they often report feeling "terrible" or sensing "impending doom." Other side effects include dyskinesias, occasional oculogyric crisis, and mild alpha-blocking activity; these increase in frequency with increasing doses.

As an adjuvant, droperidol is most frequently given for its antiemetic properties, which occur at very low doses, 0.25 to 0.50 ml, or 0.6 to 1.2

mg for a 70-kg patient. It is useful in the emergency department and the operating room as an antiemetic, and in these low doses it is virtually devoid of side effects. At any dose, it is not an analgesic.

Droperidol appears in fixed dose with fentanyl as Innovar (50 μg of fentanyl and 2.5 mg droperidol per ml); this combination forces a higher dose of the butyrophenone than is customary in this country and makes prolonged CNS depression likely compared with the shorter duration of analgesia provided by the fentanyl.

DISSOCIATIVE AGENTS

Phencyclidine and ketamine are the two agents that were developed as dissociative agents. Phencyclidine (PCP, "angel dust") was abandoned by medical practitioners because of its extremely high incidence of adverse reactions, and similar problems with ketamine may limit its use.

Ketamine

Ketamine (Ketelar, Ketaject) is a water-soluble arylcycloalkylamine that has a pH of about 4. About 40 seconds following an intravenous dose, intense analgesia and amnesia are produced [52]. Hypnosis ("eyes closed") may be absent, and involuntary muscle movements are not uncommon. Respiration is usually only transiently and slightly depressed. Pharyngeal reflexes are said to be spared, although ketamine will not prevent aspiration. Ketamine is a bronchodilator, but bronchial secretions are stimulated.

The cardiovascular system is stimulated; heart rate, blood pressure, and cardiac output usually increase with its use. These effects are probably due to sympathetic stimulation, and ketamine itself is a direct cardiac depressant. A patient who is surviving only because of maximal central sympathetic outflow should be expected to suffer cardiac depression following ketamine induction. Pretreatment with diazepam will lessen the cardiovascular stimulation of ketamine.

Ketamine increases cerebral blood flow and raises intracranial and intraocular pressures. In our case 2 above (the Mo-ped rider) ketamine would be contraindicated as an agent prior to intubation because of the patient's presumed increased intracranial pressure (ICP). Ketamine crosses the placenta but, aside from increased fetal tone, in low doses it appears not to affect the neonate adversely.

Emergence from ketamine can be an exciting time, particularly in adults. Elderly patients may be confused and disoriented long after a single dose of ketamine; adolescents may awaken even wilder than their baseline state. Children and infants seem to tolerate ketamine relatively well, perhaps because they are perpetually dissociated and don't notice a difference. Diazepam is often used in conjunction with ketamine because it seems to smooth the emergence.

Ketamine may act by dissociating the limbic and thalamoneocortical systems to produce sedation, amnesia, and marked analgesia. Its involvement with the kappa receptors has already been alluded to. Ketamine markedly alters the visual and auditory evoked potentials. Metabolism is complex and occurs primarily at the liver, where it is broken down into four different metabolites.

The usual intravenous induction dose is 1 to 2 mg/kg in a healthy individual, which will produce unconsciousness for 10 to 30 minutes and analgesia for less than an hour. Intramuscularly, ketamine has a relatively rapid onset in 3 to 4 minutes in a dose of about 4 to 6 mg/kg; this can be an effective mode of induction while supporting the cardiovascular system of children who could not tolerate a reduction in systemic vascular resistance—those with right-to-left shunts as in tetralogy of Fallot. A much smaller intravenous dose, 0.25 mg/kg, may produce short-lived but intense analgesia used to accomplish a short, painful procedure such as external skeletal manipulation. An antisialagogue such as atropine or glycopyrrolate is often given in addition to the ketamine to minimize secretions.

For the patient in case 1 above, the woman with COPD, pulmonary edema, and impending cardiorespiratory collapse, if any form of intravenous induction were contemplated to accomplish an intubation, ketamine would almost certainly be the drug of choice. As noted above, any of the barbiturates would probably ring this woman's death knell; even etomidate might depress her cardiovascular system unduly. Ketamine in a small dose, maybe as little as 0.3 mg/kg, would certainly render her amnestic for the event; any adrenergic stimulation from the ketamine would help support her blood pressure and might even lead to some bronchodilation. Caution is advised, however: this woman is a set-up to collapse completely from any pharmacologic intervention. She is existing on a thread and may already be secreting catecholamines maximally, in which case the direct cardiac depressant qualities of ketamine might even further compromise her situation. Discretion is the better part of valor; perhaps an awake intubation would be in her best interest. See Chapter 15 for a further discussion of ketamine.

NEUROMUSCULAR RELAXANTS

Neuromuscular relaxation, or muscle paralysis, is an important part of anesthesia and emergency department care; endotracheal intubation can be facilitated, metabolism slowed, and patients kept from harming themselves or others through judicious use of muscle relaxation. It must be kept in mind, however, that although the drugs discussed in the following section offer nothing in the way of analgesia, hypnosis, or amnesia, they can render the patient completely unable to communicate his pain, fears, or awareness. Two things must always be done for a paralyzed patient: he must be ventilated and rendered amnestic for the experience. Except in the most extreme cases of cardiovascular compromise, a paralyzed patient should *al-*

ways be sedated, tranquilized, or anesthetized to the point of amnesia to prevent experience or memory of the sensation of complete paralysis, which has been described as horrifying.

Muscle relaxants are divided into two classes—depolarizing and nondepolarizing; both classes are used commonly in the emergency department. This section will begin with a brief review of neuromuscular physiology and how muscle relaxation is tested clinically; each of the commonly used relaxants will then be discussed in turn.

Neuromuscular Physiology

Both the nerve and muscle cells that form the neuromuscular junction normally exist, or "rest," in a polarized condition with the inside negatively charged with respect to the outside of the cell. When a neural stimulus exceeds its "threshold," an action potential is created and propagates down the motor neuron as the entire axon depolarizes toward the myoneural junction. At this motor end-plate, the axonal depolarization causes a sudden, discrete release of vesicles of acetylcholine into the synaptic cleft, where simple diffusion carries them across to the muscle cell. If enough vesicles reach the receptors on the muscle, that is, if the muscle membrane threshold is reached, the muscle cell itself depolarizes, bound calcium is released by the sarcolemma in the muscle, and actin is allowed to interact with myosin to cause the muscle cell to shrink, or contract. For each motor end-plate unit, this occurs in an all-or-none fashion. The acetylcholine that was released into the synaptic cleft is removed by diffusion, by reuptake into the presynaptic nerve cell, or by enzymatic degradation by acetylcholinesterase.

Muscle relaxation, or "paralysis," can occur at a number of places along this pathway. The entire neural axis can be rendered relatively insensitive to stimuli that would ordinarily result in muscle tone, as in deep general inhalational anesthesia. The neural axis may be interrupted at a spinal cord or major nerve plexus level, as in regional (spinal, axillary, epidural, and so forth) anesthesia. The motor end-plate itself may be altered; false transmitters may occupy the receptor and cause the muscle to depolarize initially, contract, and then become flaccid, or the false transmitter may occupy and inactivate a receptor in either a competitive or noncompetitive fashion.

In the case of receptor blockade, the clinical manifestation of muscle relaxation is correlated with number of post-synaptic muscle receptors that are occupied by the relaxant. There is a huge margin of safety: Nearly 80 percent of the receptors may be inactivated before a detectable and presumably unsafe amount of paralysis is developed. When between 90 and 95 percent of all receptors are occupied, neuromuscular transmission is at a complete standstill, and total paralysis ensues. It is apparent that of a hundred receptors, clinically useful muscle relaxation occurs in that narrow band of involvement of between 80 and 95 receptors. Remember that a patient will be clinically totally flaccid whether there is enough relaxant available to occupy just 95 percent, or 500 percent, of the receptor population.

The degree of muscle paralysis can be more or less scientifically tested with a peripheral nerve stimulator (PNS). This device generates an electrical current, usually at about 90 volts, 30 mas, and between 30 and 100 Hz. Any peripheral nerve can be transcutaneously stimulated by the PNS; the two most commonly used are the facial nerve along its course to the periorbital muscles and the ulnar nerve along its course to the muscles of the forearm and hand. Usually two different types of stimuli can be generated by the PNS: a tetanic stimulus that is a sustained supramaximal current at about 50 Hz, and a train-of-four, which is a supramaximal current delivered twice per second for 2 seconds.

The characteristics of the muscle blockade produced by a depolarizing agent such as succinylcholine differ from those produced by a nondepolarizer such as pancuronium. The degree of blockade from the depolarizer is most accurately judged by response to tetanic stimulation: The muscle paralysis will parallel the diminution to tetanic contraction. The nondepolarizing blockade can be ascertained by response to the train-of-four, or fade to tetanus. A more detailed account of this testing process and a discussion of the so-called phase II block of succinylcholine can be found elsewhere [2, 3, 7]. Remember that the degree of muscle blockade can be easily and quickly tested in cases of doubt; this is particularly important for patients with neurologic problems in which movement in response to stimuli is an important clinical finding.

Depolarizing Muscle Relaxants

Succinylcholine. Succinylcholine (Quelicin, Anectine) and decamethonium (Syncurine, which is no longer in use) are drugs that occupy, activate, and then inactivate the postsynaptic receptor. The initial activation causes a short-lived and disorganized series of muscle fiber contractions that appear clinically as fasciculations. Although they appear harmless, fasciculations may create havoc; in addition to muscle pain, they are associated with increased intraocular pressure, increased intracranial pressure, and increased intragastric pressure. They are associated with an acute increase in serum potassium level, particularly in patients with preexisting cell damage such as burns, crush injuries, or on-going cell wasting or damage from neural, especially spinal cord, damage. These increases have the potential to exacerbate preexisting injuries—for example, an open eye may be caused to exude its contents owing to the increased intraocular pressure, parts of the intracranial contents may be further compressed or herniated owing to the increase in intracranial pressure, and the reflux of gastric contents may be aspirated into the lungs. The succinylcholine-associated hyperkalemia may be so great and so abrupt that it results in cardiac arrest. "A little sux" to facilitate endotracheal intubation may be exactly the wrong thing to give.

Many of these noxious side effects may be attenuated to a greater or lesser degree by prior administration of a small dose of a nondepolarizing agent that is termed precurarization. No attempt will be made to summarize the controversy surrounding this issue; there are staunch supporters of the concept that such pretreatment will sufficiently abate fasciculations and their sequelae that succinylcholine can be used safely in most situations [53], although there can be associated problems [54]. In any event, if precurarization is done, the dose of succinylcholine needs to be increased by 30 to 50 percent.

The personal opinion of the author is to weigh the advantages and disadvantages of the use of succinylcholine. As will be seen below, it is certainly the fastest-acting relaxant that currently exists, although by less than a minute; succinylcholine therefore represents the agent that will most quickly result in paralysis, allowing the physician to open the jaw, visualize the vocal cords, and endotracheally intubate a patient. If in the author's judgment the patient is *most* at risk from a respiratory problem such as ongoing aspiration, facial or airway trauma resulting in ineffective bag-mask ventilation, or severe hypoxia and cardiovascular collapse, he will not hesitate to use the agent most likely immediately to facilitate the intended intubation: succinylcholine. In this setting, almost certainly the luxury of time to precede succinylcholine with precurarization is lacking, and the arguments surrounding precurarization are, in the author's opinion, for the most part moot. However, if the patient appears able to tolerate another 90 to 120 seconds with out the endotracheal tube, and there is a reason for avoiding succinylcholine, the author will choose a nondepolarizing agent and administer it in a fashion to promote its earliest onset of action (see below).

Succinylcholine is degraded by pseudo (or "plasma") cholinesterase. In normal individuals this beta elimination is so fast that it precludes some of the delivery of the drug to the muscle receptors; hence, a relative "overdose" is given to flood the plasma cholinesterase and allow the succinylcholine to get to the muscle cells. Its onset of action is fast; within about 45 seconds of a dose of 1 mg/kg, a patient should be totally paralyzed. Slow IV administration or slowed circulation times, as in diminished cardiac output, will delay the onset of the drug.

Patients with abnormally low levels or abnormal types of pseudocholinesterase will demonstrate evidence of the usual overdose that is given to normal patients; their paralysis will be prolonged and irreversible while the succinylcholine is eliminated by other forms degradation. Any patient who does not show evidence of return of neuromuscular function within about 10 minutes of an appropriate dose of succinylcholine should be suspected of carrying an abnormal level or type of pseudocholinesterase.

Table 5-4. Pharmacology of neuromuscular relaxants

Drug	Intubating dose (mg/kg)	Onset (sec)	t½ Beta (min)	Duration (min)
Succinylcholine	1	< 60	< 10	< 10
Pancuronium	0.06–0.1	180	120	60
Tubocurarine	0.5	180	90	40
Metocurine	0.3	180	300	40–60
Atracurium	0.3–0.5	120	20	30
Vecuronium	0.1–0.15	90–120	60	20–30

Note: The intubating dose listed will result in the fastest onset possible with the given drug without "priming" (see text) and without unduly prolonging the duration of action. Specific side effects may be expected to result from these dosages (see text); duration of action will likewise vary with patient age and the presence of renal and/or hepatic failure. The figures given are a compilation of sources [1–3,7,54–63], tempered by personal experience.

A second dose of succinylcholine may cause profound bradycardia, and if a second dose is anticipated, it should always be preceded by a vagolytic dose of atropine, which is about 0.4 mg to an adult. The potency of succinylcholine can only be ensured if it is kept refrigerated.

Nondepolarizing Agents

Pancuronium. Pancuronium (Pavulon) will be presented as the prototypic agent, not because it was developed first (curare) or has the fewest side effects (vecuronium) or the fastest offset of action (vecuronium), but because it is probably the most commonly used nondepolarizing agent outside of the OR. In general, the use of nondepolarizers is devoid of most of the hazards associated with succinylcholine; increases in intragastric, intracranial, and intraocular pressures and hyperkalemia are not associated with paralysis induced by these agents. Their onset of action and duration of action are both longer than those of succinylcholine; the action of the nondepolarizers may be "reversed" using acetylcholinesterase inhibitors, as discussed below. Doses for each agent are listed in Table 5-4.

Pancuronium competitively inhibits the action of acetylcholine at the postsynaptic receptor; the muscle receptor occupied by a nondepolarizing agent is rendered ineffective, and muscle contraction is never initiated, so fasciculations are not induced. The onset of action of pancuronium is dose dependent; a dose just large enough to result eventually in complete muscle relaxation, which is about 0.01 mg/kg, takes about 3 minutes to become apparent and another 2 minutes to become complete. Thus, after an initial dose, it would be about 5 minutes before optimal intubating conditions would be met; this contrasts with 45 to 90 seconds for succinylcholine. The beta elimination of pancuronium is about 60 to 100 minutes; thus a fairly large intubating dose that would have a relatively rapid onset would not abate on its own (i.e., without neuromuscular relaxant reversal—see below) for several hours. Such a duration of action contrasts sharply with that of succinylcholine, which is about 5 minutes. The primary route of elimination of pancuronium is renal excretion, and in anuric patients the duration of action of pancuronium may be quadrupled. A second route of elimination is hepatic, and the duration of action of pancuronium may be doubled in patients with cirrhosis. In any event, pancuronium is the longest acting of all the nondepolarizers in current use. Its long-term potency is preserved best if it is kept refrigerated.

The primary side effect of pancuronium results from its "vagolytic" activity; it increases heart rate and, indirectly, cardiac output and blood pressure. For patients in whom tachycardia would be poorly tolerated, such as those with tight mitral stenosis, pancuronium might be an inappropriate first-choice relaxant.

The primary metabolite of pancuronium is itself an active nondepolarizing muscle relaxant. Hence, after repeated doses, the relative duration of action of pancuronium as measured by peripheral nerve stimulation will be seen to increase as more and more of this metabolite accumulates.

D-Tubocurarine. D-Tubocurarine (curare) has an onset of action similar to that of pancuronium; its beta elimination is slightly faster, and it is between one-third (personal experience) and one-seventh [7] as potent. Curare is eliminated more than twice as fast in patients with renal failure as pancuronium because the bulk of D-tubocurarine is eliminated in the bile.

The major side effects of curare are an associated ganglionic blockade and a dose-related release of histamine. The histamine can lead to significant clinical problems including hypotension, tachycardia, and bronchospasm; unfortunately, these sequelae may occur in susceptible individuals at doses commonly used. With the advent of the newer nondepolarizers, the use of this oldest agent has decreased dramatically.

Metocurine. Metocurine (Metubine) has much less of the cardiovascular side effects characteristic of either pancuronium (vagolysis, tachycardia) or curare (histamine, hypotension) [55]. Its duration of action is similar to that of curare, and it is about half as potent as pancuronium, or twice as potent as curare. Metocurine is largely eliminated in the bile, making it a suitable agent for use in patients with renal failure.

Atracurium. Atracurium (Tracrium) is the next newest nondepolarizer and has the next fastest beta elimination. Its onset of action is slightly faster than that of the three agents mentioned above but still significantly slower than that of succinylcholine. Its beta elimination, however, is significantly faster, at about 30 minutes. It is about one-fifth as potent as pancuronium.

The elimination of this drug depends in part on nonenzymatic but temperature-dependent Hoffman elimination; hence, for patients suffering both renal and hepatic failure, its pharmacokinetics are nearly normal.

Unfortunately, the use of atracurium in doses that would rapidly produce intubating conditions may be associated with significant histamine release, hypotension, and tachycardia; these effects have limited the usefulness of this drug [56]. Its long-term potency is preserved only if it is refrigerated.

Vecuronium. Vecuronium (Norcuron) has the fastest onset and offset, and offers the most cardiovascular stability of all the nondepolarizers. Although its metabolism and excretion are primarily hepatic (thus liver disease may severely increase its beta-elimination half-life), even renal failure may somewhat prolong its action. Despite a beta elimination of nearly an hour, in normal patients its duration of action is less than 30 and probably closer to 20 minutes.

Even in doses approaching threefold normal, it has been found to be virtually without direct or indirect cardiovascular effect. Unlike atracurium, associated histamine release is so rare as to be reportable [57]; tachycardia and hyper- or hypotension do not accompany its use [56, 58]. Like all nondepolarizers, increases in intracranial, intraocular, and intragastric pressures do not accompany its use [59, 60].

Because it is relatively unstable in solution, especially at room temperature, it is supplied, unlike all other nondepolarizers, in a lyophilized form that requires diluting before administration. *Vecuronium and sodium thiopental are not physically compatible*; their combination results in an insoluble solution that will clog up and stop almost any IV apparatus. The potency of vecuronium is virtually identical to that of pancuronium; its onset of action from a large intubating dose approaches 90 seconds.

The "Priming Principle". Recent literature on anesthesia has detailed a technique for decreasing the time to onset of the nondepolarizers [55, 61–64]. Although priming with a small dose of the agent about 3 minutes prior to giving the intubating dose may significantly decrease the time needed for complete paralysis, the technique is not without its own pitfalls.

Because of the variability of patient sensitivity to muscle relaxants, even a dose as little as one-tenth the anticipated intubating dose may produce enough paralysis to jeopardize a patient, setting up the possibility of aspiration [53]. Further, in the emergency department if there is time for a 3-minute priming dose, there is time to precurarize the patient and use succinylcholine instead. Even with the priming technique, the time to complete paralysis with the nondepolarizers is never as fast as that with succinylcholine.

Thus if faced with a patient in whom the physician wants to insert an endotracheal tube *as quickly as possible* and who is not a candidate for succinylcholine, for whatever reason, the usual approach is to use vecuronium and push the dose to about twice the normal amount—say, 0.15 or 0.2 mg/kg. The patient will be totally paralyzed in about 60 seconds, but the paralysis will remain unreversible, under those conditions, for at least an hour. The same dose of pancuronium would probably result in at least moderate tachycardia, intubating conditions in something like 2 minutes, and paralysis lasting 2 to 4 hours.

Neuromuscular Relaxant Reversal

The action of all nondepolarizers may be terminated prematurely by the use of acetylcholinesterase inhibitors, but only if no more than about 95 percent of muscle receptors are occupied by the blocker. Recall that one of the mechanisms by which the action of acetylcholine is terminated is enzymatic destruction; if the destroying enzyme were itself eliminated, relatively more of the acetyl choline would remain in the synaptic cleft to compete with the neuromuscular blocking agent for the muscle receptor. The acetylcholinesterase inhibitors (neostigmine [Prostigmine], edrophonium [Tensilon and Enlon], pyridostigmine [Mestinon and Regonol]) are not without their own side effects, their unopposed stimulation of muscarinic receptors leads to tracheobronchial and salivary secretion, bradycardia, and bronchoconstriction. These undesirable effects may in turn be controlled by the concomitant use of an antimuscarinic blocking agent such as atropine or glycopyrrolate (Robinul). Be aware that because the onset of action of glycopyrrolate is later than that of edrophonium, glycopyrrolate (in a dose of about 0.3 mg in a 70-kg adult) needs to be given about 5 minutes prior to the edrophonium to "cover" its side effects.

Generally, the use of neuromuscular reversing agents is unusual in the emergency department. These drugs should be kept in mind, however, in the event that paralysis by a nondepolarizing agent needs to be prematurely abated. For example, if vecuronium were used to facilitate the intubation of the Moped rider in case 2, and the neurosurgeon wanted to examine the patient's responses, neuromuscular blockade could be very quickly terminated once an appropriate number of receptors were unoccupied. See Miller [7] or Dripps [3] for further information on neuromuscular reversal. Appropriate dosages are listed in Table 5-5.

INHALATIONAL AGENTS

Occasionally inhalational agents are administered in the emergency department, and the following section outlines briefly the basic pharmacology of the vapors in current anesthetic use. Three specific situations will be discussed: the use of nitrous oxide as an adjunct for analgesia, the treatment of refractory status asthmaticus, and the treatment of refractory status epilepticus.

Table 5-5. Pharmacology of muscle relaxant reversal agents

Drug	Usual dose (mg/kg)	Dose/70 kg (mg)	Onset (min)	t½ Beta (min)
Edrophonium	0.5–1	35–70	3–5	110
Neostigmine	0.04–0.07	2.5–5	5–10	80
Pyridostigmine	0.15–0.3	10–20	7–15	110

Note: The cholinesterase inhibitors commonly used to reverse the effects of nondepolarizing muscle relaxants are listed. Their use is nearly universally accompanied by the use of an antimuscarinic drug such as glycopyrrolate or atropine to reduce side effects (see text).

Pharmacology

The delivery of supplemental oxygen by means of nasal cannulae, face mask, or endotracheal tube is discussed in Chapter 2. A more detailed account of the pharmacology of inhalational anesthetics than is given in this chapter can be found elsewhere [1–3, 7]. Such features as the concentration and second gas effects, different delivery systems, minimum alveolar concentration, and mechanisms of action will not be discussed in this chapter.

Uptake and Distribution. Inhalational anesthetics are delivered into the alveoli by one of a variety of systems; a discussion of this is beyond the scope of this chapter. However they are delivered, the vapors arrive in the alveoli, diffuse across the alveolar membranes, and are dissolved in the blood. They travel in this form through the body and diffuse back out of the blood stream into tissues of lower concentration.

This process is analogous to that characteristic of the intravenous agents, although an additional barrier—the alveolar apparatus—is interposed. The vessel-rich group of organs receives the earliest and highest concentrations of the vaporous agent; included in this group is the brain, in which the predominant effect of these vapors is produced.

Numerous factors affect the amount of the vapor and the speed with which it can be delivered. Intuitively, the more vapor that is delivered to the alveoli, the more and faster it will reach its site of action, and thus the higher the *inspired concentration,* in general, the faster the onset of action. If an alveolar concentration of 1 volume percent of an agent is needed to render the brain insensitive to pain (which is true of isoflurane, for example), and only 1 volume percent is delivered to the alveoli, it will take a long time to reach an effective brain concentration. However, if the inspired concentration is transiently increased to 3 or 4 volumes percent, the diffusion down the various gradients will be hastened, and the brain concentration of the agent will rise much more quickly; this process of introducing a higher-than-maintenance concentration is commonly referred to as *overpressure.*

The *minute ventilation* also affects the amount of agent delivered to the alveoli: The more of the former, the more of the latter. If an inspired concentration of 1 volume percent is delivered to a patient with a minute ventilation of 2 liters/min, a total of 200 ml of agent will be sent to the alveoli. If 1 volume percent is delivered to a patient being hyperventilated at 10 liters/min, 1 liter of agent will be delivered.

Likewise, the *cardiac output* affects the rate at which the agent builds up in the alveoli: If the rate of delivery into the alveoli is relatively greater than the amount that can be taken away through the blood stream, the *concentration* of the drug in the alveoli will build up more quickly. A tenet of inhalational anesthesia is that the *effect* of the vapor is related to the concentration in the brain, which is most closely related to the alveolar concentration; hence, the higher the *alveolar* concentration, the greater the effect of the drug. It would seem that with a diminished cardiac output the onset of action of an inhaled drug would be delayed, as it is in the case of intravenous agents. In fact, in the case of inhalational agents, the alveolar concentration and onset of action are increased with a lower cardiac output because the alveolar concentration rises more quickly since the drug is not being picked up and carried away in the blood stream.

The *solubility* of the agent in the various tissues also affects its rate of absorption. A soluble agent will quickly disappear from the alveolus, and its alveolar concentration will thus not rise quickly. Even though the agent is disappearing into the blood stream quickly, the all-important alveolar *concentration,* which correlates with the effect of the drug, is kept low, and the onset of action of the vapor will be delayed.

The solubility of the anesthetic vapors is measured by the blood-gas, tissue-blood, and oil-gas partition coefficient. Of these, the blood-gas coefficient gives a good indication of the speed with which an agent escapes from the alveoli, and the oil-gas coefficient indicates the tendency of the agent to dissolve into fat, which tends to delay the offset of the drug after its inhalation has been discontinued. An agent with a *high* blood-gas coefficient is very soluble and thus does readily enter the blood stream. Such an agent would be expected *not* to come rapidly to high alveolar concentrations, and its onset of action would be delayed. Ether is just such a drug; ether anesthetic induction is expected to take a very long time. On the other hand, an agent that is very insoluble would *not* leave the alveoli and would quickly build up to a high alveolar, and hence a high brain level, resulting in fast induction. Such an agent is nitrous oxide, which is 25 times less soluble than ether in blood.

Offset of Action. The effects of the inhalational agents are terminated as the process of uptake is reversed; the drug diffuses out of the brain, into the blood, out of the blood, and into the alveoli and is eliminated during exhalation. As would be expected, the more insoluble agents are eliminated more quickly. If the agent has been administered for a long period of time (hours), the oil-gas partition coefficient may come into play; drugs with a high coefficient can be expected to have been sequestered in vessel-poor fat cells, and the ultimate elimination of these drugs, halothane being the prime example, will be delayed.

Metabolism. For all intents and purposes, the biotransformation of the inhalational anesthetics plays very little part in their elimination. Nitrous oxide is probably not metabolized; isoflurane is metabolized to a very small extent. Less than 5 percent of enflurane is metabolized, mostly via the kidneys, but 15 to 20 percent of halothane may be metabolized in the liver. A description of some of the potential deleterious effects, particularly of halothane on the liver and enflurane on the kidneys, can be found in Miller's work [7].

Nitrous Oxide

Nitrous oxide is a very insoluble vapor of limited efficacy. Whereas with the more potent fluorocarbon inhalational anesthetics discussed below, which are effective in concentrations of less than 2 volumes percent, nitrous oxide cannot be given in concentrations high enough (105 percent) to provide surgical analgesia. Nonetheless, it is an adjunct of unsurpassed popularity and limited toxicity. Its effectiveness in the emergency department as an analgesic for outpatient procedures has been described by Stewart [64]; several potential problems with its use will be presented.

The combination of nitrous oxide with intravenous agents, particularly narcotics, has been advocated [64]. Of utmost concern in this setting is airway control; the combination of nitrous oxide and narcotics is additive, and injudicious use may deprive a patient of his intrinsic airway protection. In the operating room, scrupulous attention is paid to airway control, both to ensure adequate minute ventilaton and to obviate airway aspiration. Most anesthesiology departments have guidelines governing the number of hours after eating or drinking that should pass before a stomach is considered empty enough to reduce the possibility of aspiration during an elective anesthetic, even if general anesthesia is not anticipated. Nitrous oxide is a mild direct cardiac depressant. It has a propensity to diffuse into closed gaseous spaces and has been shown to increase rapidly the volume of a preexisting pneumothorax. It will diffuse into the lumen of the gastrointestinal tract, into the middle ear, and into any air trapped in the central nervous system, as after a pneumoencephalogram. It will enlarge the volume of aspirated bubbles in air emboli. It will support combustion. After it is discontinued, it may be responsible for diffusion hypoxia [7, 65]. Its use has been associated with high ambient levels of nitrous oxide, and scavenging of waste gases has been advocated [66].

Potent Anesthetic Vapors

Halothane (Fluothane) is the oldest of the potent vapors, enflurane (Ethrane) is next, and isoflurane (Forane) is the newest. Each can result in surgical planes of anesthesia in concentrations near 1 volume percent. The solubility of these agents is much higher than that of nitrous oxide, and their onset and offset of action is slower. They are more lipid soluble, and prolonged use will result in prolonged offset of action.

These potent vapors are all direct bronchodilators; halothane has the reputation for being slightly more efficacious and is the least "pungent." All three are cardiac depressants, vasodilators (isoflurane especially), and analgesics. Halothane and isoflurane will stop epileptiform activity and enflurane may incite it. Indeed, at very high concentrations (4 to 5 percent endtidal volume, which would lead to profound cardiovascular depression), halothane may render an electroencephalogram (EEG) isoelectric or "flat." At doses above about 2 percent, enflurane may produce an EEG pattern during which epileptic acivity can be incited.

Status asthmaticus is a life-threatening situation in which conventional forms of therapy including hydration, endotracheal intubation, positive endexpiratory pressure, intravenous methylxanthines, inhalational bronchodilators, steroids, and antibiotics may be ineffective. All three of the common potent inhalational anesthetics are bronchodilators, and the use of halothane in status asthmaticus has been studied [67]. Its effectiveness was found to be far from conclusive, arrhythmias were generated, and the efficacy of this form of therapy has been questioned [7]; still, if all other avenues of therapy have been unsuccessfully attempted, this potent inhalational agent may be worth considering.

Status epilepticus is another life-threatening emergency for which two of the potent inhalational anesthetics may have definite benefit. As noted above, halothane and isoflurane will stop epileptogenic activity and are uniformly effective in stopping status epilepticus. The usual protocol is to administer the anesthetic in concentrations sufficient to abolish the seizure activity as monitored by EEG while other long-term forms of therapy are instituted. Total body metabolism is increased incredibly during the tonicclonic muscle activity; in an intubated and ventilated patient, this increase may be abolished through the use of a muscle relaxant pending abatement of the seizure activity by other methods.

CONCLUSIONS

This chapter has attempted to present a brief outline of the pharmacokinetics of the individual intravenous and inhalational agents that are common to both anesthesiology and emergency departments. It is hoped that this discussion will prevent several of the pitfalls that may occur with the use of these agents. Let us return briefly to the three case discussions with which this chapter opened.

Case 1

Remember that frail, elderly woman in severe respiratory compromise, with a history of COPD? She clearly is in shock from whatever cause and will probably reach complete cardiorespiratory compromise if something isn't done soon. This was a real patient whom the author was called to see emergently for airway management. In fact, her underlying problem turned out not to be pulmonary at all; she was in the throes of an acutely evolving myocardial infarction and was in "cardiac asthma" as her pump failure resulted in florid pulmonary edema with bronchoconstriction.

After a quick assessment it was felt that the very first thing that needed to be done for this woman was to get her intubated; it was presumed that she had a "full stomach," so aspiration precautions were needed. The two methods of intubating in this case would be an awake intubation, probably blind nasal, or quick IV induction and intubation perhaps facilitated by neuromuscular paralysis. Because of her diminishing ability to cooperate as she fought harder and harder to breathe and became increasingly hypoxic, and because it was felt that she would be underoing per-endotracheal tube bronchoscopy in the near future, which mandates a larger endotracheal tube than might be comfortably passed nasally, the author opted to intubate her after an intravenous induction.

After preoxygenating the patient with a bag-valve mask apparatus, and with suction and intubation equipment available, 35 mg of ketamine were given IV push followed immediately by 60 mg of succinylcholine while cricoid pressure was administered; simultaneously, the head of the bed was lowered. Within 45 seconds an easy oral intubation was accomplished with an 8.0-mm oral endotracheal tube. During the induction and intubation the vital signs were stable, and the blood gas measurements improved dramatically after 100% oxygen was administered; the mechanics of breathing were improved somewhat after neuromuscular paralysis, which was maintained by the later administration of vecuronium.

Out of concern for awareness, 5 mg of diazepam was given IV push about 15 minutes after the ketamine dose. The patient's cardiovascular function promptly deteriorated to the point where dopamine had to be given to raise her blood pressure above 60 systolic, although her tissue perfusion appeared to be improved. Eventually her status stabilized, and she was extubated after a day or two; after an appropriate work-up, operable coronary artery disease was discovered, and she underwent a multivessel coronary artery bypass graft (CABG) with an uneventful recovery.

Case 2

What physician, working in an emergency department, hasn't seen a young ex-motorcycle rider with altered mental status? This person represents a hazard to himself as he begins to flail around; he must be presumed to have a potentially injured cervical spine, increased intracranial pressure, and a full stomach. It seems to be accepted by many of our trauma surgeons that these patients are managed best if they are paralyzed and intubated. Further diagnostic work-up, which nearly universally means CT scanning, can then be carried out.

The author's approach to these patients is to try to find out how likely cervical injury is and to try to assess jaw mobility. It is very uncommon for such patients to have an acute jaw fracture that would result in a complete inability to open the jaw after neuromuscular paralysis. For this patient, the initial approach might again be to round up all equipment and have the assistant, most appropriately the trauma surgeon or neurosurgeon, apply gentle axial head traction with the head in a neutral position. with a second assistant providing cricoid pressure, oxygen is supplied by bag-valve mask (passive ventilation when possible); an intravenous induction of sodium thiopental, 5 mg/kg, is immediately followed by neuromuscular relaxation through one of the following routes:

1. Succinylcholine without precurarization, if it is thought that airway problems surmount all others;
2. Succinylcholine 2 to 3 minutes after precurarization;
3. Vecuronium, 0.15 mg/kg, but care is needed to ensure that there is ample IV fluid running to keep the sodium thiopental from mixing with the vecuronium and causing a precipitate inside the IV tubing.

In this patient option 3 was used and the patient was intubated under direct vision without difficulty. It should be noted that the first two options for paralysis will result in a patient who will begin to move around quickly after intubation or who will be able to breathe for himself in the event the physician *can't* intubate. This particular person developed cardiovascular hyperdynamics shortly after intubation and was kept paralyzed with incremental doses of vecuronium, later changed to metocurine. He was kept sedated during the ensuing CT scans with increments of diazepam to a total of 15 mg; the hemodynamics also stabilized.

Case 3

The patient who was brought to the emergency department after his colonoscopy was a man who is, in essence, anesthetized. He has had 7 mg of midazolam and 14 mg of morphine sulfate. With his cardiovascular problems (angina, hypertension, and aneurysm) probably the last thing that is wanted is to arouse his sympathetic nervous system. The author delivers patients like this all the time but takes them from the operating room to the postanesthesia care unit (PACU, i.e., recovery room), where they recover. Two options are possible with this man:

1. The effects of the narcotic may be reversed by using either the pure antagonist naloxone, in which case all hemodynamic hell may break loose, or an agonist-antagonist, in small increments. The physician may wish to try to reverse the midazolam with physostigmine or aminophylline, but probably he or she will be stuck with its effects for another hour or two.

2. The clinician may wait for the normal hepatic metabolism to gradually reverse the effects of the intravenous agents, offer supplemental oxygen, and tell the endoscopist and the patient's wife that it will take time, maybe 2 to 3 hours, but eventually the patient will wake up. His ventilation can be monitored in part by pulse oximetry. In the mean-

time, he is very unlikely to suffer a ruptured aneurysm or a myocardial infarction.

One of the things that could be done is obtain an arterial blood gas measurement; if the patient really is dangerously hypercarbic, the physician might want to opt to reverse the narcosis gently with a small dose of an agonist-antagonist, such as 1 to 2 mg of nalbuphine, which could be repeated every 5 minutes until satisfactory minute ventilation is restored.

ACKNOWLEDGMENTS

The author wishes to acknowledge the invaluable assistance of C. Craig Moldenhauer, particularly in the sections on narcotics, agonists, and agonist-antagonists, and of Dr. David Arkin, for assistance with Fig. 5-2.

REFERENCES

1. Gilman, A. G., Goodman, L., and Gilman, A. (eds.). *The Pharmacologic Basis of Therapeutics.* New York: Macmillan, 1980.
2. Stoelting, R. K. *Pharmacology and Physiology in Anesthetic Practice.* Philadelphia: Lippincott, 1987.
3. Dripps, R. D., Eckenhoff, J. E., and Vandam, L. D. *Introduction to Anesthesia: The Principles of Safe Practice.* Philadelphia: Saunders, 1977.
4. Dundee, J. W., and Wyant, G. *Intravenous Anesthesia.* London: Churchill Livingstone, 1974.
5. Hug, C. C., Jr. Pharmacokinetics of drugs administered intravenously. *Anesth. Analg.* 57:704–723, 1978.
6. McIntyre, K. M., and Lewis, A. J. (eds.). *Textbook of Advanced Cardiac Life Support.* Dallas: American Heart Association, 1983. P. 102.
7. Miller, R. G. (ed.). *Anesthesia.* New York: Churchill Livingstone, 1981.
8. Fragen, R. J., Shanks, C. A., and Molteni, A. Effects of Etomidate on hormonal responses to surgical stress. *Anesthesiology* 61:652–656, 1984.
9. Wagner, R. L., and White, P. F. Etomidate inhibits adrenocortical function in surgical patients. *Anesthesiology* 61:647–651, 1984.
10. Lowenstein, E., et al. Cardiovascular response to large doses of intravenous morphine in man. *New Engl. J. Med.* 281:1389–1393, 1969.
11. deCastro, J., et al. Comparative study of cardiovascular, neurological and metabolic side-effects of eight narcotics in dogs. *Acta Anaesthesiolog. Belg.* 30:6–90, 1979.
12. Flacke, J. W., et al. Histamine release by four narcotics: A double-blind study. *Anesth. Analg.* 66:723–730, 1987.
13. Flacke, J. W., et al. Comparison of morphine, meperidine, fentanyl, and sufentanil in balanced anesthesia: A double-blind study. *Anesth. Analg.* 64:897–910, 1985.
14. Reves, J. G., et al. Additive negative inotropic effect of a combination of diazepam and fentanyl. *Anesth. Analg.* 63:97–100, 1984.
15. Tomicheck, R. C., et al. Diazepam-fentanyl interaction—hemodynamic and hormonal effects in coronary artery surgery. *Anesth. Analg.* 62:881–884, 1983.
16. Estafanous, F. W., ed. *Opioids in Anesthesia.* Woburn, Ma.: Butterworth, 1984.

17. Freye, E. *Opioid Agonists and Antagonists and Mixed Narcotic Analgesics.* Heidelberg: Springer Verlag, 1987.
18. Martin, W. R. History and development of mixed opioid agonists, partial agonists and antagonists. *Br. J. Clin. Pharmacol.* 7:273S–279S, 1979.
19. Flacke, J. W. Antagonism of opioid analgesics with nalbuphine and naloxone. *Sem. Anesth.,* in press.
20. Goodman, R. R., and Pasternak, G. W. Multiple Opiate Receptors. In M. Kuhar and G. Pasternak (eds.), *Analgesics: Neurochemical, Behavioral and Clinical Perspectives.* New York: Raven Press, 1984. Pp. 69–96.
21. Pasternak, G. W. Multiple morphone and enkephalin receptors and the relief of pain. *J.A.M.A.* 259:1362–1367, 1988.
22. Kaufman, R. D., Gabathuler, M. L., and Bellville, J. W. Potency, duration of action and pAO$_2$ in man of intravenous naloxone measured by reversal of morphine-depressed respiration. *J. Phamracol. Exp. Ther.* 219:156–161, 1981.
23. Schwartz, J. A., and Koenigsberg, M. D. Naloxone-induced pulmonary edema. *Am. Emerg. Med.* 16:1294–1296, 1987.
24. Andree, R. A. Sudden death following naloxone administration. *Anesth. Analg.* 59:782–784, 1980.
25. Azar, I., and Turndorf, H. Severe hypertension and multiple atrial premature contractions following naloxone administration. *Anesth. Analg.* 58:524–525, 1979.
26. DesMarteau, J. K., and Cassot, A. L. Acute pulmonary edema resulting from nalbuphine reversal of fentanyl-induced respiratory depression. *Anesthesiology* 65:237, 1986.
27. Estilio, A. E., and Cottrell, J. E. Naloxone, hypertension, and ruptured cerebral aneurysm. *Anesthesiology* 54:352, 1981.
28. Flacke, J. W., Flacke, W. E., and Williams, G. D. Acute pulmonary edema following naloxone reversal of high-dose morphine anesthesia. *Anesthesiology* 47:376–378, 1977.
29. Gillman, M. A. The hypertensive response to naloxone—a commentary. *S. Afr. Med. J.* 66(15):551–552, 1984.
30. Levin, E. R., et al. Case report: Severe hypertension induced by naloxone. *Am. J. Med. Sci.* 290:70–72, 1985.
31. Michaelis, L. L., et al. Ventricular irritability associated with the use of naloxone hydrochloride. *Ann. Thorac. Surg.* 18:608–614, 1974.
32. Partridge, B. L., and Ward, C. R. Pulmonary edema following low-dose naloxone administration. *Anesthesiology* 65:709–710, 1986.
33. Prough, D. S., et al. Acute pulmonary edema in healthy teenagers following conservative doses of intravenous naloxone. *Anesthesiology* 60:485–486, 1984.
34. Taff, R. H. Pulmonary edema following naloxone administration in a patient without heart disease. *Anesthesiology* 59:576–577, 1983.
35. Tanaka, G. Y. Hypertensive reaction to naloxone. *J.A.M.A.* 228:25–26, 1974.
36. Mills, C. A., et al. Cardiovascular effects of fentanyl reversal by naloxone at varying arterial carbon dioxide tensions in dogs. *Anesth. Analg.* 67:730–736, 1988.
37. Bonnet, F., et al. Naloxone therapy of human septic shock. *Crit. Care Med.* 13:972–975, 1985.
38. Halpern, J. S. Naloxone: A study of its use in shock. *J. Emerg. Nurs.* 10:222–225, 1984.
39. Montastruc, J. L., Richard, J. P., and Cathala, B. Naloxone fails to reverse blood pressure in shock: A double blind study in man. *J. Pharmacol.* 16:313–314, 1985.
40. Peters, W. P., et al. Pressor effect of naloxone in septic shock. *Lancet* 1(8219):529–532, 1981.
41. Gal, T. J., DiFazio, C. A., Moscicki, J. Analgesic and respiratory depressant activity of nalbuphine: A comparison with morphine. *Anesthesiology* 57:367–374, 1982.

42. Romagnoli, A., and Keats, A. S. Ceiling effect for respiratory depression by nalbuphine. *Clin. Pharmacol. Ther.* 27:478–485, 1980.

43. Gal, T. J. Morphine antagonism with nalbuphine. *Anesth. Analg.* 66:97–98, 1987.

44. Dundee, J. W. *Intravenous Anesthetic Agents.* London: Edward Arnold, 1979.

45. Bidwai, A. V., et al. Reversal of diazepam-induced postanesthetic somnolence with physostigmine. *Anesthesiology* 51:256–259, 1979.

46. Bourke, D. L., Rosenberg, M., and Allen, P. D. Physostigmine: Effectiveness as an antagonist of respiratory depression and psychomotor effects caused by morphine or diazepam. *Anesthesiology* 61:523–528, 1984.

47. Spaulding, B. C., et al. The effect of physostigmine on diazepam-induced ventilatory depression: A double-blind study. *Anesthesiology* 61:551–554, 1984.

48. Wangler, M. A., and Kilpatrick, D. S. Aminophylline is an antagonist of lorazepam. *Anesth. Analg.* 64:834–836, 1985.

49. Garber, J. G., et al. Physostigmine–atropine fails to reverse diazepam sedation. *Anesth. Analg.* 59:58–60, 1980.

50. Pandit, U. A., et al. Physostigmine fails to reverse clinical, psychomotor or EEG effects of lorazepam. *Anesth. Analg.* 62:679–685, 1983.

51. Sleigh, J. W. Failure of aminophylline to antagonize midazolam sedation (Letter). *Anesth. Analg.* 65:540, 1986.

52. White, P. F., Way, W. L., and Trevor, A. J. Ketamine—its pharmacology and therapeutic uses. *Anesthesiology* 56:119–136, 1982.

53. Miller, R. D. The advantages of giving D-tubocurarine before succinylcholine. *Anesthesiology* 37:568, 1972.

54. Rogoff, R. C., Lippman, M., and Walts, L. F. An unusual sensitivity to D-tubocurarine before succinylcholine. *Anesthesiology* 41:397, 1974.

55. Brotherton, W. P., and Matteo, R. S. Pharmacokinetics and pharmacodynamics of metocurine in humans with and without renal failure. *Anesthesiology* 55:273–276, 1981.

56. Lennon, R. L., Olson, R. A., and Gronert, G. A. Atracurium or vecuronium for rapid sequence endotracheal intubation. *Anesthesiology* 64:510–513, 1986.

57. Basta, S. K., et al. Vecuronium does not alter serum histamine within the clinical dose range. *Anesthesiology* 59:a273, 1983.

58. Gallo, J. A., Cork, R. C., and Pucki, P. Comparison of effects of atracurium and vecuronium in cardiac surgical patients. *Anesth. Analg.* 67:161–165, 1988.

59. Minton, M. D., Stirt, J. A., and Bedford, R. F. Vecuronium and intracranial pressure in man. *Anesth. Analg.* 65:S101, 1986.

60. Badrinath, S., Vazeery, A. K., and Ivankovich, A. D. Effect of vecuronium on intraocular pressure. *Anesth. Analg.* 65:S10, 1986.

61. Mehta, M. P., et al. Facilitation of rapid endotracheal intubations with divided doses of nondepolarizing neuromuscular blocking drugs. *Anesthesiology* 62:392–395, 1985.

62. Miller, R. D. The priming principle (Editorial). *Anesthesiology* 62:381–382, 1985.

63. Schwarz, S., et al. Rapid tracheal intubation with vecuronium: The priming principle. *Anesthesiollgy* 62:388–391, 1985.

64. Sosis, M., Larijani, G. E., and Marr, A. T. Priming with atracurium. *Anesth. Analg.* 66:329–332, 1987.

65. Stewart, R. D. Nitrous oxide sedation/analgesia in emergency medicine. *Ann. Emerg. Med.* 14:139–148, 1985.

66. Dula, D. J., Skiendzielewski, J. J., and Royko, M. Nitrous oxide levels in the emerency department. *Ann. Emerg. Med.* 10:575–578, 1981.

67. Gold, M. I., and Helrich, M. Pulmonary mechanics during general anesthesia: V. Status asthamaticus. *Anesthesiology* 32:422, 1970.

6. Regional Anesthetic Considerations

Glenn S. Vanstrum

The history of regional anesthetics has an international flavor. During the sixteenth century Johannes Costaeus of Italy wrote on the use of cold water, snow, or ice to relieve pain from surgical incisions [1]. Others used nerve compression, opium injected through a bladder and quill, or hypnotism. It took the inventions of the glass syringe, by Pravaz of France, and the hypodermic needle, by Wood of Scotland, to set the stage for modern regional anesthesia. Koller, an Austrian, first reported in 1884 on the use of the local anesthetic cocaine as a topical application for eye surgery. Of course, the stimulant and anesthetic properties of cocaine had long been recognized by inhabitants of the Andes mountains. Also in 1884 Halstead of the United States performed major nerve blocks using cocaine and needle and syringe. Lidocaine was synthesized by Lofgren in 1943 but was not introduced clinically until 1947 by Gordh of Sweden.

Today local and regional anesthesia is widely used, in both modern emergency departments and operating rooms. In this chapter we will discuss the local anesthetics in some detail, with emphasis on the toxicity and treatment of toxic reactions. A short treatise on general considerations for nerve block will follow, and a discussion of the more commonly performed nerve blocks will conclude the chapter.

LOCAL ANESTHETICS

MODE OF ACTION

Most local anesthetics possess an aromatic, lipophilic portion connected to a hydrophilic tertiary amine through either an amide or an ester linkage [2]. As such they are weak bases with pKa values (pH at which charged species equal uncharged species) ranging from 7.5 to 9.5. It is accepted today that both ionized and unionized forms of the local anesthetic are necessary, with the uncharged species diffusing through the nerve cell membrane and the charged species causing an effect. The importance of this clinically may be seen in the reduced effect of local anesthetics in extremely acidotic tissue, e.g., the erythematous skin overlying an abscess. This effect is presumably due to the increased amount of drug present in the charged form, which is unable to penetrate the axoplasmic membrane.

Probably the most attractive theory of the mode of action of these drugs involves their binding on a receptor that is on the inner surface of the nerve cell membrane [2]. This receptor, when occupied by a local anesthetic, blocks the sodium channel, thus preventing the nerve cell from depolarizing and transmitting its signal. This sodium channel-blocking effect not only is specific for nerve cells but also includes other types of cells, such as those that define the cardiac conduction apparatus.

TYPES OF LOCAL ANESTHETICS

As mentioned above, both amide and ester local anesthetics are used today. Generally speaking, drugs in the former group, represented by lidocaine, bupivacaine, etidocaine, and mepivacaine, are chemically stable, undergo enzymatic degradation in the liver, and have a low level of antigenicity. Esters, on the other hand, represented by cocaine, chloroprocaine, tetracaine, and procaine, are relatively unstable in solution and more rapidly metabolized by cholinesterases and have a higher propensity to cause allergic phenomena. This is most probably due to the fact that para-aminobenzoic acid, a potent hapten, is a metabolite of ester anesthetics [3].

Further classification of local anesthetics involves their potency and duration of action and their physical chemical properties. Protein binding is positively related to duration of action [3]; thus, bupivacaine is 95 percent protein bound and has a duration of effect some eight times that of the short-acting procaine. More lipid soluble drugs seem to be more potent, i.e., require less drug for a given effect. The effect of pKa is variable; however, for the most part, drugs with a lower pKa such as lidocaine have a more rapid onset because more drug exists in the unionized form initially. Drugs such as bupivacaine, which have a higher pKa, have a longer onset of action [3]. The addition of bicarbonate to a local anesthetic solution may speed onset by increasing nonionized species (see below) [4].

COMMONLY USED LOCAL ANESTHETICS—AMIDES

Lidocaine

Lidocaine is a versatile amide local anesthetic that is useful for nearly all types of regional anesthesia from local infiltration to nerve block to major conduction anesthesia by the spinal or epidural route. Lidocaine does have a shorter (1 to 3 hours) duration of action than other amide anesthetics, but this action may be prolonged by the use of added epinephrine, most typically in a 1:200,000 ratio (see below). It is also an effective cardiac antidysrhythmic agent because it suppresses ectopy by selectively preventing phase 4 (diastolic) depolarization in ischemic cardiac tissue. At higher doses it suppresses the phase 0 or rapid spike phase of depolarization, probably by the same sodium channel-blocking action that gives it local anesthetic properties [2]. Thus, toxic doses slow conduction in the heart and are revealed by widened QRS and PR intervals and by bradycardia.

One should not exceed a total dose of 6.4 mg/kg, the threshold dose for CNS overdose symptoms [2]. All local anesthetics can produce depression of the CNS. At the lower symptomatic doses, however, the initial symptoms are excitatory because the inhibitory centers are blocked first [5]. Gener-

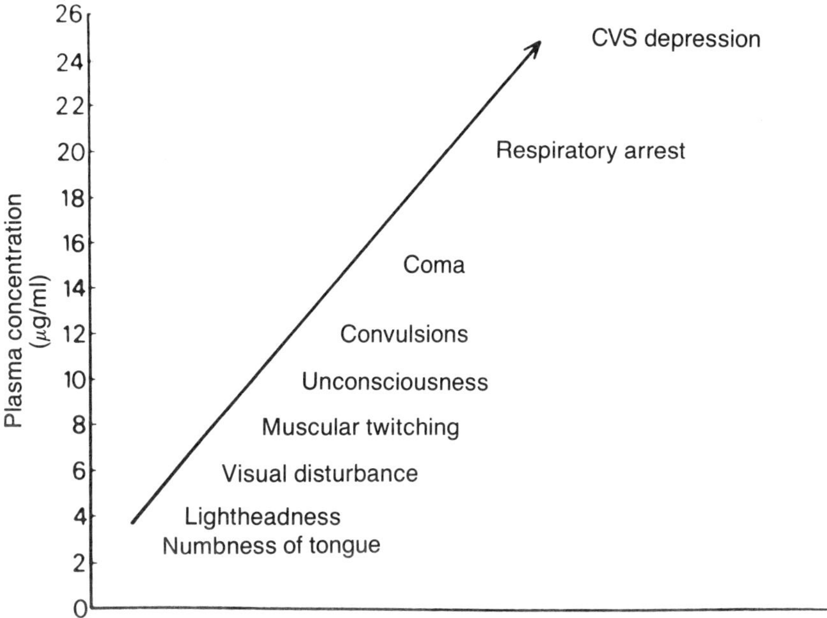

Fig. 6-1. Direct relationship between lidocaine blood concentration and symptoms. In clinical practice, although such blood levels are useful for antidysrhythmic lidocaine therapy, it is impractical to measure levels that change rapidly after regional blockade. Site of injection causes marked differences in rate of absorption and eventual serum levels as well (see text). (From M. J. Cousins and P. O. Bridenbaugh [eds.]. *Neural Blockade in Clinical Anesthesia and Pain Management.* Philadelphia: Lippincott, 1980. With permission.)

alized CNS depression occurs at higher serum levels. Cardiac collapse requires about seven times the serum levels needed to produce convulsions in sheep [6], and this is supported by clinical observations in humans. Thus, clinically, in increasing toxicity from, say, inadvertent intravascular injection, one would see a spectrum of agitation and disorientation followed by frank convulsions, followed by cardiac collapse represented by bradycardia and interval prolongation, followed by cardiac standstill (Fig. 6-1).

Treatment of lidocaine toxicity includes prompt airway management and treatment of seizures with diazepam or 50- to 100-mg increments of sodium thiopental. Generally speaking, resuscitation from lidocaine overdosage has a higher success rate than does treatment of bupivacaine overdosage. This is due to the property of lidocaine to attach rapidly and then rapidly leave sodium channels ("fast-in, fast-out") [7]. Lidocaine, like other amide anesthetics such as bupivacaine, is metabolized in the liver. Hence, the presence of liver disease or hepatic vascular congestion from right heart failure can lead to delayed metabolism and increased toxicity.

Bupivacaine

Because of its increased protein binding and subsequent prolonged duration of action (2 to 12 hours, depending on site, dosage, and other factors), bupivacaine is a valuable and commonly used local anesthetic, with a range of application similar to that of lidocaine. Because it does not cross the maternal-fetal barrier as quickly as lidocaine and because inadvertent intrathecal injection does not produce the toxic effects associated with chloroprocaine, it is an important drug for use in obstetric medicine. It has a major drawback, and that is its potential for cardiac toxicity when inadvertent intravenous administration occurs [8]. Total doses of greater than 3 mg/kg are contraindicated for this reason.

Unlike lidocaine, the cardiac toxicity noted with bupivacaine requires only about four times the dose needed to produce CNS toxicity, and studies in pregnant sheep show this margin to be even narrower [2]. A number of fatalities involving obstetric patients have led to withdrawal of Food and Drug Administration (FDA) approval for the use of 0.75% bupivacaine in obstetric patients and support the animal studies.

Cardiac collapse/convulsive activity ratios (data adapted from studies in adult sheep by Covino [9]) are as follows:

	NONPREGNANT PATIENTS	PREGNANT PATIENTS
Lidocaine	7.1	3.6
Bupivacaine	3.7	1.6

It has been proposed that the mechanism for this toxicity is due not to the rapid attachment of bupivacaine to cardiac sodium channels but rather to its much slower disengagement ("fast-in, slow-out") [7]. Bupivacaine toxicity has also been associated with both ventricular fibrillation and a torsade de pointes type of undulating ventricular tachycardia [8, 10], also unlike lidocaine. Treatment of cardiac toxicity with bupivacaine is similar to treatment of lidocaine toxicity, with prompt airway management and prevention of acidosis and hypoxia a first concern. Unfortunately, the dysrhythmias and cardiac depression that have been reported with bupivacaine have appeared resistant to various therapeutic modalities [9]. Animal studies have suggested that prompt use of multiple IV epinephrine doses (1 mg/dose) and IV bretylium (5 mg/kg q30sec for six doses), in conjunction with airway management and use of atropine and direct current (DC) shock treatment, may increase the chances for resuscitation [11]. Because of the "slow-out" nature of the bupivacaine–sodium channel relationship, prolonged resuscitation may be required. Because the CNS convulsant activity seen with local anesthetic toxicity contributes markedly to acidosis and hypoxia, prompt management of seizures by the use of IV benzodiazepines or sodium thiopental in conjunction with the above measures is important [10].

Etidocaine

Similar in many regards to bupivacaine, this amide local anesthetic is remarkable for its propensity to produce motor as well as sensory blockade in major conduction anesthesia. Hence, whenever motor block is desired, say, for orthopedic procedures, it may be useful. It is contraindicated for procedures in which motor blockade is deleterious, e.g., in obstetrics.

Mepivacaine

Like the amide anesthetic lidocaine, mepivacaine has less vasodilator effect and is slightly less toxic than the former agent. Both drugs have prolonged action when used with epinephrine. The effect of mepivacaine does last longer than that of lidocaine, probably due to the above mentioned lessened vasodilator effect.

COMMONLY USED LOCAL ANESTHETICS—ESTERS

Cocaine

Cocaine, the forerunner of all local anesthetics, is still used as a topical local anesthetic in the hospital environment. It has potent vasoconstrictor effects as well as local anesthetic effects and hence is popular for use with nasal procedures and instrumentation and for control of epistaxis. Advantages of the use of cocaine over lidocaine or bupivacaine with added epinephrine as a vasoconstrictor are not readily apparent, and the increased use of cocaine as an illicit, recreational drug has led many to abandon the added expense and trouble of dealing with a controlled substance. It is supplied in both 4% and 10% solutions (4% = 40 mg per ml), and the maximum dose for a 70-kg adult is 200 mg. Great care must be taken to avoid overdose, especially with the 10% solution, by careless and overly generous topical application. Electrocardiography (ECG), frequent blood pressure determinations, and O_2 saturation monitoring are warranted for most if not all clinical applications.

Overdose symptoms with the drug are related both to its local anesthetic action and to its property of preventing reuptake of catecholamines at adrenergic nerve terminals. Toxic manifestations include convulsions, tachydysrhythmias, hypertension, cerebral vascular accidents, and hyperthermia. Deaths from acute intoxication are not unusual, although most but not all fatalities involve street use. Treatment of overdose involves airway management and use of beta blockade. Labetelol, the combination alpha- and beta-adrenergic blocker, may also be useful [12]. Its combined alpha- and beta-adrenergic blockade prevents the unopposed alpha action permitted by sole treatment with beta blockade. Sometimes the hyperdynamic effects of cocaine may require potent IV vasodilators such as sodium nitroprusside [13]. Use of an IV benzodiazepine or IV sodium thiopental for convulsions may be necessary. Use of alkalinization, proposed for bupivacaine overdose, has not been studied. Oral overdose is uncommon, but if suspected, gastric lavage and activated charcoal should be used.

Chloroprocaine

Because chloroprocaine is rapidly metabolized by serum pseudocholinesterase, it has limited toxicity. Very little maternal-fetal transfer occurs, and it has therefore been commonly used in obstetrics. Unfortunately, it has been associated with disastrous neurologic complications resulting from inadvertent intrathecal (as opposed to the intended epidural) injection of large amounts. Much conflicting data have since accumulated, but most agree that the sodium bisulfite preservative, in conjunction with the lowered pH used in maintaining storage of the drug, is the culprit in these patients [9, 14].

Tetracaine

Tetracaine has a long duration but a slow onset of action. Use is primarily restricted to spinal anesthesia.

Procaine

Procaine is a relatively weak local ester anesthetic that has a slow onset and a short duration of action. It is useful for diagnostic spinal blocks (see Chapter 7).

GENERAL CONSIDERATIONS FOR NERVE BLOCK

ADDITION OF VASOCONSTRICTORS, BUFFERING, AND CARBONATION

Vasoconstrictors

As mentioned above, the addition of epinephrine can markedly prolong the duration of action of many of the commonly used local anesthetics. Phenylephrine and norepinephrine have also been used, although their benefits over epinephrine remain to be shown [3]. Use of epinephrine can be a two-edged sword in regard to toxicity. Although it limits systemic spread of local anesthetics and increases the intrinsic toxic thresholds of these agents, epinephrine is itself absorbed systemically and can lead to deleterious hypertension and dysrhythmias, especially in the elderly or in those with cardiac disease. Of course, one should also not use it on facial and digital appendages ("fingers and toes or tip of nose") or on the penis.

Selander and coworkers make a strong case for avoiding routine use of epinephrine for nerve blocks [15]. They demonstrated an increased incidence of nerve damage during brachial plexus blocks in patients receiving epinephrine-containing solutions and related the local neural toxicity to epinephrine-induced ischemia.

Intercostal blockade (see below) is enhanced by the addition of epinephrine. Because toxic levels of local anesthetic can most easily be achieved with this site of injection and because the addition of epinephrine not only lessens such toxicity but also prolongs the improved respiratory dynamics and patient comfort achieved with such blocks, it is often a good choice in a young patient with bruised or broken ribs.

The use of epinephrine with local anesthetics during general anesthesia must be limited carefully, especially with halothane. Halothane lowers the threshold at which epinephrine causes dysrhythmias, and most practitioners would not exceed a dose of 1 μg epinephrine per kilogram total dose (1:200,000 epinephrine solutions have 5 μg/ml). With isoflurane anesthesia 3 μ/kg is a safe limit, beyond which ventricular dysrhythmias can occur. In a patient receiving a large amount of local anesthetic with epinephrine who is not under anesthesia, in the emergency department (ED), for example, the appearance of premature ventricular contractions (PVCs) on ECG is an indicator of epinephrine toxicity.

Buffering and Carbonation

Carbonation of local anesthetics has been promoted as a means of improving rapidity of onset of local anesthetic nerve blockade by some 33 percent [16]. The diffusion of carbon dioxide through the nerve membrane theoretically lowers the axoplasmic pH, thus increasing the relative amount of charged species at the site of action [3]. Unfortunately, more recent studies have failed to confirm the clinical effect of increased rapidity of onset [17]. This failure of clinical effect may be due to intracellular buffering [3].

Buffering of local anesthetic pH by addition of sodium bicarbonate, however, has recently been shown to decrease the pain of injection of amide local anesthetics [18, 19]. Such an additive, which increases the pH of the normally acidic local anesthetic storage solution, lowered the pain of injection in one study from an average of 5 to 1, on a 1 to 10 linear analogue pain score [17].

Site of Injection and Toxicity

Although most textbook authors on local anesthetics commit themselves to firm limits on total doses of local anesthetics, it must be recognized that toxic serum levels of drug may be altered radically depending on the site at which injection takes place. Thus, a safe dose for massive local anesthetic injection in an extremity can prove toxic if given as a series of multiple intercostal blocks. There is good agreement [2] that the list shown in Table 6-1 shows the sites of increasing safety, or decreasing toxicity, of local anesthetic injection.

Table 6-1. Effect of site of injection on serum levels of local anesthetic

Highest blood levels per fixed dose

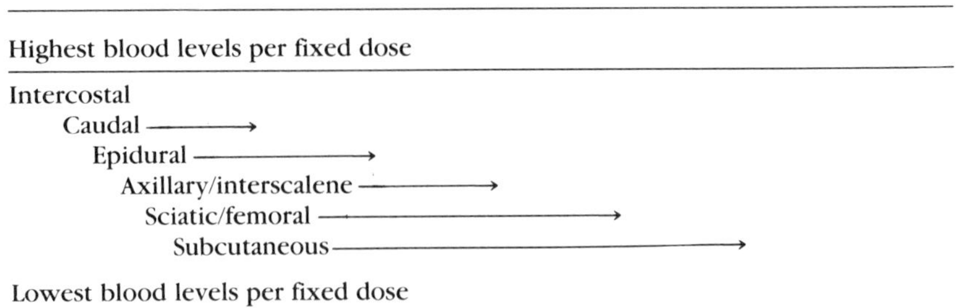

Intercostal
    Caudal ⟶
       Epidural ⟶
         Axillary/interscalene ⟶
           Sciatic/femoral ⟶
            Subcutaneous ⟶

Lowest blood levels per fixed dose

Source: Adapted from J. J. Savarese and B. G. Cavino. Basic and Clinical Pharmacology of Local Anesthetic Drugs. In R. D. Miller (ed.), *Anesthesia.* New York: Churchill Livingstone, 1986. Pp. 985–1013.

Another important consideration is the pattern of onset of nerve block. For example, an axillary or interscalene block of the brachial plexus will initially numb the shoulder because the nerves supplying the proximal limb are superficial to the centrally located nerves supplying the hand. In major regional anesthesia, the most sensitive nerve group (first and last to be anesthetized) is the autonomic system, followed by the sensory nerves, and, last, by the motor systems. Thus, a patient who has received a short-acting spinal anesthetic for outpatient surgery may have had adequate return of sensation and be discharged, only to be rushed to the ED when he or she faints in the parking lot owing to persistent autonomic blockade.

Cardiac arrest during spinal anesthesia has recently been reviewed [20] by Caplan and associates, who investigated 14 healthy patients, all but one (7 percent) of whom suffered severe neurologic damage or death as a result of the arrest. This compares with data from Seattle on out-of-hospital patients with cardiac arrest, of whom 41 percent recovered without gross neurologic deficits [21]. It is speculated that sympathetic blockade from spinal anesthesia may limit cerebral blood flow during cardiopulmonary resuscitation (CPR) because there is increased peripheral blood flow at the brain's expense during sympathectomy. The reviewers concluded that reasonable treatment of the arrests was performed but that common denominators of sedation and possibly hypoxia preceding the arrests, and the underuse of prompt, adequate doses of powerful adrenergic agents such as epinephrine may have contributed to the poor outcomes.

EQUIPMENT, AVOIDANCE OF NEURAL DAMAGE, AND TECHNIQUE

Use of short-bevel needles is important for all types of nerve blocks. Such needles, used in conjunction with a technique in which the bevel is held facing the side of the nerve, will reduce neural trauma. Just as a spinal needle will create a larger hole in the fibers of the dura if its bevel is held facing the direction in which the fibers run [22], so a block needle can

Fig. 6-2. Short-bevel needle (*left*) is favored for most nerve blocks over the standard long-bevel needle (*right*). Direction of bevel should be at right angles to the nerve fibers (see text). (From R. D. Miller [ed.]. *Anesthesia* [2nd ed.]. New York: Churchill Livingstone, 1986. With permission.)

damage nerves [23]. Katz recommends a standard long bevel needle for subcutaneous infiltration [24] (Fig. 6-2).

Eliciting a paresthesia prior to injection of local anesthetic is a two-edged sword—one can never be sure one will develop a good block without the paresthesia, yet most probably the chances of giving an intraneural injection and causing postinjection neuropathy are increased [15]. This author's solution to the problem is to elicit the paresthesia, withdraw the needle a millimeter or two, and, if the paresthesia resolves, inject at that position. Others use stimulating needles, in which a low-frequency, pulse-generated electric current is transmitted through an insulated exploring needle. The physician gives the patient a short-acting IV analgesic and then searches for motor responses elicited by the needle to isolate the nerve. Withdrawal of the needle slightly may, however, also be indicated with this technique.

Use of a ring syringe is also a good idea, because one may easily aspirate and inject with one hand, leaving the other hand free for palpation and other tasks. Intra-arterial injection is more easily recognized by aspiration than intravenous injection because the thinner venous wall may be drawn up against the needle and may yield negative results on aspiration while the needle bevel is still in the vessel. Should signs of agitation or seizures herald an intravascular injection, it is wise to take over the airway immediately with bag and mask, if the patient has an empty stomach, and give the patient IV sodium thiopental (1–3 mg/kg) or midazolam (0.01–0.03 mg/kg). Performance of a proper rapid-sequence induction with cricoid pressure and intubation is a lot to do while treating the neurologic and circulatory effects of local anesthetic overdose; hence, it should be apparent why patients are preferably kept NPO for at least 8 hours prior to major nerve blocks. Especially with lidocaine, toxic manifestations are often short lived, and intubation is often unnecessary unless the stomach is full.

Smooth technique in blocking nerves demands adequate patient rapport, care in avoiding painful stimuli, and artful titration of IV analgesics. Gentle, ongoing explanations exert a hypnotic effect on a patient and do much to allay discomfort, as does a friendly touch or hand-hold. Skin wheals should be placed with the new 30-gauge needles, not the coarser 25-gauge variety. Slow injection is much less painful than rapid, vigorous injection at any site. If a block demands "walking" the needle off a bony structure, the practitioner should be very gentle and infiltrate as he or she reaches bone because periosteum is exquisitely sensitive. If a paresthesia is required, often a small amount of benzodiazepine or narcotic given intravenously will reduce the inherent discomfort, although overzealous sedation will render a patient somnolent and incommunicative.

At all times the physician should aspirate at regular intervals while injecting local anesthetic. If one is injecting large amounts of local anesthetic near the central nervous system, as in an axillary block, special care must be taken because local anesthetic can migrate intraneurally in a longitudinal fashion to the spinal cord, and a spinal anesthetic may result [25]. Injections that are intravascular or intrathecal can be the most dangerous if they are unexpected. Hence, when injecting large amounts of local anesthetic near the spinal cord, especially with epidural injections, it is best to give a small amount of lidocaine with epinephrine as a test dose. The epinephrine will induce a tachycardia if injected intravascularly, and the lidocaine will induce a relatively short-acting spinal block if the needle is placed intrathecally. Because as little as 0.2 ml of lidocaine injected into the cervical vasculature can induce convulsions, extreme caution is demanded with head and neck blocks. A total spinal block is a complication that can be recognized by sudden loss of consciousness, apnea, bradycardia, and hypotension. It can be treated by prompt airway management (usually including intubation), volume replacement, and an IV vasoconstrictor, such as ephedrine in repeated bolus doses of 5 to 10 mg, or phenylephrine in bolus doses of 100 to 200 µg.

Monitoring

Adequate monitoring for local anesthetic use depends on the amount and type of drug to be used and the anticipated frequency of dangerous side effects. Performance of a wrist or ankle block with lidocaine is safe with careful technique, for example, in all but the rare patient who has an allergy to amide local anesthetics, and should not require other than the most basic monitoring (i.e., monitoring vital signs as needed). Performance of major leg blocks is rarely done but requires a high enough dose of local anesthetic to mandate at least IV access and ECG monitoring. Intercostal blockade, because of the high blood concentrations of local anesthetic that are rapidly achieved, demands IV access and ECG monitoring. A postblock chest radiograph to rule out pneumothorax is also suggested. Performance of intravenous block with a tourniquet (Bier block), brachial plexus block, and major conduction nerve blocks such as epidural or spinal block deserve the same level of monitoring and patient preparation as any other major anesthetic procedure. Thus, patients must be NPO for 8 hours. Preparations for positive pressure ventilation and treatment of seizures and cardiac arrest must be made, and at the bedside. ECG, blood pressure, and oxygen saturation monitoring should all be used. Oxygen supplementation must be available and should be supplied if supplemental analgesia is given. An intravenous catheter and infusion must be in place prior to the block, and, in a Bier block, it must be in the contralateral arm (thus, two IVs must be initiated for Bier block [Figs. 6-3 and 6-4]).

Even if an emergency physician does not perform nerve blocks routinely, he or she should be cognizant of the above-discussed special problems inherent in resuscitation from local anesthetic toxicity and sympathectomy. Even if one's particular hospital does not require the ED physician to respond to Code Blue situations outside of the ED, it has become increasingly common for other specialists, especially orthopedic surgeons, to give Bier blocks or brachial plexus blocks in the ED. Misplaced injections can often inadvertently migrate proximally and cause spinal anesthesia and sympathectomy, especially intercostal blocks and cervical sympathetic blocks. Failure of aspiration procedures to detect intravascular injections, faulty or improperly used tourniquets in Bier blocks, or overdose of topical cocaine can all lead to sudden cardiovascular or CNS symptoms of local anesthetic overdose.

Regional anesthesia has many advantages over general anesthesia, one of the most obvious being that nonanesthesiologists may safely use many of the techniques, especially the more distal blocks. Other advantages include the alert postprocedure patient, fewer postoperative cardiorespiratory problems, reduced endocrine metabolic stress responses, and increased postprocedure analgesia. Disadvantages of regional anesthesia include the complications discussed above as well as the incidence of ineffective block. There is no doubt that as the experience and skill of the practitioner increase, so will the incidence of successful blocks. However, one must also

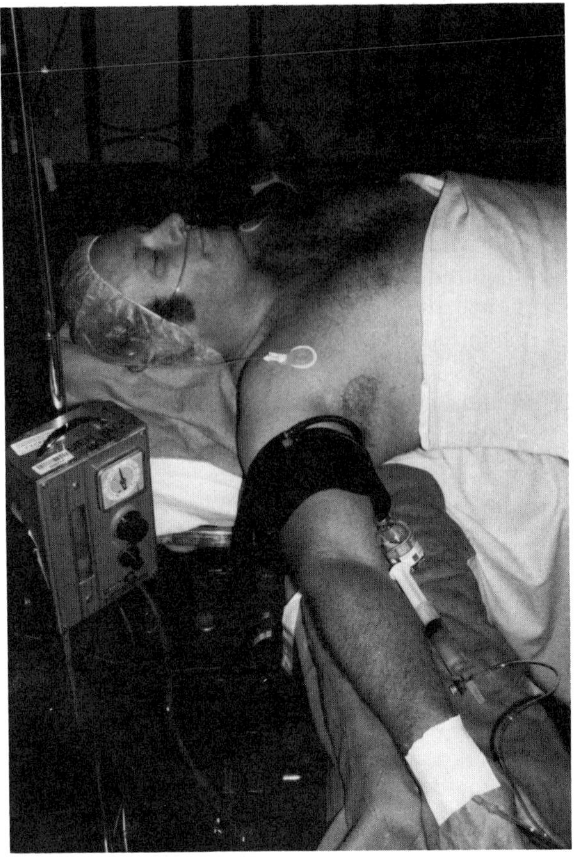

Fig. 6-3. Bier block setup. Note that intravenous lines have been started in both arms; the one in the left arm is used for sedation or resuscitation. Monitoring includes automatic blood pressure measurement, oxygen saturation monitoring, and electrocardiography (ECG). Supplemental oxygen is given by cannula.

realize that adequate time must be allowed after injection for any given block to set up. An inpatient surgeon or the demands of a busy emergency department must be kept at bay if one wishes to reap the benefits of regional anesthesia.

NERVE BLOCKS

Only those blocks that are germane to the intersection of the specialties of anesthesiology and emergency medicine are included below. More extensive discussions of these blocks and additional blocks may be found in a number of sources for the interested reader. These include Jordan Katz' *Atlas of Regional Anesthesia* [24]. Terence Murphy's "Nerve Blocks," a

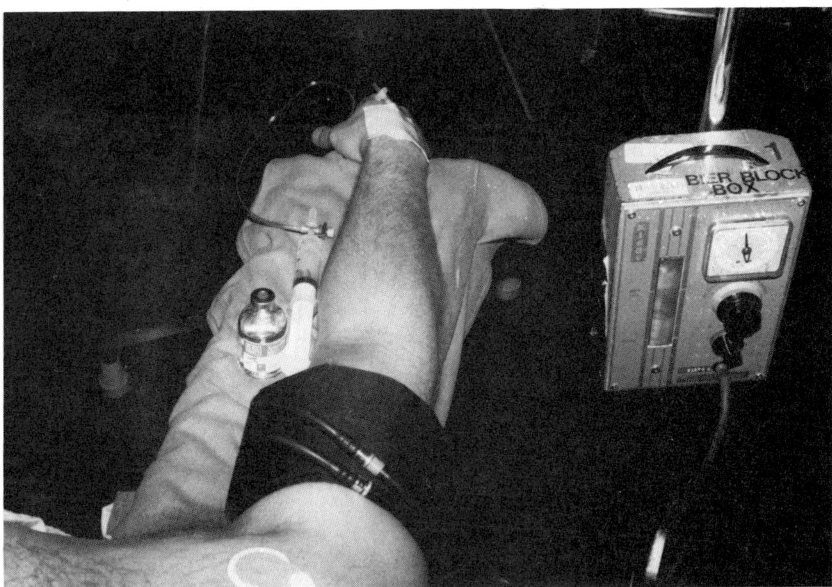

Fig. 6-4. Close-up of Bier block apparatus. Prior to inflation of tourniquet, limb is exsanguinated by wrapping it in a distal to proximal direction with Esmarch elastic (not shown). A good quality double tourniquet is a must. Initially, the proximal portion is inflated to 250 to 300 mm Hg, and 30 to 40 ml of 0.5 percent plain IV lidocaine is injected. Ten minutes later, the distal portion is inflated, and then the proximal one is released. Release of the tourniquet must be done in increments, with reinflation at intervals. Procedures lasting less than 30 minutes increase the possibility of toxicity.

chapter in Miller's *Anesthesia* [26], is another excellent reference, as is Moore's *Regional Blocks* [27]. Use of these blocks requires a thorough understanding of their potential complications and side effects, and they should be performed only by adequately trained and experienced physicians.

HEAD AND NECK BLOCKS

Trigeminal Nerve and Branches

Blocks of the trigeminal nerve are useful for repairing lacerations, for nasal fracture approximation, and for treatment of certain chronic pain problems.

Maxillary Nerve. This nerve can be blocked proximally after it leaves the middle cranial fossa, or distally after it has branched into the infraorbital nerve or joined the sphenopalatine ganglion. It supplies sensation to the nose, cheek, upper lip, and zygoma. To block the nerve proximally, a skin wheal is raised at the coronoid notch of the mandible, and a block needle is advanced to the lateral pterygoid plate. The needle is then walked off the plate anteriorly and advanced 1 cm, at which point a bolus of 3 ml of local anesthetic is slowly injected. Blockade of the sphenopalatine ganglion, an important block for nasal fracture reduction, is performed by advancing a 120-degree block needle [24] through the greater palatine foramen, located just medial to the third molar or wisdom tooth inside the mouth. The needle is advanced 3 to 4 cm, at which time a paresthesia is elicited, and 2 ml of local anesthetic is injected. Blockade of the infraorbital nerve, which supplies the lower eyelid, upper lip, and lateral nasal skin, is achieved by first palpating the infraorbital foramen, which is below the infraorbital ridge, on a vertical line through the pupil of the eye when the patient is looking straight ahead. Two or three ml of local anesthetic is injected around the foramen but not directly into the narrow canal.

Mandibular Nerve. This branch of the trigeminal nerve supplies the muscles of mastication and sensation to the jaw. Like the maxillary nerve, it can be blocked both proximally and distally, although no equivalent for the sphenopalatine ganglion exists. The proximal block is performed by inserting a block needle (after a skin wheal, of course) through the coronoid arch of the mandible just below the midpoint of the zygomatic arch, in a manner similar to the maxillary block discussed above. However, the needle is walked posteriorly off the lateral pterygoid plate in the general direction of the ear, where, about a centimeter deep to the depth of the lateral pterygoid plate, 3 to 5 ml of local anesthetic is carefully injected while continual intermittent aspiration is performed.

A more distal, and safer, mandibular nerve block can be performed at the level of the inferior alveolar nerve. After inserting a bite block, one induces mucosal anesthesia with a cotton swab soaked in local anesthetic just medial to the anterior ramus of the mandible, as palpated with the gloved hand inside the mouth, just above the last molar of the lower jaw. A 2-inch block needle is then inserted between the mucosal surface and the ramus, and, as local anesthetic is infiltrated, the needle is advanced some 2 to 3 cm. At this depth, or if a paresthesia is elicited to the tongue or teeth, 5 ml is injected slowly as the needle is withdrawn. This block also anesthetizes the lingual nerve, which runs in close proximity to the inferior alveolar nerve (Fig. 6-5).

A final distal block of the mandibular nerve can be performed at the mental nerve, which provides sensory innervation to the lower lip and the gingival surface in the lower corner of the mouth. It may be blocked in a manner similar to that used for the infraorbital nerve, at the level of its exit from its foramen at the corner of the anterior jaw, where it is readily palpable.

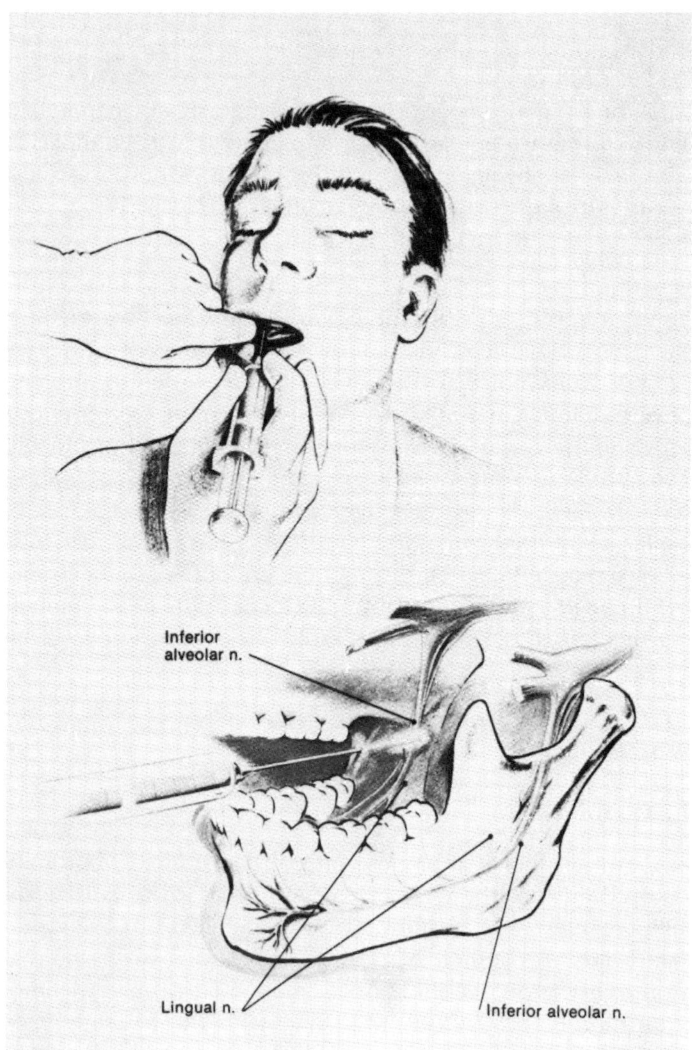

Fig. 6-5. Inferior alveolar and lingual nerve block. (From J. Katz. *Atlas of Regional Anesthesia.* Norwalk, Conn.: Appleton-Century-Crofts, 1985. With permission.)

Nose

The nose has a complex and redundant innervation, which is not surprising, given its importance in evolution as a sensory organ. Adequate block can be achieved by a combination of a subcutaneous skin wheal raised around the periphery, mucosal block by intranasal insertion of cotton pledgets soaked in lidocaine with epinephrine, and the sphenopalatine block discussed above.

Ear

Anesthetization of the ear may be performed by raising a subcutaneous skin wheal in the skin adjacent to the ear in a circumferential pattern. Block of the external ear canal may be achieved by injecting 0.25 ml of local anesthetic at four quadrants of the canal near its opening [24].

Vagal Nerve

Branches of the vagal nerve innervate the larynx and trachea (see Chapter 2). The superior laryngeal nerve, which innervates the mucous membranes of the pharynx and larynx down to the level of the vocal cords, may be blocked at its insertion into the larynx at a point between the greater cornu of the hyoid bone and the cornu of the thyroid cartilage. A 25-gauge needle is "popped" through the thyrohyoid ligament, and 2 to 3 ml of local anesthetic is injected (Fig. 6-6). The recurrent laryngeal nerve, which innervates sensation to the larynx at the level of the vocal cords and below, may best be blocked by transtracheal injection through the cricothyroid membrane. Because a forceful cough and concomitant movement of the head immediately follow this injection, it is wise to inject rapidly and remove the needle briskly (Fig. 6-7).

UPPER EXTREMITY

Brachial Plexus

Proximal blockade of the brachial plexus and the entire upper extremity can best be achieved through the interscalene approach or the axillary approach. Although techniques do exist for blocking the plexus by the supraclavicular and infraclavicular approaches [24, 26], the author has found that they lack clinical utility owing to the risk of creating iatrogenic pneumothorax. The interscalene approach is best done with the patient's head slightly hyperextended and rotated toward the contralateral side. One then lays one's finger along the strap muscles of the neck, parallel and just lateral to the lateral edge of the sternocleidomastoid muscle. One can generally palpate the groove between the anterior and middle scalene muscles by rolling the finger from side to side and using the entire length of the finger for palpation, not just the tip. Generally, the external jugular vein is present near the groove (Fig. 6-8). One then raises a skin wheal and advances a 22-gauge block needle 1 cm or so into the groove at an angle of about 30 degrees to the palpating finger. A greater angle and a deeper insertion could conceivably result in complications such as total spinal or vertebral artery injection. If this technique is followed and a paresthesia to the shoulder or arm is raised, one may inject 30 to 40 ml of local anesthetic, used with careful aspiration, in an adult with relative safety. The block invests the peripheral aspects of the brachial plexus initially, and thus the shoulder is the first area to be blocked. As such, this is an excellent anesthetic technique

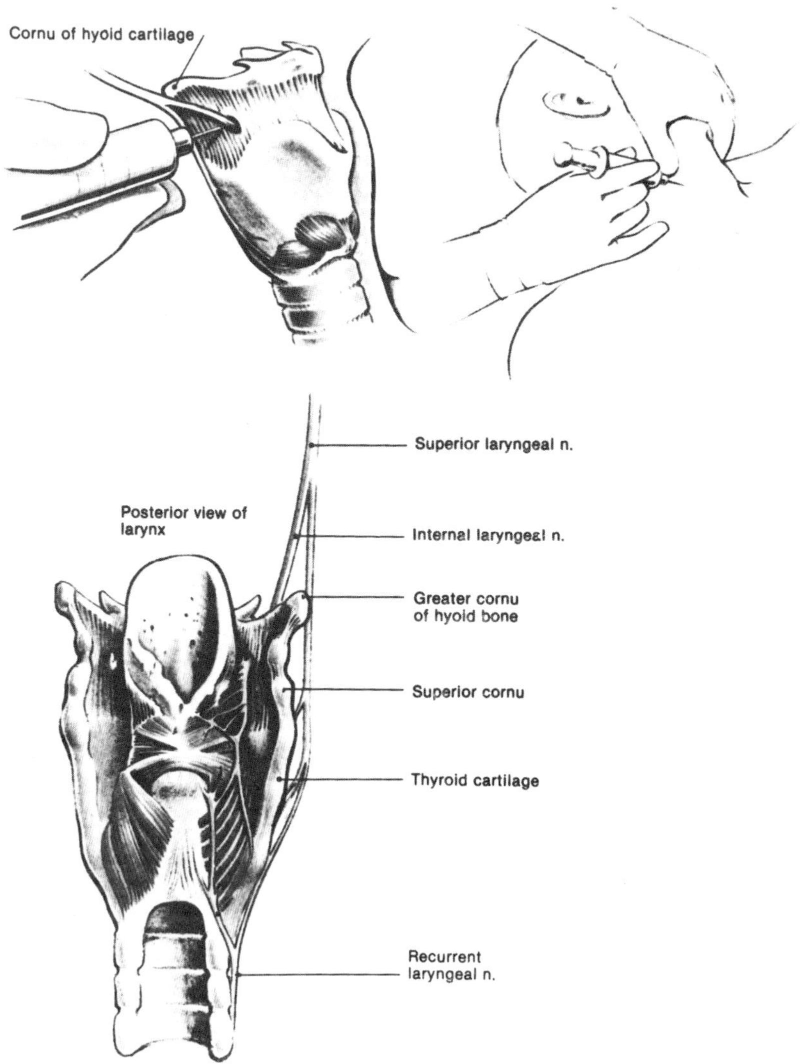

Fig. 6-6. Superior laryngeal nerve block. (From J. Katz. *Atlas of Regional Anesthesia.* Norwalk, Conn: Appleton-Century-Crofts, 1985. With permission.)

to use for relocation of an obstinate shoulder dislocation, or for shoulder surgery or ensuing postoperative pain relief. A distal upper extremity block takes 15 to 25 minutes for the agent to be absorbed. Blockade with 0.25% bupivacaine often lasts for 12 to 16 hours.

Bilateral interscalene blocks are contraindicated. The phrenic nerve may be blocked as a side effect, and although unilateral phrenic paralysis is well tolerated, bilateral phrenic blockade can be disastrous.

Block of the brachial plexus at the axillary artery requires initial abduc-

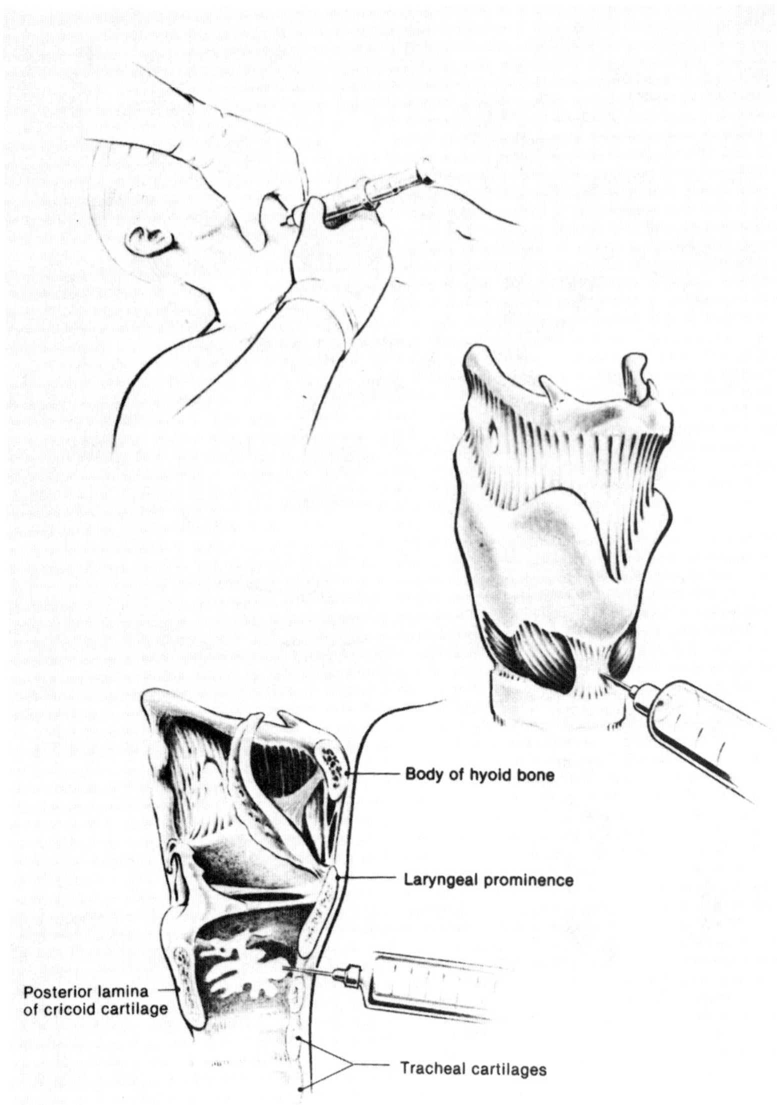

Fig. 6-7. Transtracheal nerve block of the larynx. Use of a 25-gauge needle is recommended, paying strict attention to sterile technique. Patient will cough vigorously after injection. (See text.) (From J. Katz. *Atlas of Regional Anesthesia.* Norwalk, Conn: Appleton-Century-Crofts, 1985. With permission.)

tion of the arm (Fig. 6-9). After the artery is palpated, one creates a skin wheal and advances a 22-gauge block needle attached to a syringe by means of a short length of IV connective tubing (K-50 or K-52). At this point, one may establish the block in three ways. First, one may search for the artery, which will be manifested by bright red blood in the IV tubing on aspiration. One then inserts the needle just past the point at which blood is aspirated and injects half (20 ml) of a local anesthetic dose. One then encounters the

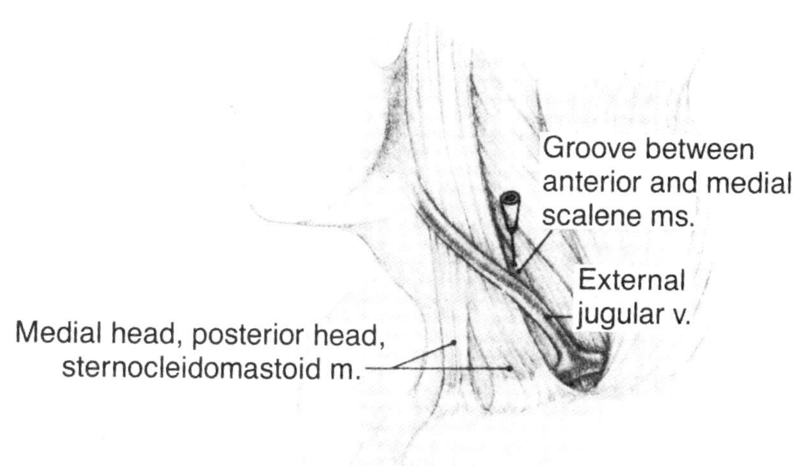

Fig. 6-8. Interscalene block of brachial plexus. Once paresthesia is encountered, needle should be withdrawn until paresthesia is resolved, then injection may be made. Monitoring and oxygen supplementation similar to that shown in Fig. 6-3 must precede this block. (From R. K. Stoelting, and R. D. Miller. *Basics in Anesthesia.* New York: Churchill Livingstone, 1984. With permission.)

point just superficial to the artery in a similar manner and injects the remaining 15 to 20 ml of anesthetic. Firm pressure distal to the injection site forces the anesthetic proximally and may improve the block. This technique is based on the assumption that the nerves, artery, and vein of the axillary region are surrounded by a sheath, and periarterial injection will thus gain access to the plexus. Difficulties with this technique are hematoma formation in patients with coagulopathy, and intravascular injection, which is especially likely if the vein is mistaken for the artery. One may subsequently get negative results on aspiration while the needle is still within the vein (see earlier under Equipment, Avoidance of Neural Damage, and Technique), and subsequent injection, especially with bupivacaine, may be disastrous. Nevertheless, this block, in skilled hands and using lidocaine or mepivacaine, is a standard procedure in anesthesiology.

A second method of axillary block is similar to the above, except that one injects the solution after a "popping" sensation indicates that the needle is within the neurovascular sheath. Arterial puncture is not sought. This technique is more difficult and more prone to failure.

A third technique has been popularized by Thompson. After review of computed tomographic studies of the axilla, he noted the presence of multiple septa investing the neurovascular sheath [28]. Because a failure rate of 20 percent has been reported [29] with the above perivascular blocks, the concept of injecting multiple small amounts of anesthetic throughout the area wherever a paresthesia occurs was developed. A 25-gauge needle is

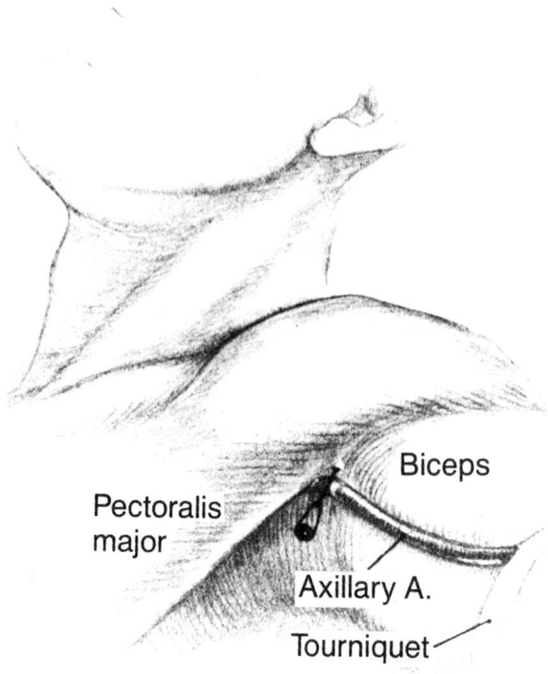

Fig. 6-9. Axillary approach to brachial plexus block. Monitoring and oxygen supplementation similar to that shown in Fig. 6-3 must precede this block. Attachment of intravenous extension tubing to needle with syringe will allow aspiration of bright red blood, indicating puncture of axillary artery. Careful infiltration on either side of artery will produce block. Proximity of axillary vessels demands careful and frequent aspiration. (From R. K. Stoelting and R. D. Miller. *Basics in Anesthesia.* New York: Churchill Livingstone, 1984. With permission.)

recommended for this, with a total dose of 20 to 25 ml of anesthetic [30]. Recent work [31] has shown that the septa offer little obstruction to the injected solution, raising questions about the rationale for the multiple-injection, paresthesia-guided technique. Problems with elicitation of paresthesias are discussed above.

Elbow Blocks. The ulnar, median, and radial nerves may all be blocked at the elbow. This block may be advantageous for forearm laceration repairs, fractures, or "rescue" of incomplete axillary block for operation. The ulnar nerve may be palpated where it courses through the groove between the medial epicondyle of the humerus and the olecranon (the "funny bone"). Five to ten milliliters of local anesthetic is injected just proximal to the groove. One should not inject the anesthetic if a patient has continued paresthesias because the nerve is tightly bound by fascia; this is the rationale for injecting proximally as well.

The radial nerve may be blocked proximal to the elbow, where it is often palpable on the lateral aspect of the junction of the middle and lower thirds of the humerus. Five to ten milliliters of local anesthetic is injected after a paresthesia is encountered. The nerve may also be blocked at the elbow, midway between the lateral edge of the biceps tendon and the lateral edge of the arm, where a paresthesia is sought and 5 to 10 ml of local anesthetic is injected.

The median nerve runs just ulnarward of the brachial artery, where it may be blocked with 5 ml of local. Paresthesia is often encountered.

Wrist Blocks. Wrist blocks are useful and are underused, especially in the emergency department. The radial nerve may be blocked just lateral or radialward to the radial artery. Three milliliters of local will achieve the block with the addition of a subcutaneous cuff deposited on the lateral and dorsal aspects of the radial side of the wrist to block skin branches that have decussated proximally. The ulnar nerve may be blocked just medial or ulnarward to the ulnar artery. Three milliliters is injected. The median nerve may be blocked at the flexion crease level of the wrist just between the flexor carpi radialis and the palmeris longus tendons. Because the nerve is tightly bound here in the carpal tunnel, 3 ml of local anesthetic must be carefully injected and paresthesia avoided to avoid nerve trauma. One must supplement the median block, as with the radial block at the wrist, by injecting a skin wheal over the proximal thenar eminence to block the superficial palmar branch.

Digital Blocks. Fingers and toes may be anesthetized either by a cuff of anesthetic deposited around the digit or by a more proximal block of the common digital nerves. The cuff technique requires avoidance of epinephrine and excessive volume (maximum 2 ml per side) because vascular compromise can be created by either. The digital nerve block can best be accomplished by creating a dorsal skin wheal on either side of the metacarpal or metatarsal. Through these skin wheals anesthetic is deposited at 2, 5, 7, and 10 o'clock positions surrounding the metacarpal or metatarsal. Most of the anesthetic is deposited on the flexor side. Skin wheals on the flexor side are extremely painful and are to be avoided. Adequate blockade of the great toe has proved clinically resistant to this author with either technique and is best combined with appropriate ankle block rescue (see below, Ankle Blocks).

LOWER EXTREMITY BLOCKS

Proximal Leg Blocks

Although rarely performed, proximal leg blocks can be useful for transport analgesia in femoral fractures or even for surgery in selected circumstances. They may be especially useful in rural or wilderness settings, where major conduction or general anesthesia is unavailable but a needle, syringe, and local anesthetic are accessible. Four major nerves must be considered—the femoral, obturator, lateral cutaneous, and sciatic nerves.

Femoral nerve block may be easily performed just below the inguinal ligament and lateral to the femoral artery. One feels a loss of resistance in popping through the fascia lata, and 10 to 15 ml of local anesthetic may be injected with or without eliciting paresthesia. Good analgesia for the middle third of femur fractures can be obtained with this block [26]. Because the obturator and lateral cutaneous nerves of the thigh run in close approximation to the femoral nerve within the psoas compartment, the needle may be directed slightly cephalad but in the same location under the ligament, and 30 ml of local anesthetic to block all three nerves can then be injected.

The obturator nerve, which innervates the medial thigh and muscles of thigh adduction, can be blocked most easily by the above technique. Alternatively, one may inject the nerve directly at a point 2 cm lateral and 2 cm caudad to the pubic tubercle, where a block needle is walked medially off the pubic bone into the obturator foramen; 10 to 15 ml of local is then injected. This block is uncomfortable for the patient, and liberal amounts of skin and periosteal local should be used.

The sciatic nerve, the largest nerve in the body, is one nerve that requires a paresthesia to ensure block by local anesthetic. It is best encountered by placing the patient in the lateral decubitus position and drawing a line between the posterior iliac spine and the greater trocanter. One then draws a line perpendicular to this line, and, at a point 5 cm caudad along this second line, one places a 10-cm block needle (a spinal needle will suffice) through a skin wheal and searches for paresthesias at a depth of 5 to 10 cm. Injection of 25 ml of local anesthetic is required to block this large nerve. A slight paresthesia is adequate, and repeated paresthesia elicitation, which may cause neurapraxia, is to be condemned.

The lateral femoral cutaneous nerve may be blocked at a point 2 cm medial to the anterior iliac crest and just below the inguinal ligament. Five to eight milliliters injected here will produce anesthesia to the lateral thigh and buttock.

Knee Blocks

Because knee blocks are traditionally thought to have a high incidence of postblock paresthesias [27], Rorie reexamined blockade of the common peroneal nerve and the tibial nerve and found only 2 of 119 patients who had transient postblock paresthesias [32]. The peroneal nerve may be blocked where it is palpable as it winds around the head of the fibula in the lateral leg. Five milliliters is required. The tibial nerve may be blocked in the upper and outer quadrants of the popliteal fossa. The saphenous nerve, the continuation of the femoral nerve, may be blocked as it courses around the medial condyle of the femur. Five to seven milliliters will anesthetize the medial portion of the lower leg and ankle.

Ankle Blocks

Ankle blocks are especially useful in emergency medicine because they have a low incidence of complications and greatly facilitate patient acceptance of such painful procedures as repair of lacerations of the sole of the foot. Block of the posterior tibial nerve, for example, will provide anesthesia to most of the sole of the foot and to the nail beds of the phalanges. It is achieved by injecting 5 ml of local anesthetic just lateral (toward the lateral malleolus) to the posterior tibial artery. This artery is generally easily palpable about a centimeter posterior to the medial malleolus. Paresthesia may be elicited but is not essential.

Sensation to the lateral foot is supplied by the sural nerve, which has the same relationship to the lateral malleolus as the posterior tibial has to the medial malleolus (running posterior to it). No artery is palpable here, as a rule, and anesthesia is effected by injecting a cuff of subcutaneous anesthesia extending from the Achilles tendon to the lateral malleolus.

Blockade of the dorsal aspect of the foot is achieved by infiltrating a similar cuff of local anesthesia anteriorly from the medial malleolus to the lateral malleolus. Anesthesia of the cleft between the great and second toes is achieved by injecting 3 to 5 ml between the tendons of the extensor hallucis longus and the tibialis anterior, at the malleolar level. This blocks the deep peroneal nerve, which runs just below the extensor retinaculum. This fascial structure will cause the sensation of a pop when the needle passes it to a point near the nerve, where paresthesia may or may not be elicited.

MISCELLANEOUS BLOCKS

Intercostal Block

An important block used to relieve pain and improve respiratory mechanics after bruising or damage to the ribs, this block is easily done if adequate attention is paid to avoidance of the principle complications, which include pneumothorax and intravascular injection. Raising the arms forward onto a padded Mayo stand with the patient in a sitting position is usually the most efficacious manner of lifting the scapula out of the way. Some authors recommend the use of the prone position with one or both arms raised above the head [24]. This position gives excellent exposure if the patient can tolerate it (Fig. 6-10).

Once a patient is positioned properly, the ribs are palpated as proximally to the spinal column as possible—usually between the posterior axillary line and the costal angle. One then injects a skin wheal over each rib and

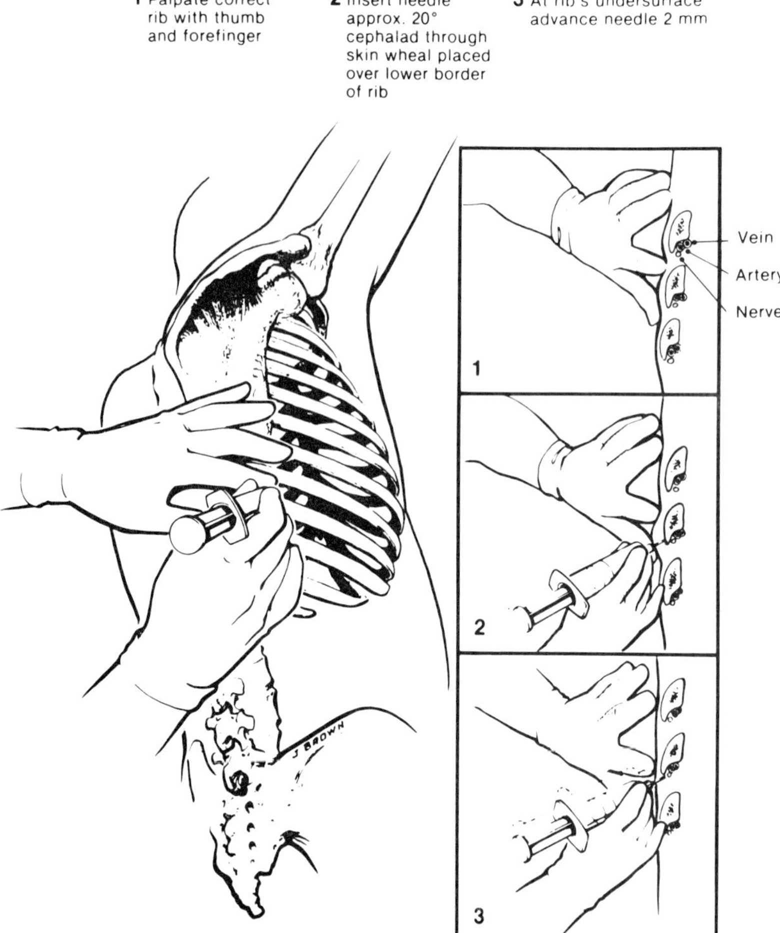

Fig. 6-10. Intercostal block. Great care must be taken to avoid intravascular injection or lung puncture. Although this block produces higher blood levels per unit of local anesthetic injected, 3 to 4 ml of 0.25 percent bupivacaine is the favored agent because it produces a longer duration of block than the safer lidocaine. Adequate block requires infiltration of one nerve above and below the injured area in addition to the nerves supplying the injured ribs; thus, block of five or six intercostal nerves is not uncommon. A postblock radiograph to rule out occult pneumothorax should be considered. (From J. Katz. *Atlas of Regional Anesthesia*. Norwalk, Conn: Appleton-Century-Crofts, 1985. With permission.)

inserts a short bevel block needle gently to the periosteum, where one injects a bit of local and then, very gently, walks off the rib in a caudal, inferior direction. This is the side of the rib opposite to the superior aspect used for thoracentesis. One should keep the syringe and needle tilted at a cephalad angle, so that when the needle does slip off the rib, it is very close to the neurovascular bundle. As the needle walks off the bone, it is advanced 2 to 3 mm, where, after careful aspiration, 4 ml of local anesthetic (usually 0.25% bupivacaine) is injected. Because even a single rib has redundant innervation from superior and inferior intercostal nerves, one should inject one to two intercostal nerves both above and below the injured ribs, as well as the intercostal nerves directly involved.

Because blood levels of a local anesthetic reach higher serum levels more rapidly with an intercostal block than with other blocks, one should not exceed 1.5 mg/kg bupivacaine (4 ml of 0.25% bupivacaine equals 10 mg per nerve; in a 70-kg patient, then, ten nerves at most should be blocked). Pneumothorax is avoided by using the short bevel block needle, by holding the needle at the proper cephalad angle at the hub, and by avoiding inadvertent deep penetration beyond the recommended 2 to 3 mm. In patients with severe rib injuries, one must remember that pulmonary mechanics may deteriorate over time and that alternative avenues of treatment such as peridural narcotics (see Chapter 7) or intubation and IV narcotics may be preferable.

Recently, a new thoracic block has been described that may prove to be of use in patients with painful thoracic conditions [33, 34]. It involves inserting a 17-gauge Tuohy needle through a skin wheal over the rib into the pleural space. If one uses a moistened glass syringe with 1 cc of air, one will note a loss of resistance as the parietal pleura is punctured. Anesthesiologists will find this technique similar to the loss of resistance encountered on entering the epidural space with the same needle. One then passes an epidural catheter into the pleural space and tapes it in place after the needle is removed. Then one can achieve good analgesia of the thoracic and upper abdominal region by simply instilling 20 ml of 0.5% bupivacaine through the catheter. Remarkable duration of anesthesia has been reported, up to 18 hours in some cases [34]. By entering the space at an acute angle (the needle placed 30 to 40 degrees to the skin and directed toward the midline), pneumothorax risk is lessened.

Paracervical Block

Although performance of suction curettage in the emergency department is controversial, it is still performed in some rural EDs by the emergency physician. Because in spontaneous abortion the cervix is by definition already dilated, one may achieve good analgesia for the curettage portion of the procedure by injecting 10 ml of short-acting anesthetic, such as lidocaine, at a depth of 1 cm into the lateral fornices on either side of the cervix.

Careful aspiration is essential for this vascular area. These blocks have been abandoned for delivery because they have been associated with fetal bradycardia.

Hernia Block

This block is useful for reduction or operative repair of inguinal hernia. One anesthetizes the ilioinguinal and iliohypogastric nerves by injecting 10 ml of local anesthetic 2 cm medial to the anterior iliac spine. This should be done at a depth that approximates the layers of the abdominal oblique musculature. Although some claim they can feel each layer of muscle, the author finds this difficult and uses a fanlike approach. If reduction of hernia is the only goal, this should suffice. If operative repair is envisioned, one should supplement the block with skin wheals from the anterior iliac spine to the umbilicus and down to the base of the penis. A cutaneous branch of the femoral nerve that innervates the inguinal region may also be blocked by injecting 5 to 10 ml just lateral to the pubic spine.

REFERENCES

1. Cousins, M. J., and Phillips, G. D. Historical Introduction. In M. J. Cousins and G. D. Phillips (eds.), *Acute Pain Management.* New York: Churchill Livingstone, 1986.
2. Savarese, J. J., and Covino, B. G. Basic and Clinical Pharmacology of Local Anesthetic Drugs. In R. D. Miller (ed.), *Anesthesia.* New York: Churchill Livingstone, 1986. Pp. 985–1013.
3. Covino, B. G. Pharmacology of local anesthetics. *Br. J. Anesth.* 58:701–716, 1986.
4. DiFazio, C. A., Carron, H., Grosslight, K. R., et al. Comparison of pH-adjusted lidocaine solutions for epidural anesthesia. *Anesth. Analg.* 65:760–764, 1986.
5. Warnick, J. E., Kee, R. D., and Yim, G. K. W. The effects of lidocaine on inhibition in the cerebral cortex. *Anesthesiology* 34:327, 1971.
6. Morishima, H. O., Pederson, H., Finster, M., et al. Etidocaine toxicity in the adult, newborn and fetal sheep. *Anesthesiology* 58:342, 1983.
7. Clarkson, C. W., and Hondeghem, L. M. Mechanism for bupivicaine depression of cardiac conduction. *Anesthesiology* 62:396–405, 1985.
8. Albright, G. A. Cardiac arrest following regional anesthesia with etidocaine or bupivicaine. *Anesthesiology* 51:285–287, 1979.
9. Covino, B. G. Recent advances in local anesthesia. *Can. Anaesth. Soc.* 33:(Suppl.) S5–S8, 1986.
10. Kasten, G. W. Amide local anesthetic alterations of effective refractory period temporal dispersion. *Anesthesiology* 65:61–66, 1986.
11. Kasten, G. W., and Martin, S. T. Comparison of resuscitation of sheep and dogs after bupivicaine-induced cardiovascular collapse. *Anesth. Analg.* 65:1029–1032, 1986.
12. Gay, G. R., and Loper, K. A. The use of labetalol in the management of cocaine crisis. *Ann. Emerg. Med.* 17:282–283, 1988.
13. McMullen, M. J. Stimulants. In P. Rosen, F. J. Baker, R. M. Barkin, et al. (eds.), *Emergency Medicine.* St. Louis: Mosby, 1988.

14. Gissen, A. J., Datta, S., Lambert, D., et al. Is chloroprocaine neurotoxic? *Reg. Anesth.* 9:38, 1984.
15. Selander, D., Edshage, S., and Wolff, T. Paresthesiae or no paresthesiae? Nerve lesions after axillary blocks. *Acta Anaesth. Scand.* 23:27–33, 1979.
16. Bromage, P. R. A comparison of the hydrochloride and carbon dioxide salts of lidocaine and prilocaine in epidural anesthesia. *Acta Anaesth. Scand.* (Suppl.) 16:55–69, 1965.
17. Cole, C. O., McMorland, G. H., Axelson, J. E., et al. Epidural blockade for Cesarean section comparing lidocaine hydrocarbonate and lidocaine hydrochloride. *Anesthesiology* 62:348–350, 1985.
18. Christoph, R. A., Buchanan, L., Begalla, K., et al. Pain reduction in local anesthetic administration through pH buffering. *Ann. Emerg. Med.* 17:117–120, 1988.
19. McKay, W., Morris, R., and Mushlin, P. Sodium bicarbonate attenuates pain on skin infiltration with lidocaine, with or without epinephrine. *Anesth. Analg.* 66:572–574, 1987.
20. Caplan, R. A., Ward, R. J., Posner, K., et al. Unexpected cardiac arrest during spinal anesthesia: A closed claims analysis of predisposing factors. *Anesthesiology* 68:5–11, 1988.
21. Longstreth, W. T., Inui, T. S., Cobb, L. A., et al. Neurologic recovery after out-of-hospital cardiac arrest. *Ann. Intern. Med.* 98(Part 1):588–592, 1983.
22. Mihic, D. N. Postspinal headache and relationship of needle bevel to longitudinal dural fibers. *Reg. Anesth.* 10:76–81, 1985.
23. Selander, D., Dhuner, K. G., and Lundborg, G. Peripheral nerve injury due to injection needles used for regional anesthesia. *Acta Anaesth. Scand.* 21:182–188, 1977.
24. Katz, J. *Atlas of Regional Anesthesia.* Norwalk, Conn: Appleton-Century-Crofts, 1985.
25. Selander, D., and Sjostrand, J. Longitudinal spread of intraneurally injected local anesthetics. *Acta Anaesth. Scand.* 22:622–634, 1978.
26. Murphy, T. M. Nerve Blocks. In R. D. Miller (ed.), *Anesthesia.* New York: Churchill Livingstone, 1986.
27. Moore, D. C. *Regional Block* (4th ed.). Springfield, Ill: Thomas, 1965.
28. Thompson, G. A., and Rorie, D. K. Functional anatomy of the brachial plexus sheaths. *Anesthesiology* 59:117–122, 1983.
29. Selander, D. Axillary plexus block: Paresthetic or perivascular. *Anesthesiology* 66:726–728, 1987.
30. Thompson, G. A. Upper extremity nerve block. American Society of Regional Anesthesiologists, Refresher Course, quoted in D. Selander. Axillary plexus block: Paresthetic or perivascular. *Anesthesiology* 66:726–728, 1987.
31. Partridge, B. L., Katz, J., and Bernirschke, K. Functional anatomy of the brachial plexus sheath: Implications for anesthesia. *Anesthesiology* 66:743–747, 1987.
32. Rorie, D. K., Byer, D. E., Nelson, D. O., et al. Assessment of block of the sciatic nerve in the popliteal fossa. *Anesth. Analg.* 59:371, 1980.
33. Reiestad, F., and Stromskag, K. E. Intrapleural catheter in the management of postoperative pain. *Reg. Anesth.* 11:89–91, 1986.
34. Covino, B. G. Recent advances in regional anesthesia. *Anesth. Analg. 1988 Review Course Lectures* 28–33, 1988.

7. Pain Management

Glenn S. Vanstrum

As discussed in Chapter 1, the scope of anesthesia includes provision of amnesia, analgesia, hypnosis, patient homeostasis, and surgical relaxation. Emergency medicine encompasses the initial period of hospital care in a wide range of specialties, including anesthesia. In both specialties, probably the major symptom complaint is pain. The lay public sees anesthesiologists' primary role as "taking away the pain" and often ignore the other aspects of the specialty. Nevertheless, provision of analgesia is a major aspect of anesthesiology. Similarly, complaints of chest pain, headache, back pain, neck pain, and so on are legion in a busy emergency department. Although pain complaints associated with acute problems such as neck trauma or myocardial infarction tend to overshadow the chronic pain problems seen in a busy emergency department, important care contributions can be made to the latter group by a physician who has a thorough understanding of the diagnosis, management, and referral of the pain patient. For example, making the diagnosis of reflex sympathetic dystrophy or establishing a headache patient who chronically abuses narcotics in the right treatment center will not only be of infinite help to the patients but will also relieve one's fellow physicians from dealing with further ED admissions for that familiar complaint, "Severe pain. Wants shot."

In this chapter we will present a brief overview of the current understanding of pain physiology, providing definitions of the acute and chronic symptom complexes. Acute pain management strategies will then be considered, followed by a discussion of certain aspects of chronic pain management. A brief consideration of cancer pain treatment will conclude the chapter.

PAIN PHYSIOLOGY AND SYMPTOM COMPLEXES

THEORIES OF PAIN

Pain may be defined as "an unpleasant sensory and emotional experience associated with actual or potential tissue damage, or described in terms of such damage" [1]. Precise physiologic description of pain has been difficult, however, and only in the last 20 years has real progress been made. A theory of pain must explain, for example, how a soldier with a severe wound who knows he will be sent home feels no pain, or how the slightest touch can cause paroxysms of agony in a person with causalgia. Before 1965, there were two unsatisfactory theories of pain, the first being the specificity theory, which held that pain is a specific sensory system like vision or hearing, with its own anatomic equipment, and the second being the pattern theory, which held that nonspecific receptors relayed intense stimuli and that no specialized pain apparatus existed [2]. Such phenomena as phantom limb pain or the failure of surgical ablation refute the first theory, and specific nerves such as the myelinated A-delta fibers and C fibers refute the second.

Melzack and Wall proposed a new theory in 1965 [2], in which they hypothesized that although definite pain pathways exist, a gate control system modulates sensory input from the skin before it evokes pain perception and response. As refined and understood today, it is clear that nociceptive activity is altered by non-nociceptive input at spinal-segmental, thalamic, and cortical levels [3]. This efferent modulation of afferent stimuli is mediated by enkephalins and endorphins (morphine-analogue natural peptides) and by adrenergic fibers and may be either inhibitory or facilitory in nature (Fig. 7-1).

As a painful stimulus becomes persistent, constant neural activity "spills over" into related neurologic structures at more rostral levels, with heightened outflow to alpha and gamma neurons and to the autonomic nervous system. At some point in time, these secondary changes become nociceptive stimuli themselves, independent of the original stimulus, and hence increasingly difficult to manage [3]. Global problems including depression become the norm, and patients change their behavioral approach to the world. Positive operant conditioning for chronic pain includes financial rewards, such as disability payments or litigation settlements, drug rewards from narcotics or tranquilizers, or familial rewards, such as relief from onerous domestic tasks. Such high cortical perpetuation of pain behavior represents the end-rostral migration of the original somatic or visceral stimulus. Generically such a condition is referred to as a central pain state.

PAIN PATHWAYS AND CLINICAL CORRELATES

At a molecular level, transmitters involved in both the nociceptive system and the pain-modulating system are of clinical interest because pharmacologic agents may be tailored to interact or compete with chemical transmitters. The very first step in activation of the primary system, i.e., the small, diffusely distributed free nerve endings, is thought to involve the release of prostaglandins, serotonin, histamine, bradykinin, and leukotriene from damaged cells, these mediators then activating or sensitizing the nociceptors [4]. Aspirin and other nonsteroidal anti-inflammatory drugs (NSAIDs) prevent pain by inhibiting the metabolism of arachidonic acid to prostaglandins [5]. Unfortunately, pharmacologic means of blocking leukotrienes and the other mediators are still undergoing evaluation. Antihistamines and antiserotonergic drugs do not seem to be efficacious.

Pain impulses are then transmitted by unmyelinated C fibers and by small A-delta myelinated fibers to the dorsal horn of the spinal cord. Blockade at the nerve may be performed by local anesthetics. Primarily at the level of the spinal cord, the pain message is relayed by polypeptide transmitters such as substance P, somatostatin, vasoactive intestinal polypeptide, and cholecystokinin [4]. The neurotoxin capsaicin has been used to destroy substance P–containing neurons, with resultant experimental nonresponsiveness to noxious stimuli [6]. Unfortunately, useful applications of modulation

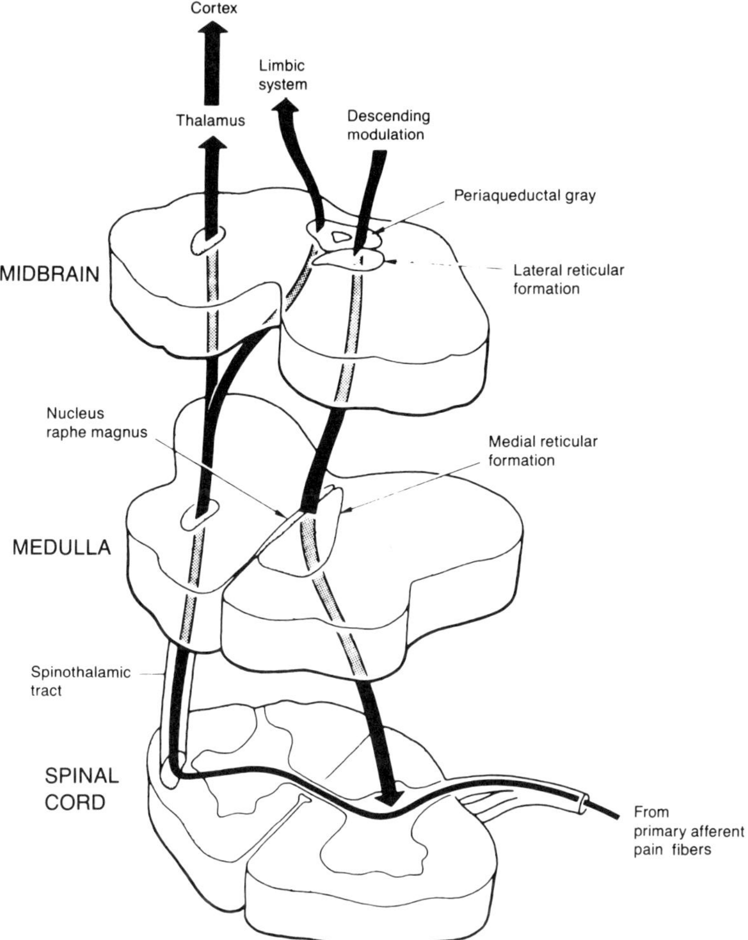

Fig. 7-1. Modulation of pain at the spinal cord, medulla, and midbrain. Note initial modulation in dorsal horn of spinal cord. Descending modulation is initiated in the periaqueductal gray matter, in the medial and lateral reticular formations, and in the nucleus raphe magnus. Descending inhibitory tracts in the dorsolateral fasciculus then impinge on the dorsal horn and release several inhibitory neurotransmitters. Note that the main afferent pain pathway ascends via the thalamus to the cerebral cortex, probably to produce the physical aspects of pain. An offshoot relays impulses to the limbic system, probably resulting in the emotional aspects of pain. (From M. J. Cousins and G. D. Philips *Acute Pain Management.* New York: Churchill Livingstone, 1986. With permission.)

of such polypeptides are still forthcoming, although substance P antagonists are undergoing clinical studies [7].

Inhibitory modulation occurs from input from non-nociceptive large myelinated sensory nerves, from serotonergic and noradrenergic cortical tonic inhibition, and from endorphinergic periventricular and periaqueductal areas. The discovery of enkephalin-mediated modulation of pain at laminias I and V of the spinal cord dorsal horn led directly to the clinical use of intrathecal and epidural morphine, one of the most exciting and efficacious pain management developments of the 1980s [8]. Transcutaneous nerve stimulation (TENS) utilizes the discovery that stimulation of myelinated nerve fibers through either high-frequency, low-intensity (nonopiate) or low-frequency, high-intensity (opiate) pathways can ameliorate pain [3]. Acupuncture also stimulates the body's pain inhibitory system.

At a cortical level, the relationship of the adrenergic system to pain via the global symptom of depression can be modulated with some success by antidepressive drugs. The use of clonidine, an alpha-2 agonist, for pain management and opiate withdrawal shows the important relation of the noradrenergic system to pain inhibition. The use of anticonvulsant drugs such as phenytoin for central pain states such as trigeminal neuralgia is another example of how central increases in nervous tone can be modified.

ACUTE VERSUS CHRONIC PAIN

It is not just a matter of convenience to separate pain into acute and chronic varieties, although the physician must recognize that there are intermediate, transition states. There is a considerable body of evidence that acute and chronic pain are two distinct entities, with the former related to the injury itself and the latter involving the global picture discussed above [9, 10]. Acute pain is "useful," "alerting" a person to pain from a remediable source; it is often accompanied by autonomic hyperactivity and is responsive to antiinflammatory and narcotic drugs. Chronic pain, on the other hand, is not amenable to acute pain drug therapy and often has a long, downward spiraling course with the patient chasing a long series of futile, alternative therapies [3].

Acute pain, while seemingly the more amenable to treatment, still offers a great challenge to the emergency physician or anesthesiologist. Because of concerns related to the acute problem itself, physicians often delay analgesic therapy. For example, many question the old surgical rule that abdominal pain should not be treated pending diagnosis [11]. Because of concern about respiratory depression, postoperative patients are undertreated [12]. There are potent forces preventing adequate pain treatment in acute situations. For example, in addition to the stressful dictates of his or her conscience, a physician stands some chance of being the target of litigation, or at least peer criticism, if a diagnosis is missed in the emergency department owing to a poor abdominal examination due to excessive narcosis, or if a patient has a respiratory arrest due to narcotics prescribed on the postoperative surgery ward. Although no one would question the legitimacy of such concerns, it would appear that we are overcompensating. A 1980 multicenter study, for example, showed that three-fourths of adult patients reported moderate to marked pain following surgery [13].

Should a patient endure extra pain as a result of such often unconscious concerns, very little damage will occur to the physician until, of course, the roles are reversed, and he or she becomes a patient and a victim of similar forces. Adequate acute pain control, which we will discuss below, requires a thorough understanding of the pharmacology of the analgesic drugs, an understanding of the cause of the pain, and, quite simply, recognition of the problem and compassion for the patient. It is a personal bias of this author that the best education in analgesia for any physician is the personal experience of a major surgical operation. If a doctor has never been a patient, he or she must constantly be aware that, to a patient, it is not just the successful outcome that is important but also the arriving there without agony.

Chronic pain requires a different approach altogether. Unlike acute pain, there is often no likely cure, and the patient has to be reconciled with adaptation to the pain. Complex behavioral problems must be dealt with, and use of such tools as patient-physician contracts is essential. There is an important role for diagnostic and therapeutic nerve blocks by anesthesiologists, but such therapy must be combined with an integrated behavioral and pharmacologic approach. Inpatient pain clinics have increased in number in response to this need, and it behooves any emergency department to establish a referral link with such a clinic.

Cancer pain is a special category that combines the characteristics of both acute and chronic pain. It has been estimated that 25 percent of all cancer patients die without adequate pain control [14]. These persons occasionally present to the emergency department in search of relief, and although most have private physicians, input from a knowledgeable emergency physician can have a large effect on management. Optimal treatment requires accurate diagnosis of the source of the pain; pain due to bony metastasis, for example, will respond better to radiation than to narcotics as a rule. In addition, other principles of pain management such as adequate initial treatment, avoidance of prn dosing, and tiered use of prostaglandin inhibitors followed by weak and then strong narcotics should be observed [15]. Consideration of an anesthesiology consultation for celiac plexus block should be made in those patients with appropriate gastrointestinal cancer pain.

ACUTE PAIN MANAGEMENT

TRAUMA

As in all aspects of medicine, one must guide a course between the Scylla of errors of commission and the Charybdis of errors of omission. Steering one's course in trauma pain management, as discussed in Chapter 12, is no exception. Therapy must be tailored to the patient. A patient in extremis often will best benefit from oxygen, intubation, and operation. Only when a patient's condition is stabilized and blood pressure starts to rise should titration of narcotics or ketamine begin. In a patient with isolated rib trauma, such a spare approach is clinically unwarranted and, from the patient's point of view, totally unacceptable. Multiple rib fractures or lateral thoracotomy operations cause great pain with each breath, and patients tend to splint that thoracic region, with associated atelectasis and diminished PO_2. Inability to cough well leads to retained secretions and a propensity for pneumonia. Titration of intravenous narcotics in this setting, often left to nursing personnel, is often inadequate. For example, a common order is "Demerol, 50 to 75 mg IM q3–4 h prn pain." Nurses consistently start at the lower dose and the longer time interval and, because of the fears discussed above, only very hesitantly increase the dose. The short duration of action of meperidine, from 2.5 to 3 hours, and the fact that the dosing is prn will surely lead to periods of extreme pain.

More rational use of narcotics would involve a titrated drip narcotic, patient-controlled analgesia (PCA), in which a patient can initiate the IV injection of a small periodic bolus of narcotic from a special infusion device, or non-time-contingent round-the-clock dosage. PCA devices may well be the delivery mode of the future, because major advantages over other methods of delivery have been demonstrated in many areas, including shortened hospital stays [16]. Intercostal blockade, even with bupivacaine, is only temporary, although the new technique of interpleural administration of local anesthetics [17] (see Chapter 6) offers continuous analgesia.

Intrathecal (spinal) and epidural injections of morphine are also excellent therapeutic options for the clinical problem of acute pain. Intrathecal injections of 0.5 to 1.0 mg of preservative-free morphine offer up to 24 hours of pain relief, even if injected in the lumbar region. Morphine is sufficiently water soluble that it migrates from the site of injection to the injured thoracic region. Epidural catheter placement and either bolus injection of 3 to 7 mg of preservative-free morphine q6–12h or a continuous drip of 80 to 120 µg/hour of fentanyl results in dramatic pain relief and improved respiratory dynamics in these patients. Side effects of narcotics used in this manner include urinary retention, nausea and vomiting, itching, and, most important, respiratory depression secondary to rostral diffusion of more water-soluble narcotics such as morphine (fentanyl, being lipid soluble, is less likely to cause this). Such respiratory depression often is delayed by many hours from the original injection [8] and thus mandates hourly, or even half-hourly, respiratory rate checks by nursing staff. Although it is anesthesiologists who should administer such blocks and follow such patients, it is the emergency physician who may initiate the anesthesiology consult and who may have to assist, unfortunately, with narcotic reversal in a patient with respiratory arrest who received a relative overdose of spinal or epidural narcotic. Gentle titration of 50 to 100 μg (⅛ to ¼ ml) increments of naloxone is preferable in such a situation to a more heavy-handed use of naloxone, which may be appropriate in the patient who presents to the emergency department with heroin overdose. It is clear that reversal of opiates that have been administered therapeutically for pain can result in serious hyperdynamic sequelae, including pulmonary edema and ventricular fibrillation [18, 19] (see Chapter 5).

Delayed respiratory arrest due to intrathecal or epidural narcotics may be limited by taking care in dosing. Elderly patients, who have an increasingly diminished sensation of pain, should be given less narcotic, and young, strong males with well-developed thoracic muscle mass need correspondingly more drug. The reported respiratory arrests invariably involve the use of spinal narcotics in elderly patients with relatively minor injuries or operations [20].

Even if a patient requires prolonged intubation after thoracic trauma or operation, and many do, the use of peridural narcotics can assist the eventual weaning from the ventilator. Contraindications to the technique include localized infection, anticoagulation, and intracranial mass lesions.

Nonthoracic trauma includes neurologic trauma, orthopedic injuries, and abdominal trauma. Use of any analgesic agent other than aspirin and the nonsteroidal anti-inflammatory drugs (NSAIDs) is contraindicated in the nonventilated neurally injured patient because most analgesic drugs lead to arterial PCO_2 retention, increased cerebral blood flow, and concomitant increased intracranial pressure (ICP) (see Chapter 13). In a patient who is ventilated mechanically the use of narcotics does not lead to increased PCO_2 or ICP and furthermore is recommended in treating hypertension related to catecholamine discharge secondary to pain.

Orthopedic trauma produces deep bony pain that is more amenable to treatment with narcotics such as morphine or hydromorphone (Dilaudid) than meperidine. Large amounts of blood may be lost from long bone and pelvic fractures, and one must titrate narcotics carefully because they can unmask compensated hypovolemia through their propensity to decrease systemic vascular resistance.

Acute abdominal visceral trauma, like orthopedic trauma, can lead to unrecognized hypovolemia; hence, careful titration should be observed in the use of narcotic analgesics. Many prefer meperidine because it has less propensity to induce biliary spasm and other constrictive sequelae in the smooth bowel musculature.

MYOCARDIAL INFARCTION AND ISCHEMIA

In general, pain from the visceral regions is different from pain in the somatic and cutaneous regions. It is dull, aching or boring, and not well localized. It is accompanied by a sense of malais and often is associated with autonomic changes. Visceral pain may present as referred pain (or, as in German, "transferred pain" or "übertragener Schmerz"), which occurs as pain in the dermatomes associated with the region of the spinal cord where afferent fibers from the viscera decussate [21]. Thus, in the specific case of myocardial infarction or ischemia, pain may be radiated to the jaw and left arm as well as through the precordium. Braunwald and others [22] make the observation that in myocardial infarction a patient tends to be restless in response to the pain, whereas in angina a more immobile state occurs.

Although the primary goal in myocardial infarction is prevention of dysrhythmia and minimization of necrosis of myocardial muscle mass, alleviation of pain is a related important objective. Nitrates reduce myocardial pain through venous dilatation and resulting decreased preload and heart work indices and through coronary arterial dilatation. Unlike sodium nitroprusside, which has a propensity for creation of a "coronary steal," in which the normal end arteries dilate and receive increased blood flow at the expense of narrowed, diseased arteries, nitroglycerin seems to dilate the large epicardial vessels in a uniform manner, thus reducing ischemia and, as a result, pain (see Chapter 4). Sublingual nifedipine in a dose of 10 mg can also dilate the coronaries and achieve pain relief.

Physicians are familiar with the use of morphine for cardiac pain. Like nitroglycerin, it dilates the venous bed and induces vagotonic slowing of the heart rate, effects that augment the direct pain-alleviating enkephalin-receptor analogue effect of morphine. Avoidance of tachycardia is important in myocardial ischemia because perfusion depends on diastolic filling times, which are shortened in tachycardic states. When a patient presents with myocardial ischemia and hypotension, any of the above pain treatment modalities present problems unless the hypotension is due to hypovolemia, which is easily correctable. Some use a combination of dopamine and nitroglycerin with good results in this situation.

Interestingly, the linkage of the enkephalinergic and adrenergic nervous systems has been suggested by the decreased systemic vascular resistance brought about by the use of intrathecal morphine in potentially ischemic cardiac surgery patients [23]. Intrathecal morphine has the potential for clinical use in hyperdynamic myocardial infarction patients who have unremitting chest pain.

Emergency physicians are well aware that chest pain, however vague, must be treated with respect because myocardial infarction or ischemia may be less than obvious. Anesthesiologists, who may be faced with an anxious patient to be prepared for elective operation who has new onset of precordial pain, would do well to consider this experience of emergency physicians. Because the risk of surgery in a patient with a recent or ongoing infarction is elevated [24], any evidence of a changed pattern of chest pain or a 20-minute period of chest pain in the preoperative period should precipitate a myocardial infarction work-up prior to elective surgery, with serial enzyme and ECG monitoring.

GASTROINTESTINAL DISORDERS

Visceral pain from gastrointestinal disorders that do not involve the peritoneum is poorly located. Use of meperidine to alleviate such pain is often recommended because it may have a lesser propensity than narcotics such as morphine or hydromorphone to cause biliary tree spasm or other increased smooth muscle tone. All narcotics, of course, cause constipation, which may aggravate many gastrointestinal medical and surgical conditions. This is a fact that the lay public rarely appreciates. Because stretching and distention of the viscera stimulate pain much more than cutting or stabbing, the side effect of constipation may be worse for the patient than the initial pain that prompted narcotic use in the first place. This is especially true for less acute conditions. A transition to NSAIDs or aspirin after 48 hours will often be beneficial, for example, in postherniorrhaphy patients.

In acute bowel obstruction, patients often complain of terrible pain. Because of the enormous loss of volume into the edematous bowel wall and lumen (which may often require 5 to 10 liters of crystalloid resuscitation), use of narcotics for such patients may precipitate hypotension or even cardiac arrest; hence, simultaneous repletion of volume status with narcotization is important (see Chapter 10). The best treatment for such pain is often general anesthesia and surgical operation.

OTHER ACUTE STATES

Childbirth is painful, especially in elderly primigravidas. If an emergency physician must perform acute delivery, use of lidocaine for episiotomy is probably the only modality appropriate. Cesarean section can be performed emergently under local anesthetic, although this procedure is not optimal and may lead to a good deal of pain for the mother and some risk of local anesthetic overdose. Epidural and spinal anesthetics are the mainstays of obstetric anesthesia, although the gamut runs from no anesthesia to general anesthesia (see Chapter 9).

Invasive procedures such as tube thoracostomy are discussed in Chapter 12. A plea is again made here for adequate local anesthesia for all such procedures when time permits.

There is evidence that premature infants and newborns do feel pain, and anesthesia should be administered for all painful procedures in such patients as tolerated [25].

ACUTE PAIN AND PREHOSPITAL CARE

Pain management in the prehospital phase of care is of great importance. Narcotic titration, in the case of myocardial infarction unresponsive to sublingual nitroglycerin or in the setting of acute trauma, may be carried out under the aegis of the base station physician. Certainly such treatment requires careful prior training of paramedics in many of the points discussed above as well as close ongoing communication. Use of morphine should be cautious; 1- to 2-mg IV increments should be followed by measurement of vital signs, paying close attention to volume status, especially in trauma patients. As stated previously (see Chapter 5), overdose of narcotic in a cardiac patient may respond to naloxone reversal with dangerous hyperdynamic sequelae that are not usually observed when naloxone reversal is used in the narcotic addict.

Local anesthetics are not generally used by prehospital personnel, although their use has been recommended in certain disaster situations (see Chapter 15). Use of the lidocaine skin wheal is invaluable for difficult intravenous access cases because the pain of a failed start may lead to increased vasoconstriction and disappearance of veins. This technique (best used with a 30-gauge needle) is underutilized by paramedics and in EDs in this author's opinion. Some of the more aggressive air ambulance programs include field placement of a tube thoracostomy. As discussed in Chapter 12, infiltration of the site with lidocaine takes very little time and should be done unless the patient is in extremis.

CHRONIC PAIN DIAGNOSIS AND MANAGEMENT

Both anesthesiologists and emergency physicians need a good understanding of the differential diagnosis of chronic pain. The former group plays a diagnostic role in administering differential spinal blocks and in assessing the value of specific nerve blocks for such conditions as reflex sympathetic dystrophy. The latter group needs to have an idea of a patient's best options for referral, based on the diagnosis, and a means of identifying the chronic ED-abusing patient from the acute pain patient who needs prompt action.

Treatment modalities for chronic pain have been extensively reviewed elsewhere [3, 4, 15]. Here we shall focus on those problems that relate directly to the interface of anesthesia and emergency medicine. These include postlumbar puncture headache, reflex sympathetic dystrophy and causalgia, herpes zoster, low back pain, and certain aspects of central pain states.

HEADACHE

The differential diagnosis of headache has been reviewed thoroughly by Henry in Rosen's *Emergency Medicine* [26]. Headaches that include double vision, unstable vital signs, such as a high fever or extreme hypertension, focal neurologic defects, or depressed mental status mandate immediate attention because they are often symptoms of acute neurologic catastrophe. Most headaches permit a more leisurely approach, whether they are vascular, traction, or tension headaches, or inflammatory headaches. A special type of headache is the postlumbar puncture headache, which presents from several days to several months after lumbar puncture, usually in younger patients, and is notable for increasing in severity with the upright position. Often these headaches occur after a large-bore lumbar puncture for a myelogram (18- to 20-gauge needle) or a diagnostic lumbar puncture for a neurologic work-up with measurement of cerebrospinal fluid (CSF) pressures (22-gauge needle). These headaches can and do occur, however, after the 26-gauge lumbar puncture used by most obstetric anesthesiologists. Whatever the size needle is used, it is important to place the bevel at right angles to the longitudinal dural fibers, thus limiting the number of lacerated fibers and the resulting dural hole size. Postlumbar puncture headaches are very rare after the age of 50.

The most prevalent theory explaining these common headaches is that leakage of CSF through the dural rent left by the needle causes lowered CSF pressure and resultant traction on the pain-sensitive perineural structures [27]. Others claim that there is compensatory dilatation of the cerebral vasculature in response to the decreased CSF pressure from the leak, this in turn causing the headache in a manner similar to a migrainous headache [28].

Whatever the exact cause, it is important to distinguish these headaches from garden-variety tension or migrainous headaches because efficacious, permanent short-term treatment exists. Unfortunately, patients may languish for as long as a year before spontaneous relief occurs [29]. The key to diagnosis is eliciting a history of exacerbation with the upright position and relief with the horizontal position. The symptom complex may include nonspecific symptoms such as nausea and vomiting, dizziness, and auditory or visual disturbances.

Interestingly, chronic headaches with no history of lumbar puncture may be related to this complex [30, 31]. These headaches have a postural component as well as a throbbing nature, aggravation by ambulation, normal psychological profile, and failure of conventional treatment modalities [31]. Most important, they appear to respond to the same treatment modality as postlumbar puncture headaches—epidural blood patch.

The epidural blood patch, first reported in 1960 by Gormley [32], has been widely used and accepted in anesthesiology as a safe and effective method of treatment for the troublesome and often incapacitating headaches that follow spinal anesthesia. Unfortunately, the technique has not been used to the same degree for postspinal headaches caused by diagnostic or myelographic procedures, most probably due to a lack of familiarity by the involved specialists [29]. The procedure involves the placement of a 17-gauge Tuohy needle or an 18-gauge short-bevel needle in the epidural space, ideally at the same level as the prior site of lumbar puncture. The lateral decubitus position, sterile technique, and local anesthetic infiltration with a 30-gauge needle are used, with some extra local anesthetic infiltrated through the deeper ligamentous structures. A "loss of resistance" is then utilized to recognize the encounter with the epidural space. This technique relies on the fact that the potential space just outside the dura has a negative atmospheric pressure. Thus, if one connects a saline-lubricated glass syringe to the Tuohy needle and exerts constant gentle pressure on the plunger of the syringe as the needle is advanced in a millimeter by millimeter fashion, when the bevel of the needle enters the epidural space the plunger will suddenly give way, and the operator will feel a "loss of resistance." At that point no further advancement is warranted. Indeed, further advancement will result in a subdural or standard lumbar puncture ("wet tap"), creating an even larger dural rent.

After placing the needle correctly, one performs sterile venipuncture of 10 to 20 ml of blood and slowly injects this into the epidural space. Relief of symptoms is usually dramatic, although on rare occasions a second epidural blood patch must be performed [33]. Supine positioning for 30 minutes should follow, and excessive straining should be avoided for 24 hours. The technique is contraindicated in anticoagulated, septicemic, or locally infected patients and in patients with blood dyscrasias [29]. Complications are generally rare and self-limited, even if the blood is inadvertently injected into the subarachnoid space [34].

Although this technique is best performed by anesthesiologists, who have a large experience in the art of epidural injections from their familiarity with obstetric anesthesia, it is important for emergency physicians and other specialists who perform diagnostic spinal taps to be aware of the blood patch as a treatment option for postural headaches that they may have caused unwittingly. If a patient is discharged from the ED after a negative lumbar puncture, he or she should be advised to seek help if a persistent headache should occur later.

Classification and treatment of headaches are summarized in Table 7-1 [35]. The classification into three groups is useful because the general treatment modalities are quite different. Vascular headaches do respond to ergot preparations, caffeine, beta blockers, and centrally active modifiers of the adrenergic system such as clonidine or tricyclic antidepressants. Muscle contraction headaches have less specific treatments and often require standard chronic pain management strategies, such as behavior operant conditioning modification, treatment of depression, and the like. Traction and inflammatory headaches, which can often be identified by the marked exacerbation of pain on rotation of the head, include dangerous diagnoses such as subacute intracerebral hematomas and other mass-occupying lesions, headache radiating from eye, ear, nose and throat disorders, and infections, and the low-pressure CSF headaches mentioned above. Goebel has published a valuable summary of the diagnosis and treatment of headache [35].

There is no greater annoyance to the emergency physician than a patient who demands narcotics for his "migraine." In a busy ED it is rare for a physician to have the time to do more than make sure that no neurologic or infectious catastrophe is present and then either give the patient the narcotic injection or not. There is no easy solution to this problem. It is helpful for hospital emergency departments to keep track of known narcotic abusers and to communicate aliases, and so on. It is essential to refer these patients to chronic pain clinics and physicians who are interested in such problems (see Chapter 1). If such patients are known repeaters and do not take advantage of such referrals, it may be appropriate to refuse

Table 7-1. Classification and treatment of headache

Vascular headache	Muscle contraction headache	Traction and inflammatory headache

Migraine
  Classic
  Common
  Complicated
    Hemiplegic
    Ophthalmoplegic
Cluster (histamine)
Toxic vascular
Hypertensive
	Depressive equivalents and conversion reactions
	Cervical osteoarthritis
	Chronic myositis
		Mass lesions (tumors, hematomas, cerebral hemorrhage)
		Diseases of the eye, ear, nose, throat, teeth
		Arteritis, phlebitis (cranial neuralgias)
		Occlusive vascular disease
		Atypical facial pain
		Temporomandibular joint disease

Suggested treatment		

Ergot derivatives
Sedation
Methysergide
Cyproheptadine
Propranolol
Clonidine
Lithium
Platelet antagonists
Analgesics
Antihypertensives
Behavioral conditioning
	Common analgesics
	Sedation
	Antidepressants
	Physical therapy
	Behavioral conditioning
		Appropriate consultation
		Therapy of underlying disease:
		  Antibiotics
		  Anticonvulsants
		  Corticosteroids
		  Miotics
		  Surgery

Source: J. Goebel. The chronic headache. *Ear Nose Throat J.* 66:384, 1987. With permission.

narcotics. If such a patient is a first-time admission, he or she may well have a painful headache that does not respond to ergots and may require narcotics. In this case, however, it is important to make proper referral and to keep track of future ED admissions to ensure that the patient is not taking advantage of the system.

REFLEX SYMPATHETIC DYSTROPHY

The syndrome of reflex sympathetic dystrophy (RSD), also known as causalgia, algodystrophia, shoulder-hand syndrome, and post-traumatic arthrosis, is a painful condition that arises in an extremity after serious or trivial injury and appears to involve a positive feedback loop between the sympathetic nervous system and the extremity. The injury causes aberrant afferent activity that causes a disturbance in the spinal cord and eventually in the lateral and ventral gray matter, thus triggering reflex sympathetic activity [36]. The resultant efferent sympathetic activity leads to vasoconstriction, temperature changes, and, eventually, dystrophic changes in soft and bony tissue. Such changes in turn result in further afferent activity and further sympathetic stimulation until, if it is left untreated, severe osteoporosis and muscle wasting leave the limb frozen and nonfunctional and the patient with a nontreatable, severe, central pain problem.

Roberts has proposed that wide dynamic-range neurons, or myelinated A-fiber neurons, which have abnormal persistent sensitization, may be the cause of the feedback loop [37]. This concept explains how movement or touch, which stimulate only non-nociceptive fibers, can elicit pain and vasoconstriction.

Signs and symptoms of RSD include a cold limb, the temperature of which may be quantified by the new technique of thermography, constant burning pain, allodynia (painful sensation with touch alone as the stimulus), altered hair growth or sweat gland production, and characteristic shiny, smooth skin changes. The burning pain and the decreased temperature of the limb are the hallmarks, however. Early diagnosis is essential to prevent the full-blown causalgia picture described above. Often the initial symptoms appear within 1 to 4 weeks after injury and may be confused with direct problems due to the injury itself. For example, swelling accompanies the initial symptoms and may cause cast pain. Simple bivalving of a cast in the ED will not suffice in such a case, whereas recognition and appropriate referral of a patient with an asymmetrically cold limb and atypical burning pain may lead to gratifying results.

Treatment success of RSD is directly related to the rapidity with which the diagnosis is made. Treatment of RSD that has been left untreated for a year or more has a uniformly dismal success rate, although the pain is such that all modalities are exploited nevertheless. Sympathetic blockade, either by stellate ganglion block for the upper extremity or lumbar sympathetic block for the lower extremity, is an important first line of treatment [38, 39]. Often three to four blocks per week must be performed before permanent improvement occurs. The technique for these blocks has been well described elsewhere [40] and is probably best left to anesthesiologists specializing in pain management. Other modalities include systemic corticosteroids, in a dose of 10 mg prednisone tid for up to 12 weeks [41] or a series of regional intravenous blocks (Bier block, see Chapter 6) with guanethidine [42] or the new serotonin antagonist, ketanserin [43].

The variety of treatment options available simply underscore the fact that if the condition is left untreated, no modality will be consistently effective. Thus it is important for emergency physicians and other specialists to consider this syndrome as a diagnostic possibility whenever they are confronted with subacute or chronic burning limb pain and dystrophic and thermal abnormalities on physical examination.

HERPES ZOSTER

Herpes zoster attacks are marked by painful lesions that occur in a dermatomic distribution. Generally, pain is the first sign or symptom, after which the skin lesions appear. Traditional treatment includes narcotic and non-narcotic analgesics. Sympathetic block has been shown to increase the healing time of the lesions [44].

LOW BACK PAIN

Initial treatment of low back pain emphasizes conservative management including bed rest. Excessive rest, which may lead to muscular atrophy, however, may be deleterious. Neurologic defects involving focal sensory or motor findings or incontinence mandate prompt neurosurgical consultation. Campana has done an excellent review of this problem [45]. Prevention of low back pain depends on proper lifting techniques that avoid twisting, weight bearing at a distance from the axial skeleton, or bending of the back (thus leg extension is used to lift). Prevention also depends on proper lifting mechanics, abdominal conditioning, and tightening of the abdominal musculature while lifting (see Chapter 12).

Epidural steroids may be required for severe, incalcitrant, chronic low back pain [46]. Should a myelogram or other diagnostic study reveal extrusion of a disk or spinal stenosis with nerve root compression, spinal surgery, such as lumbar laminectomy, foraminotomy, or disectomy, may be indicated, especially after failure of conservative treatment. Discussion of the controversies and complexities of diagnosis and treatment of chronic low back pain is beyond the scope of this chapter. As in all chronic pain states, a multidisciplinary approach that addresses behavioral as well as physiologic aspects of the problem is essential.

CENTRAL PAIN STATES

Pain states in which the peripheral afferent nerve supply does not appear to be intact are termed *central pain states.* Included in this category are tic douloureux, postherpetic neuralgia, denervation dysesthesia, anesthesia dolorosa, and phantom limb pain [40]. Such conditions do not lend themselves to traditional analgesic therapy, perhaps because they are caused by central nervous epileptiform abnormal nervous activity. Episodic disorders such as tic douloureux respond to anticonvulsants such as carbamazepine (Tegretol) in a dose of 200 to 1500 mg/day, or phenytoin (Dilantin), 100 mg tid. The other central pain states listed tend to have a more relentless presentation, and, although anticonvulsants are worth trying, tricyclic antidepressants and neuroleptic drugs [47, 48] may be required.

PAIN CLINIC MULTIDISCIPLINARY APPROACH

Understanding that most emergency physicians and anesthesiologists do not work with chronic pain patients, we shall summarize the basic treatment philosophies of most pain clinics. This will assist, we hope, in better referral practices and a better knowledge of what type of care a patient can expect to receive at such a clinic.

Because many chronic pain patients have complex operant conditioning apparatus that have evolved in their domestic environments, inpatient management is often an important initial aspect of pain clinics. At the outset, patients are made aware that complete cure of their pain is doubtful but that the goal of adjustment to the pain is more realistic. Initial formal pain psychological evaluation is undertaken using such tools as the McGill pain questionnaire and the Minnesota Multiphasic Personality Inventory. Diagnostic nerve blocks are performed when indicated. These include the diagnostic spinal block, in which an anesthesiologist follows a patient's pain through the course of a short-acting spinal anesthetic or administers different concentrations of anesthetic to achieve different levels of block [40]. Pain relief, or the lack thereof, is noted with placebo injection, sympathetic block (recall that this is the earliest and last nervous system affected by a spinal anesthetic), or sensory and/or motor block. If a patient still has pain when the affected area is totally blocked, the pain is central, whether psychological or organic in origin. If sympathetic block relieves the pain, a variation of reflex sympathetic dystrophy is suspected. If placebo relieves the pain, again, the pain may be psychogenic in cause. Because naloxone can reverse the effects of placebo, and the endorphin system has been involved with the placebo effect [49], it is important to realize that psychogenic pain is still "real" pain, not "imaginary" pain. If sensory blockade relieves the pain, a true somatic nociceptive source is suspected. This may require further diagnostic blockade, such as trigger point injection or nerve root block.

Once the pain and the patient's psychological response to the pain have been well evaluated, a treatment management plan is formulated. Fundamental to this plan is the role of the contract, in which specific opinions, recommendations, and limits to treatment are written, signed, and dated by both patient and physician. The contract should include discussion of medication use, daily pain diaries, schedules for therapies, and the physician's responsibilities in regard to disability claims and legal interactions [3].

Medication management is crucial to the success of the pain program. One practitioner should manage all medications, and prn dosing should be avoided. Often optimal utilization of non-narcotic drugs in combination with nondrug techniques such as TENS, acupuncture, psychological adaptation techniques, and active rehabilitation of painful joint and muscle conditions can markedly reduce or eliminate narcotic drug use, with its problems of tolerance, addiction, somnolence, constipation, and the like. Epidural steroid injections are useful for certain types of back and lower extremity pain.

Rarely, surgical intervention is indicated, although for noncancer chronic pain this therapy is usually condemned because most pain pathways have multiple decussations. Even if short-term relief occurs, often the same or worse pain returns 6 months later.

CANCER PAIN

Cancer pain, as mentioned above, is a special category because often the prognosis is poor and the pain extreme. Brigden and Barnett have reviewed the topic thoroughly [15]. As in other chronic pain management methods, the pain must be diagnosed accurately because cancer patients have many pains from multiple sources. In the case of certain gastrointestinal cancers, such as stomach or pancreatic cancer, celiac plexus block with phenol may provide long-lasting profound relief [50]. Similarly, cervical and lumbar sympathetic blocks may provide relief for appropriate cancers.

Medication management for cancer pain involves optimal use of nonnarcotic medications such as NSAIDs and adding oral narcotics such as codeine when necessary. Phenothiazines may extend the analgesic and sedative effects of narcotics and provide important antiemetic effects. Nausea and vomiting are pernicious signs in cancer, occurring both from the effect of the antimetabolites used in treatment and as side effects of narcotics. Antiemetic drugs include various phenothiazines such as droperidol (Inapsine) or promethazine (Phenergan) or unique drugs such as trimethobenzamide (Tigan). Recently, restrictions on availability for cancer patients of the antiemetic THC, the active ingredient in the plant marijuana, have been relaxed.

Drugs such as propoxyphene napsylate (Darvon-N) and pentazocine (Talwin) are best avoided; aspirin works better than the former, and the latter's agonist-antagonist actions confound further narcotic treatment. Meperidine, with its short half-life and CNS irritability due to its first-order metabolite, is also a troublesome drug for chronic pain treatment. Often morphine, whether oral or parenteral, is needed, especially in patients with varying pain; methadone, with its long half-life, may be better suited for stable malignant pain.

Avoidance of parenteral medication requiring hospitalization and encouraging maximum patient participation in care and treatment decisions, as emphasized by the hospice movement, are essentials for achieving an optimal quality of life for patients with limited life spans. Neurosurgical ablation is considered only in patients with life expectancies of less than 6 months because distressing side effects related to nerve regeneration occur near that time.

The use of epidural narcotics for cancer pain has been explored. Malone and coworkers reported on 15 patients with malignant intractable pain who were given epidural morphine for up to 190 days through tunneled indwelling catheters [51]. They concluded that tolerance did not seem to be a problem, side effects were minimal, and patient acceptance was high.

REFERENCES

1. International Association for the Study of Pain Subcommittee on Taxonomy. Pain terms: A list with definitions and notes on usage. *Pain* 6:249, 1979.
2. Melzack, R., and Wall, P. D. Pain mechanism: A new theory. *Science* 150:971–979, 1965.
3. Perlman, S. L. Modern techniques of pain management. *West. J. Med.* 148:54–61, 1988.
4. Fields, H. L., and Levine, J. D. Pain—mechanisms and management. *West. J. Med.* 141:347–357, 1984.
5. Moncada, S., and Vane, J. R. Mode of action of aspirin-like drugs. *Adv. Intern. Med.* 24:1–22, 1979.
6. Yaksh, T. L., Farb, D. H., Leeman, S. E., et al. Intrathecal capsaicin depletes substance P in the rat spinal cord and produces prolonged thermal analgesia. *Science* 206:481–483, 1979.
7. Engberg, G., Svensson, T. H., Rosell, S., et al. A synthetic peptide as an antagonist of substance P. *Nature* 293:222–223, 1981.
8. Cousins, M. J., and Mather, L. E. Intrathecal and epidural administration of opioids. *Anesthesiology* 61:276–310, 1984.
9. Ty, T. C., Melzack, R., and Wall, P. D. Acute Trauma. In P. D. Wall and R. Melzack (eds.), *Textbook of Pain*. New York: Churchill Livingstone, 1984. Pp. 209–214.
10. Bonica, J. J. The relation of injury to pain (Letter). *Pain* 7:203–207, 1979.
11. Leonard, F. Pain control: Anesthesia and analgesia. In P. Rosen et al. (eds.), *Emergency Medicine* (2nd ed.). St. Louis: Mosby, 1988. Pp. 295–307.
12. Mather, L. E., and Phillips, G. D. Opioids and adjuvants: Principles of use. In M. J. Cousins and G. D. Phillips (eds.), *Acute Pain Management*. New York: Churchill Livingstone, 1986. Pp. 77–103.
13. Cohen, F. L. Postsurgical pain relief: Patient's status and nurses' medication choices. *Pain* 9:265, 1980.
14. Foley, K. M. The treatment of cancer pain. *N. Engl. J. Med.* 313:84–95, 1985.
15. Brigden, M. L., and Barnett, J. B. A practical approach to improving pain control in cancer patients. *West. J. Med.* 146:580–584, 1987.
16. Ross, E. L., and Perumbeti, P. PCA: Is it cost effective when used for postoperative pain management? *Anesthesiology* 69(3A):A710, 1988.
17. Covino, B. G. Interpleural regional anesthesia. *Anesth. Analg.* 67:427–429, 1988.
18. Azar, I., and Turndorf, H. Severe hypertension and multiple atrial premature contractions following naloxone administration. *Anesth. Analg.* 58:524, 1979.
19. Schwartz, J. A., and Koenigsberg, M. D. Naloxone-produced pulmonary edema. *Ann. Emerg. Med.* 16:1294–1296, 1987.
20. Glass, P. S. A. Respiratory depression following only 0.4 mg of intrathecal morphine. *Anesthesiology* 60:256–257, 1984.
21. Procacci, P., and Zoppi, M. Heart Pain. In P. D. Wall and R. Melzack (eds.), *Pain*. New York: Churchill Livingstone, 1984. Pp. 309–318.
22. Braunwald, E., Alpert, J. S., and Ross, R. S. Acute Myocardial Infarction. In K. J. Isselbacher, R. D. Adams, and E. Braunwald, et al. (eds.), *Principles of Internal Medicine*. New York: McGraw-Hill, 1980. Pp. 1125–1136.
23. Vanstrum, G. S., Bjornson, K. M., and Ilko, R. Postoperative effects of intrathecal morphine in coronary artery bypass surgery. *Anesth. Analg.* 67:261–267, 1988.
24. Rao, T. L. K., Jacobs, K. H., and El-Etr, A. A. Reinfarction following anesthesia in patients with myocardial infarction. *Anesthesiology* 59:499–505, 1983.
25. Berry, F. A., and Gregory, G. A. Do premature infants require anesthesia for surgery? *Anesthesiology* 67:291–293, 1987.
26. Henry, G. L. Headache. In P. Rosen, F. J. Baker, R. M. Barkin, et al. (eds.), *Emergency Medicine* (2nd ed.). St. Louis: Mosby, 1988. Pp. 279–293.

27. Spielman, F. J. Post-lumbar puncture headache. *Headache* 11:280–283, 1982.
28. Sechzer, P. H., and Abel, L. Post-spinal anesthesia headache treated with caffeine. *Curr. Ther. Res.* 26:440–448, 1979.
29. Olsen, K. S. Epidural blood patch in the treatment of post-lumbar puncture headache. *Pain* 30:293–301, 1987.
30. Gaukroger, P. B., and Brownridge, P. Epidural blood patch in the treatment of spontaneous low CSF pressure headache. *Pain* 29:119–122, 1987.
31. Parris, W. C. V. Use of epidural blood patch in treating chronic headache: A report of six cases. *Can. J. Anaesth.* 34:403–406.
32. Gormley, J. B. Treatment of post-spinal headaches. *Anesthesiology* 21:565–566, 1960.
33. Casement, B. A., and Danielson, D. R. The epidural blood patch: Are more than two ever necessary? *Anesth. Analg.* 55:89–90, 1983.
34. Wilkinson, H. A. Lumbosacral meningismus complicating subdural injection and "blood patch." *J. Neurosurg.* 52:849–851, 1980.
35. Goebel, J. A. The chronic headache. *Ear, Nose Throat J.* 66:383–397, 1987.
36. Lewis, R., Racz, J. A., and Fabian, G. Therapeutic approaches to reflex sympathetic dystrophy of the upper extremity. *Clin. Issues Reg. Anesth.* 1:1–6, 1985.
37. Roberts, W. J. A hypothesis on the physiological basis for causalgia and related pains. *Pain* 24:297–311, 1986.
38. Wang, J. K., Johnson, K. A., and Ilstrup, D. M. Sympathetic blocks for reflex sympathetic dystrophy. *Pain* 23:13–17, 1985.
39. Linson, M. A., Leffert, R., and Todd, D. P. The treatment of upper extremity reflex sympathetic dystrophy with prolonged continuous stellate ganglion blockade. *J. Hand Surg.* 8:153–159, 1983.
40. Murphy, T. M. Treatment of Chronic Pain. In R. D. Miller (ed.), *Anesthesia* (2nd ed.). New York: Churchill Livingstone, 1986. Pp. 2077–2109.
41. Christensen, K., Jensen, E. M., and Noer, I. The reflex dystrophy syndrome response to treatment with systemic corticosteroids. *Acta Chir. Scand.* 148:653–655, 1982.
42. Bonelli, S., Conoscente, F., Movilia, P. G., et al. Regional intravenous guanethidine vs. stellate ganglion block in reflex sympathetic dystrophies: A randomized trial. *Pain* 16:297–307.
43. Davies, J. A. H., Beswick, T., and Dickson, G. Ketanserin and guanethidine in the treatment of causalgia. *Anesth. Analg.* 66:575–576, 1987.
44. Grosslight, K. R., Rowlingson, J. C., and Boaden, R. W. Herpes zoster and reflex sympathetic dystrophy. *Anesth. Analg.* 65:309–311, 1986.
45. Campana, B. C. Cervical Hyperextension Injuries and Low Back Pain. In P. Rosen (ed.), *Emergency Medicine.* St. Louis: Mosby, 1988. Pp. 799–816.
46. Carron, H., and Toomey, T. C. Epidural Steroid Treatment for Low Back Pain. In M. Stanton-Hicks and R. A. Boas (eds.), *Chronic Low Back Pain.* New York: Raven Press, 1982. Pp. 192–198.
47. Watson, C. P., Evans, R. J., Reed, K., et al. Amitryptiline vs. placebo in postherpetic neuralgia. *Neurology* 32:671, 1982.
48. Ward, N. G., Bloom, V. L., and Friedel, R. D. The effectiveness of tricyclic antidepressants in the treatment of co-existing pain and depression. *Pain* 7:331, 1979.
49. Reuler, J. B., Girard, D. E., and Nardone, D. A. The chronic pain syndrome: Misconceptions and management. *Ann. Intern. Med.* 93:588–596, 1980.
50. Brown, D. L., Bulley, K., and Quiel, E. L. Neurolytic celiac plexus block for pancreatic cancer pain. *Anesth. Analg.* 66:869–873, 1987.
51. Malone, B. T., Beye, R., and Walker, J. Management of pain in the terminally ill by administration of epidural narcotics. *Cancer* 55:438–440, 1985.

8. Pediatric Anesthesia in Emergency Medicine

H. Shannon Carson III

The first steps in diagnosis and preoperative care taken by the emergency physician can often play a significant role in later medical, surgical, and anesthetic management. Early diagnosis, prompt fluid resuscitation, and appropriate laboratory evaluation can mean better care, fewer complications, and shorter hospital stays for all types of pediatric patients.

AGE RANGES

Discussion of pediatric patients is made easier by dividing them into groups to identify problems characteristic of various age ranges.

Preterm

Preterm patients are born before the thirty-seventh week of gestation and are usually of low birth weight. Their organ systems are immature and unable to function properly in an extrauterine environment. Their metabolic pathways are yet to be completely developed, and they will not tolerate the same drugs in the same dosages that other patients do. They do not have the same stress response. Almost everything about them physiologically and pharmacologically is very different from all other age groups seen in pediatric practice.

Term Infants

Term infants are born between the thirty-eighth and forty-third weeks of gestation. Their organ systems have developed the ability to make a rapid transition to compensated, mature, extrauterine function. This transitional state is very delicate, however, and is easily reversed, halted, or prolonged by various insults such as hypoxemia or acidosis.

Newborn

The newborn period is the first 24 hours after birth. This is an extremely delicate time, and transitional cardiopulmonary changes normally occur very rapidly. Physiologic stress easily interrupts the delicate transitional cardiorespiratory changes taking place.

Neonate

The term *neonate* refers to the first 30 days of life. Heart and lung transition continues, and rapid maturation occurs also in hepatorenal and metabolic status. This is still a critical time during which there is relatively poor tolerance to physiologic stress.

Infant

The term *infant* is applied to individuals in the first 12 months of life. Most of the transitional state is normally complete in 3 to 4 months, and these patients have mature systemic function. They start to respond to physiologic stresses, surgery, anesthesia, and the various routinely used drug groups pretty much the same as adults. They are still very different from adults, mostly because, although their bodies are very small, their heads and surface-to-volume ratios are relatively large.

The Young Child

Young children are aged 1 through 6. This group is physiologically and pharmacologically like adults. Anatomically these children are still small but no longer threateningly tiny. They are a separate group mostly because they have prominent separation anxiety. This is a real source of trauma for the patient, parent, and physician and demands special treatment considerations by the anesthesiologist and emergency physician. Five- or six-year-olds are an intermediate subgroup and may act either like young children or older children.

Older Children

This term covers children aged 7 through puberty. These children are usually the easiest patients in every way. They have mature systems, good stress response, reasonable size, and receding separation anxiety. Usually some type of communication may be directed to them, and they will understand to some extent what is being explained. They have yet to deal with the hormonal and emotional upheavals of adolescence or the multisystemic declines beginning in adulthood.

Adolescent

Adolescence covers the time from puberty through the teenage years. For the purposes of this chapter only, adolescents will be considered comparable to adults.

PHARMACOLOGY

The body composition of pediatric patients differs from that of the adult. Premature infants, neonates, and infants have a higher percentage of body water than adults, and the ratio of intracellular fluid to extracellular fluid is higher. Most of these compartmental differences disappear by 1 year of age.

Neonates have a higher gastric pH at birth than adults. The pH is around 4 for several days and decreases to adult levels slowly. Gastrointestinal absorption is less complete in the neonate than in the adult.

Drugs bind less well to neonatal serum proteins, and neonates have decreased serum albumin levels [1]. Therefore, there is more free or unbound drug available, and in many cases, drug doses are smaller because of this

[2]. Additionally, increases in bilirubin may displace drugs from albumin-active sites and make more free drug available for systemic effect [3]. Protein binding reaches adult levels by approximately 1 year of age. The blood-brain barrier is poorly developed in neonates, and higher drug levels exist in the central nervous system than in adults [4, 5].

Several metabolic pathways are immature in the neonate. These include the oxidative and reductive systems in the liver. Some conjugating pathways are also immature. Generally, these pathways mature quickly and reach near-adult levels after 2 to 3 months. A number of drugs may have prolonged action in the neonate. Examples include morphine, diazepam (Valium), and pancuronium.

PREMEDICATION

Often pediatric patients in the emergency department go straight to surgery. A consideration of premedication and thoughtful, psychological preparation is important for emergency physicians. Clear documentation of the premedication given is extremely important for the anesthesiologist who sees the patient later.

The traditional pharmacologic premedication protocols (Table 8-1) were used to decrease anxiety, sedate the patient, dry secretions, decrease gastric volume, and increase gastric pH. Pharmacologic premedication in pediatric patients has largely been replaced by two important developments. First, thorough patient and parent teaching programs can prepare the patient and the parents psychologically for the hospital experience and decrease much of their fear and anxiety. Second, parents are now allowed to be present for anesthetic induction or such procedures as suturing in the emergency department. This effectively eliminates the need for premedication in certain

Table 8-1. Premedication[a]

Atropine	0.01–0.02 mg/kg	IM
Glycopyrrolate	0.005–0.01 mg/kg	IM
Morphine	0.1 mg/kg	IM
Meperidine	1 mg/kg	IM
Codeine	1 mg/kg	po
Diazepam	0.1–0.4 mg/kg	po
Midazolam	0.05–0.1 mg/kg	po
Chloralhydrate	50–100 mg/kg[b]	po
Cimetidine	7.5 mg/kg	po
Innovar	0.04 ml/kg	IM

Note: Commonly used doses at Children's Hospital and Health Center, San Diego, California.
[a]Infants generally receive only anticholinergics.
[b]Not to exceed 1.0 gm total.

age groups. Good psychological preparation helps all parents and most patients over age 2. Parental presence for induction or emergency department procedures is most helpful for patients 1½ to 6 years old. Infants can usually be separated from parents atraumatically. Older children are usually cooperative after a reasonable interview and proper explanation. However, most patients aged 1½ to 6 have prominent separation anxiety. Allowing parents to be present for anesthetic induction or for emergency department procedures obviates or eliminates this very strong source of emotional stress for patient and parent alike.

Anticholinergic premedicant drugs are still advocated by many to decrease secretions and vagal tone. These drugs seem most reasonable in the neonate and young infant, in whom bradycardia is most poorly tolerated. Tables 8-2 and 8-3 contain appropriate doses for these and other premedication agents.

Pulmonary aspiration of gastric contents continues to be an infrequent but serious problem. Although the pediatric incidence of aspiration may be less than that in adults, it still merits considerable concern, particularly in those patients at increased risk. These include patients with a full stomach, difficult airway, or bowel obstruction.

Table 8-2. Pediatric doses

Muscle relaxants	Intubation	Halothane maintenance	Isoflurane maintenance
Pancuronium	0.1 mg/kg	0.04 mg/kg	0.02 mg/kg
Curare	0.7 mg/kg	0.28 mg/kg	0.14 mg/kg
Metocurine	0.4 mg/kg	0.16 mg/kg	0.08 mg/kg
Succinylcholine	1.0 mg/kg		
Pancuronium/metocurine	0.02/0.08 mg/kg		
Pancuronium/curare	0.02/0.144 mg/kg		
Atracurium	0.4 mg/kg	0.1–0.2 mg/kg	
Vecuronium	0.1 mg/kg	0.02–0.4 mg/kg	

Reversal of muscle relaxants

Neostigmine 1 mg/ml and glycopyrrolate 0.2 mg/ml, mix equal volumes and give 0.1 ml/kg

Edrophorium 1 mg/kg

Atropine 10 μ/kg

Narcotics	Balanced anesthesia	Cardiac	Maintenance infusion
Fentanyl	2–10 μ/kg	10–50 μ/kg	3–4 μg/kg/hr
Morphine	0.2 mg/kg	2 mg/kg	
Meperidine	1–2 mg/kg	—	
Codeine	—	—	

Table 8-2 (continued)

Sedatives/hypnotics	IV	IM	Rectal
Thiopental	5 mg/kg	—	40 mg/kg
Methohexital	2 mg/kg	7–10 mg/kg	30 mg/kg
Ketamine	1–2 mg/kg	4–8 mg/kg	—
Diazepam	0.1–0.4 mg/kg		

Cardiovascular	Dose	CPR	Dose
Dobutamine	2–10 μ/kg/min	Epinephrine	5–10 μ/kg
Dopamine	2–10 μ/kg/min	Lidocaine	1 mg/kg
Epinephrine	0.1–1.0 μ/kg/min	Atropine	10 μ/kg
Isuprel	0.1–0.5 μ/kg/min		
Neo-Synephrine	1–10 μ/kg/min		
Norepinephrine	0.1–1.0 μ/kg/min		
Nitroprusside	1–10 μ/kg/min		
Nitroglycerin	1–10 μ/kg/min		
Hydralazine	0.1–1.0 mg/kg		

Miscellaneous	Dose	Remember
Aminophylline	5 mg/kg loading	$15 \times$ wt (kg) in 250 ml =
Aminophylline	0.5 mg/kg/hr	1.0 μ/kg/min/minidrop
Ampicillin	25 mg/kg	
$CaCl_2$	10–20 mg/kg	
Dantrolene	2.5–4.0 mg/kg IV prophylactic	
Dantrolene	3–10 mg/kg IV divided doses	
Dexamethasone	0.2 mg/kg	
Droperidol	20 μ/kg	
Cefazoline	25 mg/kg	
Gentamicin	2 mg/kg	
Furosemide	0.25 mg/kg	
Lidocaine	20–50 μ/kg/min	
$NaHCO_3$	1 meq/kg	
Narcan	1–10 μg/kg	
Physostigmine	30–40 μ/kg	
Propranolol	0.01–0.1 mg/kg	
Solucortef	5 mg/kg	
Solumedrol	1 mg/kg	
Verapamil	0.1 mg/kg divided doses	

Commonly used doses at Children's Hospital and Health Center, San Diego, California

Table 8-3. Guidelines for approximate estimation of drug dosages in children

Age	Fraction of adult dose
7 yr	½ (0.5)
1 yr	¼ (0.25)
1 mo	⅛ (0.125)
Newborn	⅒ (0.1)

Source: J. Ryan. *A Practice of Anesthesia in Infants and Children.* New York: Appleton-Century-Crofts, 1986. With permission.

Histamine H_2 receptor antagonists such as cimetidine and ranitidine effectively decrease gastric volume and increase gastric pH. Cimetidine 7.5 mg/kg may be given preoperatively. Complications are infrequent. It is metabolized by the same liver enzyme systems as lidocaine, diazepam, propranolol, and warfarin (Coumadin) and may alter serum concentrations of these drugs [6].

Metoclopramide (0.05 to 0.10 mg/kg) has received some attention in the adult literature for use as premedication. It is too early to tell if it will achieve much use in pediatric medicine. It decreases dopamine levels in the basal ganglia and is a peripheral cholinergic agonist, facilitating gastric emptying. It is contraindicated in mechanical small bowel obstruction, and its peripheral cholinergic effects may be antagonized by concomitant use of atropine or glycopyrrolate.

GENERAL ANESTHETICS

Anesthetic agents have been fully discussed elsewhere in this book. Only pediatric differences will be highlighted in this chapter. The volatile agents are occasionally used in the emergency treatment of status asthmaticus or status epilepticus that is refractory to conventional therapy. Emergency physicians should also note their use in disaster medicine.

The systemic effects of nitrous oxide are the same in pediatric patients as in adults, and its indications and contraindications are virtually the same from cradle to grave.

The three volatile agents in current use are halothane, isoflurane, and enflurane. The oldest, halothane, is the most widely used in pediatric practice because it smells the best and is the smoothest for inhalation inductions. It is the least irritating to the airway, resulting in less coughing, breath holding, and laryngospasm. This nonirritant characteristic leads to faster, smoother inductions even though the other two agents are less soluble in blood (see Chapter 5). It is also the cheapest of the three agents at the present time.

In healthy adults the uptake of the anesthetic agent is such that the alveolar concentration is 50 to 60 percent of the inspired concentration after 15 to 20 minutes. Infants, however, will reach 70 to 80 percent of the inspired concentration during the same amount of time [7], probably because their alveolar ventilation is about 150 cc/kg as opposed to 60 cc/kg in adults. Therefore, infants become anesthetized much faster than adults and may suddenly achieve unacceptable levels of cardiorespiratory depression when rapid inhalation inductions are used.

It has been widely believed that MAC values (minimum alveolar concentration—the ED_{50} of an anesthetic gas, see Chapter 5) are inversely proportional to age. Recently, some published data indicate that MAC is highest during infancy (1 to 6 months old) and decreases with both increasing and decreasing age. Neonates were reported to have smaller MAC values [7]. Preterm babies had even smaller values, and some studies of fetuses show values even less than those of preterm infants.

As mentioned earlier, the volatile agents may cause more hypotension in the neonate and young infant than in older patients. Generally, the reason given is the poor contractile properties of the neonatal myocardium during the period of transitional circulation.

These agents may also cause a greater decrease in heart rate than in adults owing to the higher degree of vagal tone present in infancy. Because of this, it has been traditionally taught that atropine should be given to neonates, infants, and children before proceeding with anesthetic induction. It is probably reasonable to use atropine preinduction in neonates and infants when planning an inhalation induction with halothane or (emergency physicians take special note) when succinylcholine will be used. Older children usually do not have an unacceptable slowing of the heart rate during proper induction with halothane, except in the presence of airway compromise and hypoxemia, and probably do not need routine preinduction atropine.

The reported incidence of prepubertal halothane hepatitis has been much less than that in the adult population. The National Halothane Study showed a virtual absence of halothane hepatitis before puberty [8]. Some authors believe that the metabolism of halothane may partially change at puberty to include a higher percentage of reductive metabolites, thus leading rarely to so-called halothane hepatitis. Others have shown that infants metabolize less halothane than adults. Whatever the reason, the reported incidence is much lower in the pediatric population [9]. However, any history of hepatitis or other liver disease elicited by the emergency physician should be prominently displayed and communicated to the anesthesiologist.

Ketamine may be used in much the same way in pediatric practice as in adults. In addition, Berry has recently popularized the "stun" dose of ketamine, 3 mg/kg IM, given to the uncontrollable fighting patient. Within a few minutes the patient becomes quite docile. Some appear "dissociated" from their surroundings. One may then proceed with an intravenous or inhalation induction [10]. Additionally, emergency physicians might then proceed with minor procedures such as a laceration repair with local anesthesia. Of course, the physician must utilize proper monitoring methods, have proper resuscitative skills and equipment available, and understand that children with a full stomach are not candidates for this technique. Ketamine is a sympathomimetic, and it increases intracerebral pressure. It is relatively contraindicated in the patient with a possible head injury.

Barbiturates are widely used as pediatric induction agents in much the same way and in the same dosages used in adults. In addition, rectal methohexital (30 mg/kg) and rectal thiopental (40 mg/kg) are commonly used as induction agents.

Neonates are more sensitive to nondepolarizing muscle relaxants than older patients, but this characteristic is counterbalanced by their larger volume of distribution, resulting in clinical doses equivalent to those used in older patients on a per weight basis [11]. The elimination half-life is generally shorter, thus giving these drugs a shorter duration of action in infants. In contrast, however, premature infants may have much longer elimination times for the traditional relaxants such as pancuronium.

Infants generally require a higher dosage of succinylcholine than adults [12], possibly due to their larger volume of distribution and a larger extracellular fluid compartment. The incidence of bradydysrhythmias is higher in children than in adults when they are given succinylcholine. Also, there is a 20 to 40 percent incidence of myoglobinemia and myoglobinuria in infants given succinylcholine [13]. The incidence of myoglobin release after infancy is reported to be very low.

Infants up to 6 months of age have a plasmacholinesterase activity about half that of the adult [14]. Theoretically, this characteristic might affect the metabolism of ester-type local anesthetics and succinylcholine (see Chapter 5). Neonates also have decreased hepatic and renal clearances of local anesthetics of the amide type. Myelinization is far from complete at birth. Most motor neurons are myelinated by 1 year of age, but others are not myelinated until brain growth is completed at puberty. Thus, many of these fibers may be blocked by lower concentrations of local anesthetics than are used in the adult, in whom the full myelin barrier is present. Neonates and infants have decreased plasma binding of local anesthetics, thus potentially creating more free plasma levels of drug. Counterbalancing all the above factors is the large volume of distribution in the neonate and infant that results in the same per kilogram doses as are used in adults (see Chapter 9). Treatment of local anesthetic overdose or accidental intravascular injection in the neonate or infant is the same as that in the adult. Adequate oxygenation and prevention of aspiration remain the central concerns. Cardiovascular collapse may be a serious problem, especially with bupivacaine.

AIRWAY AND FLUID MANAGEMENT

PEDIATRIC AIRWAY

A number of anatomic differences occur in the pediatric airway. The infant tongue is relatively larger in proportion to the rest of the mouth. The epiglottis is narrower and shorter, and the larynx is higher in the neck. The narrowest portion is the cricoid cartilage, as opposed to the vocal cords in adults. Infants are obligate nasal breathers and are unable to breath well orally for several months. The small diameter of the infant larynx makes it more vulnerable to small amounts of circumferential edema. For example, 1 mm of edema in the 4-mm larynx will cause a 75 percent reduction in the cross-sectional area. Since airway resistance increases by the radius to the fourth power, the work of breathing will rise drastically.

This makes endotracheal tube size selection critically important because tight-fitting tubes may cause unacceptable degrees of mucosal edema at the level of the cricoid. Table 8-4 shows the recommended sizes of endotracheal tube for the various ages and proper depths of placement. Charts and tables are only approximate guidelines, and final proper sizing dictates easy insertion to the proper depth and an audible leak at about 20 cm H_2O pressure.

The best check for proper depth of insertion is direct visualization of the insertion distance and careful avoidance of any movement until taping and securing are complete. Listening for quality of breath sounds bilaterally is not as useful for determining proper depth in the small patient, because breath sounds, especially large positive pressure breaths, are easily transmitted to the other lung field and even to the abdomen (see Chapter 1). Table 8-4 also shows guidelines for the proper depth of insertion for each age group. Table 8-5 shows the simple formulas for remembering depth approximations in patients through the age of 10 years.

Depth is particularly critical in the first year. The newborn's vocal cords-to-carina distance is 4 cm. Thus, a midtracheal placement is 2 cm past the

Table 8-4. Endotracheal tube sizes

Age	Inner diameter	Outer diameter	Insertion depth (cm)
Preterm to 1500 gm	2.5	3.4	6–7
Preterm 1500–3000 gm	3.0	4.1	8–9
Term 3400 gm	3.0	4.0	10
	3.5	4.8	
Neonates to 6 mo	3.5	4.8	10
6–18 mo	4.0	5.4	11
18 mo–3 yr	4.5	6.1	12–13
3–4 yr	5.0	6.8	13–14
5 yr	5.5	7.4	15
6 yr	6.0	8.1	16
8 yr	6.5		18
10 yr	7.0		20

Common tube sizes used at Children's Hospital and Health Center, San Diego, California.

Table 8-5. Endotracheal tube depth at incisors (cm)

Oral	10 + age (yr) (to 10 years old)
Nasal	14 + age (yr) (to 10 years old)
Neonatal	8–10 cm (oral)
Preterm	5 + wt (kg) (oral)

vocal cords. If the placement is not proper, extension or flexion of the head may move the tube up or down enough to result in either an endobronchial placement (with hypoxemia, arrhythmias, or bucking) or extubation with possibly tragic outcome. It is useful to remember that the tip of the tube goes in the same direction as the nose. Thus, in extending the head, the nose goes cephalad and so does the tip of the tube. Many pediatric intensive care physicians prefer to err on the side of slightly deeper placement because the potential complications of a low-riding tube are rarely life threatening, and pulling the tube back 1 cm is easier than the converse situation, whereas if a high-riding endotracheal tube comes out of the trachea, emergency reintubation is necessary. Although the infant triples his weight by age 12 months, the vocal cords-to-carina distance increases only by 1 cm, from 4 to 5 cm.

Laryngoscopy and visualization of the larynx is much the same in the older pediatric patient as in the adult. In infants the tongue, as mentioned before, is relatively larger, and the larynx is higher in the neck. Regardless of this, only minor modifications of technique are needed to make pediatric laryngoscopy amenable to almost everyone who is reasonably skilled. Because the occiput is so prominent, the head needs no further ventral displacement, and doing so may make matters worse. Instead, placing a small folded towel or pad under the neck will stabilize the head and bring the airway angles into proper position. Also, as in the adult, the use of a stylette may be helpful. Slight cricoid pressure will gently depress the larynx, bringing it into better view.

Any of the commonly used laryngoscope blade designs are acceptable. Both straight and curved blade designs are available in small sizes. The two most commonly used styles are the Miller design and the Macintosh design. The Miller is straighter and narrower and has a shallower flange than the Macintosh design. Although it probably gives a less complete view of the larynx, the Macintosh design stabilizes the tongue better and holds the mouth open wider, thus giving more room for entry. Choosing one or the other style is largely a matter of personal preference except in the preterm infant and the newborn, in whom a Miller size 0 may be preferable. Given the proper conditions, proper equipment, and proper positioning as discussed above, the great majority of pediatric patients are very little more challenging to intubate than adults. The reputation for difficulty in pediatric and infant laryngoscopy is usually derived not from the patient's anatomy but from poor positioning, suboptimal conditions, or lack of proper equipment.

Several groups of patients have abnormal anatomy that makes exposing and securing the airway more difficult. The most celebrated of these groups are patients with Pierre Robin syndrome, Treacher Collins syndrome, Goldenhar's syndrome, cystic hygroma, and acute epiglottitis. Defects in these conditions may be severe, and securing the airway in some may be impossible, requiring tracheostomy. Proper positioning and proper equipment are extremely important for even the most experienced personnel. Optimal intubating conditions in these groups usually mean a well-conducted general anesthetic with adequate relaxation. This may require transport to the operating room and immediate availability of surgeons if emergency tracheostomy is needed.

Intubation Techniques

Several techniques have been suggested for use in patients not amenable to routine direct vision laryngoscopy. These include:

1. *Blind oral intubation.* The endotracheal tube is styletted and shaped like a J ("hockey stick") with the same predicted radius of curvature as the approach to the unseen larynx. The laryngoscope is used to hold the mouth open and provide access. The styletted endotracheal tube is advanced slowly in the midline around the anterior bend toward the estimated area of glottic opening. Listening for breath sounds through the endotracheal tube or watching for the moisture column in the tube will enable one to push the endotracheal tube off the stylette into the larynx when the tube rests in the glottic opening. Spontaneous respirations and insufflation of anesthetic gases and oxygen greatly facilitate this procedure since the patient will then be less likely to become hypoxemic or awaken enough to go into laryngospasm during the period of instrumentation.

2. *Blind nasal intubation.* This technique differs little from that in adults. Proper conditions usually dictate a general anesthetic or a depressed level of consciousness because cooperation will be impossible in most children. The nasally placed endotracheal tube is slowly advanced using various head and neck positions (assuming cervical spine fracture has been ruled out) until the larynx is entered as judged by breath sounds and the moisture column in the endotracheal tube. Here again spontaneous ventilation and insufflation of anesthetics and/or oxygen may give more time for performance of the technique.

3. *Retrograde intubation.* In infants or children a 20-gauge IV catheter is used to enter the airway percutaneously through the cricothyroid membrane. A 0.021 inch guidewire is threaded through the catheter cephalad into the pharynx, where it may be grasped with Magill forceps or hemostat. An endotracheal tube is then threaded over the guidewire into the larynx and the guidewire removed. This technique in children also generally requires adequate general anesthesia. It is complicated, time consuming, and difficult in infants owing to poor development of the cricothyroid mem-

brane. The general elasticity of the tissues in the small patient makes this procedure very difficult.

4. *Fiberoptic intubation.* This technique is the same as that used for adults, and, as smaller fiberoptic instruments become available, smaller endotracheal tubes will fit over the fiberoptic scopes. An endotracheal tube is fitted over the fiberoptic instrument, and the instrument is guided into the larynx. The endotracheal tube then may be slid over the scope into the larynx and trachea. Present limitations of bronchoscope size preclude use with endotracheal tubes smaller than 4.5 mm. This technique also requires considerable experience electively before emergency or difficult placements can be performed reliably.

5. *Cricothyroidotomy.* This is basically the same procedure as that performed in adults but is more difficult because the airway is smaller. The tissues are softer and more elastic, and tissue planes may be more difficult to discern. In this technique the head is extended, the trachea stabilized, and the cricothyroid membrane pierced with a 14- or 16-gauge IV catheter. The catheter is advanced caudally over the needle into the trachea. A 3-mm endotracheal tube adapter is connected to the catheter, and oxygenation is carried out until the airway is secured by other means.

Surgical cricothyroidotomy entails a transverse incision down to and through the cricothyroid membrane, insertion of a dilator, and then insertion of a tracheostomy tube or endotracheal tube. This gives better flow rates than catheter cricothyroidotomy but takes longer to perform. It may be quicker to perform than a surgical tracheostomy but may have more long-term complications, especially in the infant (see Chapter 1).

6. *Tracheostomy.* In any of the above syndromes, or when a difficult airway is suspected or diagnosed electively, surgical tracheostomy may be necessary when all else fails.

THE CHILD WITH UPPER AIRWAY OBSTRUCTION

Careful observation and examination of the child with acute upper airway obstruction may give clues to the diagnosis or the location of the obstruction. During normal inspiration negative intrapleural pressure tends to expand the intrathoracic airway and to constrict the extrathoracic trachea and larynx. Conversely, during normal expiration, the intrathoracic structures become a little smaller, and the extrathoracic airway dilates.

Mild changes in diameter occurring for any reason are relatively more important in the small airway of the neonate or infant because resistance varies inversely by the radius to the fourth power. To repeat, 1 mm of edema in a 4-mm diameter airway will decrease the surface area by 75 percent and increase resistance 16 times. Turbulent airway flow makes these numbers even worse. When symptoms such as stridor and retractions are predominantly inspiratory, epiglottitis, croup, or laryngeal foreign body may be suggested.

Expiratory symptoms such as prolonged or forced expiration or wheezing may be more consistent with intrathoracic obstruction such as a vascular ring, asthma, or endobronchial foreign body.

Acute Epiglottitis

Acute epiglottitis is usually due to a *Haemophilus influenzae* type b infection in a child 2 to 6 years old. Such patients present with a rapidly progressive course of fever, stridor, and dysphagia. In severe stages the child may have a high fever, appear toxic and dehydrated, and may prefer to sit forward with the head in the sniffing position, mouth open, and drooling. The child will not talk, cough, or move.

Moderate symptoms in the earlier phases of the process include stridor and an exquisitely sore throat, but the patient may not appear toxic, may not have retractions at rest, and may have good alveolar air entry bilaterally.

Because of the much heralded tendency for sudden complete airways obstruction in epiglottitis, the diagnosis must be confirmed quickly when this process is suspected. Once confirmed, intubation should be performed under controlled circumstances.

In children with mild or moderate symptoms lateral neck x-rays may be performed and may be helpful in diagnosis. Advanced cases should be taken directly to the operating room for laryngoscopy and control of the airway.

Diagnosis can be made in a number of ways. Children with early mild symptoms may cooperate by opening the mouth, sticking out the tongue and panting, thus possibly showing a swollen epiglottis. The lateral neck x-ray may show the swollen blurred epiglottis and loss of the radiolucent area anterior to the epiglottis.

Most authorities recommend that all patients with suspected or confirmed acute epiglottitis be taken to the operating room for diagnostic laryngoscopy and, if confirmed, immediate intubation. Also most everyone today recommends anesthesia for laryngoscopy and intubation because it provides much easier conditions and better control. It also avoids the potentially fatal complete airway obstruction that can occur when the child is stimulated or given laryngoscopy while awake. The anesthetic may be started with rectal methohexital or with inhalation agents such as nitrous oxide and halothane. The child may prefer to start sitting up or on the side. Use of CPAP (continuous positive airway pressure) during the induction improves ventilation in most cases. With a proper induction the airway will improve in all but the severest of cases. Most anesthesiologists start the IV during the induction. Some brave anesthesiologists administer succinylcholine to facilitate the laryngoscopy.

An alternative technique consists of starting an IV and utilizing a barbiturate-relaxant sequence for laryngoscopy and intubation. This technique has found favor only in certain institutions whose physicians in the emergency department and intensive care unit (ICU) are extraordinarily skilled, well equipped, and amply insured.

Oral intubation should be performed with an endotracheal tube 0.5 to 1 mm smaller than normal, and the leak around the tube should be measured. Proper sizing dictates a leak at 20 to 25 cm of water peak positive pressure.

Some physicians prefer to switch to a nasotracheal tube at this time. Nasal tubes are more comfortable and may be more secure. However, they are also harder to suction and are associated with sinus infections.

Blood cultures should be taken and the patient started on ampicillin and chloramphenicol. The latter drug is usually discontinued later if the organism is susceptible to ampicillin.

Management differs regarding sedation and ventilation. Some protocols call for restraints, intravenous sedation, and spontaneous ventilation. Others advocate sleep, paralysis, and mechanical ventilation.

Laryngotracheobronchitis (Croup)

Children with croup are usually 6 months to 3 years old and have experienced a gradual progression of symptoms over several days associated with an upper respiratory infection. Fever is usually low grade. The white blood cell counts are usually only mildly elevated. The patients do not appear toxic, cough spontaneously, do not drool, and have no trouble swallowing. Hoarseness is characteristic, as is the barking character of the cough.

Lateral neck radiographs usually show a normal epiglottis and supraglottic structures. The chest x-ray shows the tapered narrowing of the sublottic area that is called the steeple sign.

Viral laryngotracheobronchitis is usually benign and predictable. Treatment is supportive and noninvasive in all but the severest cases. Humidified oxygen, intravenous hydration, and aerosol racemic epinephrine (0.15 to 0.30 ml racemic epinephrine in 3 to 5 ml normal saline) every 1 to 2 hours are usually adequate. Symptoms severe enough to require aerosol racemic epinephrine warrant admission because of the possibility of "rebound" obstruction. Intubation is usually reserved for those patients showing severe retractions and poor alveolar air entry that is refractory to maximal aerosol epinephrine therapy.

Foreign Body Aspiration

Foreign body aspiration is very common in the 1- to 4-year-old age group, and the presenting symptoms vary widely. Five percent of foreign bodies are laryngeal or tracheal, and obstructive symptoms may be severe and potentially lethal. The other 95 percent are endobronchial and present as pneumonia, asthma, or chronic cough that is poorly responsive to reasonable therapy. An exhalation chest x-ray may show the characteristic mediastinal deviation away from the affected side.

FLUID THERAPY

Although surgical fluid management in pediatric patients bears many similarities to that used in adult medicine in terms of fluid types, medical maintenance, and replacement of losses, there are significant differences in body fluid compartments, metabolic rate, use of glucose, tolerance of anemia, and rate of dehydration in the neonate.

As discussed earlier, the preterm baby has approximately 76 percent total body water, whereas the term infant has 70 percent and the adult has 60 percent. The ratio of the extracellular to intracellular fluid is 1.4 in neonates as opposed to 0.5 in adults. The newborn infant becomes dehydrated at the rate of approximately 10 percent in 24 hours compared to 4 percent in the adult.

Metabolic rates are higher in the newborn and infant. The glucose and water requirements are higher. The newborn and small infant tolerate starvation poorly and cannot rapidly metabolize glucose stores. Hypoglycemia is an ever present danger, and glucose should be maintained in the 80 to 120 mg/dl range and monitored frequently, especially in the stressed, hypothermic or septic neonate. (See Table 8-11 for differences in oxygen requirements between newborns and adults.)

There are many formulas in the literature for deriving medical and surgical fluid requirements. There are inaccuracies in all. They ignore normal biologic variability and varying patient conditions and usually only apply to maintenance therapy and not replacement of ongoing losses. It is important to recognize that most patients come to surgery or to the emergency department with a fluid deficit. This may be due to bleeding, vomiting, or trauma, or from being NPO. The effects of anesthetics and many analgesic drugs such as narcotics on the cardiovascular system, particularly on the venous capacitance vessels, make even a normally hydrated patient relatively hypovolemic while under anesthesia. The importance of replacing losses (and accurate documentation of replacement) in the emergency department in patients headed for surgery should be obvious. Neonates and small infants under anesthesia need a relatively high filling pressure to maintain good cardiac output. All formulas are at best rough guidelines and must sometimes be drastically modified or even ignored when physical findings, laboratory data, or monitoring indicate the need for further therapy.

Developing a dose-response mentality toward fluid management will enable the user to administer fluids according to a reasonable calculation of needs and then to measure patient response and act accordingly. Tables 8-6 and 8-7 show a recommended modified formula for maintenance and replacement fluids based on age, weight, and degree of surgical trauma. Note that replacement during the first hour is higher than that given in traditional formulas. Fluid overload in babies and children is possible but rare, and inadequate fluid therapy has been much more common with the older formulas.

Table 8-6. Guidelines for fluids for patients age 3 and under: lactated Ringer's solution

---

1. First hour—hydrating solution, 25 ml/kg, plus item 3 below
2. All other hours, plus item 3 below
   Maintenance fluid = 4 ml/kg
   Maintenance + trauma = basic hourly fluid
   4 ml/kg + mild trauma, 2 ml/kg = 6 ml/kg/hr
   4 ml/kg + moderate trauma, 4 ml/kg = 8 ml/kg/hr
   4 ml/kg + maximal trauma, 6 ml/kg = 10 ml/kg/hr
3. Blood replacement with blood or 3:1 volume replacement with crystalloid

---

Source: Modified from F. A. Berry (ed.), *Anesthetic Management of Difficult and Routine Pediatric Patients.* New York: Churchill Livingstone, 1986. With permission.

Table 8-7. Guidelines for fluids for patients age 4 and over: Ringer's lactate

---

1. First hour—hydrating solution 15 ml/kg, plus item 3 below
2. All other hours, plus item 3 below
   Maintenance fluid = 4 ml/kg
   Maintenance + trauma, basic hourly fluid
   4 ml/kg + mild trauma = 2 ml/kg = 6 ml/kg/hr
   4 ml/kg = moderate trauma, 4 ml/kg = 8 ml/kg/hr
   4 ml/kg + maximal trauma, 6 ml/kg = 10 ml/kg/hr
3. Blood replacement with blood or 3:1 volume replacement with crystalloid

---

Source: Modified from F. A. Berry (ed.), *Anesthetic Management of Difficult and Routine Pediatric Patients.* New York: Churchill Livingstone, 1986. With permission.

Pulmonary aspiration of gastric contents has been a much publicized and ongoing problem in anesthesia. However, it has not received the same attention in emergency medicine. Patients are kept NPO for a period of time before elective surgery and anesthesia to minimize gastric contents and decrease the incidence of aspiration. Gastric emptying times are shorter in neonates, infants, and small children than in adults. For this reason as well as the fact that they lose body fluids relatively faster than adults, children have traditionally not been kept NPO preoperatively as long as adults. The literature seems to be in a state of flux in this area, and opinions and practice vary considerably, recently tending toward more flexibility and common sense in NPO protocols. Present recommendations at some centers include no solids for at least 8 hours and then clear liquids only until being placed NPO as follows:

Infants	2 hours
Small children	3 hours
Children	4 hours
Children over 10 years old	6 hours

The above recommendations apply only to healthy patients for elective surgery. Children with unusual anxiety or pain or those scheduled for emergency surgery should always be treated as having a full stomach regardless of NPO status.

Note that the formulas in Tables 8-6 and 8-7 require replacement of routine preoperative deficits with hydrating solutions in the first hour.

Pathologic preoperative losses requiring fluid replacement may include blood loss, third-space losses, bowel fluid losses, or vomiting as in pyloric stenosis. These losses must be estimated by the patient's findings on examination, hemodynamics, laboratory data, and urinary output. Gastric fluid loss usually involves loss of sodium chloride and hydrogen ion, and replacement commonly is half-strength or full-strength saline. Bowel losses are high in sodium and commonly are replaced with Ringer's lactate solution. Third-space losses from trauma or gastrointestinal obstruction are usually replaced with Ringer's lactate solution, and blood loss may be replaced with combinations of crystalloid and blood components as needed.

Any approach must be modified by the patient's condition and the response to therapy. More or less fluid may be needed based on frequent assessment of laboratory data, hemodynamics, and urinary output. After 2 or 3 hours of operative or resuscitative time, the formulas must frequently be discarded and therapy given on a strictly individualized basis according to patient status and physiologic response.

Glucose in Fluid Management

The use of glucose in operative and resuscitative fluid replacement has received a great deal of attention since the early 1980s, and, with the exception of the newborn and small infant, the glucose controversy probably applies to pediatric medicine as well as to adults. As previously mentioned, glucose levels must be monitored very closely in the newborn and small infant and must be rigorously maintained in the normal range. These patients cannot mobilize glucose stores well to combat hypoglycemia. Also they may be more adversely affected by hyperglycemic states than their older counterparts. The earlier literature on glucose administration focused on concerns of possible increased organ system damage when the patient was exposed to anesthetics and other drugs in a fasting state (the usual preoperative fasting state). Although some recent studies have focused on concerns with glucose-induced hyperosmotic states and osmotic diuresis, the most important issue for emergency physicians and anesthesiologists has been the finding of increased central nervous system damage and mortality in several laboratory models when cerebral ischemia occurs in hyperglycemic laboratory models. Except for neonates and small infants, the normal metabolic response to trauma and surgery is hyperglycemia. Glucose administration increases this already higher than normal blood glucose level. Some authorities postulate that providing glycolytic substrate to ischemic cerebral tissue may increase anaerobic metabolism to lactic acid, making the resulting acidosis worse than would occur if no glucose were administered for fueling the anaerobic pathway [15].

As a result of these studies and widespread generalizations made from them, many clinicians are using nonglucose-containing solutions for emergency resuscitation and operations possibly complicated by focal or global cerebral ischemia (craniotomy, cardiopulmonary bypass, trauma, shock). Some clinicians have gone further and abandoned the routine use of glucose solutions in all cases. It goes without saying that more studies on all human organ systems are needed to verify and quantify this area of concern.

Blood Transfusion

Table 8-8 shows hematocrit values at various ages. Note that a newborn is anemic if the hematocrit is less than 45 but that at 3 months of age the hematocrit may normally be as low as 30. Thereafter the normal range shifts upward as the bone marrow begins to catch up with patient growth.

Indications for blood transfusion in pediatric medicine have changed drastically. Doctors have traditionally disregarded the myriad complications of transfusion (anaphylaxis, hepatitis, and so on) and pretty much transfused everyone when the hematocrit fell to 30. This practice disregarded much good research on physiologic response to anemia. It also resulted in needless patient morbidity and mortality and wasted a precious and finite natural resource. The widespread AIDS phenomenon in the 1980s had led to public rejection of blood transfusion, forcing the field of medicine to make transfusion safer and to use bank blood much less often. When blood volume is kept normal, healthy children can tolerate a hematocrit of 20 or even lower reasonably well, satisfying tissue oxygen needs by increasing cardiac output. Many clinicians now recommend transfusion much less often and only in settings of decompensated shock, massive sudden blood loss, or predicted ongoing unacceptable losses.

Table 8-9 shows the blood volume of various age groups. Calculations of blood volume and acceptable losses based on the patient's hematocrit are easily made to predict when the amount of blood loss might indicate the need for transfusion. Blood loss smaller than the maximum allowable amount is generally replaced with lactated Ringer's solution in a ratio of three parts solution to one part of lost blood.

Table 8-8. Normal hematocrit

	Mean	Range
Premie	45	40–50
Newborn	54	45–65
3 months	36	30–42
1 year	38	34–42
6 years	38	35–43

From F. A. Berry (ed.), *Anesthetic Management of Difficult and Routine Pediatric Patients.* New York: Churchill Livingstone, 1986. With permission.

Table 8-9. Blood volume (ml/kg)

Preterm	100
Term	90
Infancy	80
Childhood	70
Adult	65–75

VASCULAR ACCESS AND MONITORING

Vascular access techniques for administering fluids and medicines and for invasive monitoring are probably the most challenging technical area of pediatric anesthesia. These techniques are at times a major hurdle for even the most experienced pediatric specialist. Size considerations notwithstanding, there are few differences in the approach to venous access in patients aged 2 and older. The advantages, disadvantages, location, and relative sizes of their veins mirror those of the adult. This discussion will emphasize the differences in approach required in the infant and the neonate.

VASCULAR ACCESS IN INFANTS

The most difficult group is the 9- to 15-month-old infants who have tripled their birth weight and have excess subcutaneous fat over their neck, arms, hands, and feet. Newborns are smaller but have much less subcutaneous tissue, rendering their peripheral veins and arteries more visible and accessible.

All the usual veins may be used for cannulation. Some neonates and some chubby 12-month-olds will have no visible peripheral veins. However, both the fifth interdigital vein in the hand and the saphenous vein at the ankle have a reasonably constant anatomic location. Placing a tourniquet may render these veins palpable, if not visible. Even if not easily palpable, the fifth interdigital vein may be cannulated with a 22- or 24-gauge catheter by percutaneous entry dorsally midway between the fourth and fifth metacarpals. Varying the entry to one side or the other and the depth of insertion may allow successful venipuncture. Likewise, the saphenous vein lies just anterior to the medial malleolus in the neonate and infant just as in the adult. Blind percutaneous attempts here with varying paths of entry will frequently be successful.

Fiberoptic light sources are frequently used by neonatal specialists to transilluminate the hands, wrists, and feet of neonates to find veins and arteries and to guide them in their insertion of catheters. These lights are invaluable in small infants, neonates, and premature infants. Some light sources generate a lot of heat and can easily burn the skin with prolonged contact. They should not be left in contact with the skin if they are hot.

Scalp veins are also frequently used as a third choice after the upper and lower extremity veins.

The femoral vein may be used just as it is in the adult. Its advantages are it location and size when a larger vein is needed quickly. However, it is hard to keep sterile and may be disrupted with repeated flexion of the thigh. Cases of septic arthritis of the hip joint have been reported secondary to femoral venipuncture.

The umbilical vein is easily cannulated at birth but becomes inaccessible to catheterization after a very few hours. It is accessible by cutdown for 2 to 3 days. Its usefulness is pretty much restricted to the first few days of life. The umbilical vein catheter passes through the ductus venosus into the inferior vena cava and then to the right atrium. It may fail to pass and become wedged in the liver. Should hyperosmolar solutions (sodium bicarbonate or glucose) be injected into the wedged catheter, scarring of the portal vein may occur.

The subclavian, femoral, and jugular veins have the same anatomic relationships in babies, children, and adults, and, with appropriately matched smaller sizes of equipment, they are nearly as accessible in babies as in adults.

Thus, in order of desirability in infants, routine intravenous placement would use a dorsal hand vein, then a saphenous vein at the ankle, and third, a scalp vein. The brachial or cephalic vein at the antecubital space, the femoral vein, and percutaneous central venous catheter placement are less desirable for routine intravenous use. Last in desirability would be a cutdown.

Central venous pressure (CVP) catheter placement requires appropriately matched sets of smaller sized introducer needles, guidewires, dilators, and catheters. With the appropriate equipment, the percutaneous insertion technique involving the external jugular, internal jugular, subclavian, and femoral veins are pretty much the same as in the adult. Although the anatomic relationships are the same, the structures are smaller and shallower, and the surrounding landmarks, especially the sternocleidomastoid muscle in the neck, may be less developed. The relative advantages and disadvantages of each site are the same as those in the adult. One important caveat involves the final position of the catheter tip. Catheters lying in the right ventricle cause arrhythmias and may perforate the heart. Catheters lying low in the right atrium may also perforate the heart. Catheters introduced from the left neck or the left subclavian position, with final placement in the superior vena cava, may erode into the right pleural space or into the mediastinum. Proper catheter tip placement is probably at the superior vena cava–right atrial junction or high in the right atrium.

Emergency physicians are sometimes faced with an infant or small child needing prompt resuscitation who seemingly is without immediate venous access. Vital therapy may be delayed during attempted cutdown or CVP placement. Intraosseus infusion is an old technique that has aroused some increased interest in the last few years. This technique is simple and quick, and all fluids and drugs used intravenously can be given in comparable doses.

Needles with stylets, such as bone marrow (Jamshidi) or larger spinal needles, are best; they are placed in the flat anteromedial surface of the tibia one or two finger breadths below the tibial tubercle. A screwing motion may facilitate passing through the bone until a decrease in resistance denotes marrow entry. Free inflow of fluid and ability to aspirate marrow confirm proper placement, and resuscitation may then begin [16, 17].

Balloon tip flotation catheters as small as 2 Fr allow monitoring of pulmonary artery pressure in almost any size patient. The 3.5 Fr size is a thermodilution catheter that gives cardiac output and allows easy calculation of systemic vascular resistance (see Chapter 6).

BLOOD PRESSURE MONITORING

Blood pressure monitoring is now routinely done by automated devices that take the pressure at varying preset intervals. For routine cases they have the advantage of time cycling and convenient digital readouts. They work by oscillometry and may not be accurate at lower perfusion pressures. It is important to use the proper size cuff. Table 8-10 shows the commercially available cuff sizes for various age groups.

Intra-arterial pressure monitoring in the pediatric patient aged 2 and older is just as safe and easy and uses the same locations as in the adult. Twenty-gauge catheters may be used in the radial and femoral positions. Twenty-two-gauge catheters may be used in the posterior tibial or dorsalis pedis positions.

The infant arterial tree will also usually accept a 22-gauge catheter in the radial position and a 20-gauge catheter in the femoral position. Percutaneous placement of 24-gauge catheters is common in preterm and term neonates in the radial or posterior tibial position. Fiberoptic light source transillumination is very helpful in these small patients.

Table 8-10. Blood pressure cuff sizes

	Width (cm)
Preterm ($<$ 1500 gm)	2.1
Preterm (1500–2500 gm)	2.8
Term (2500–4000 gm)	3.8
Infant (to 6 mo)	4.6
Infant (6–12 mo)	6
Child (to 6 yr)	7.6–8.25
Child (6–12 yr)	10
Adult	13

The umbilical arteries are utilized commonly at birth. The catheter is inserted through the umbilical artery into the hypogastric artery and should be positioned at L3–4 just above the bifurcation of the descending aorta. Complications of the umbilical artery catheter include bleeding, sepsis, and emboli. Renal emboli may produce hypertension, and mesenteric artery emboli may produce bowel infarction.

Twenty-four-gauge catheters are also used commonly in the radial or posterior tibial position in preterm patients, newborns, or neonates. Fiberoptic transillumination aids in placement in these patients.

The temporal artery has been used in the past in certain situations. It does give preductal blood gas values when right-to-left shunting through the ductus arteriosus is present. Preductal oxygen tension values may be desirable in monitoring the proper arterial oxygen tensions in preterm infants who are at risk for retinopathy of prematurity. It should be noted that preductal arterial gas measurements may also be obtained from the right radial arterial position. The temporal artery location is difficult to place, hard to secure, usually short lived, and too flexible for reliable blood gas sample withdrawal. Furthermore, the literature contains reports of central nervous system embolization secondary to flushing these catheters, and they are not commonly used at this time.

RESPIRATORY MONITORING

Respiratory monitoring includes the traditional arterial blood gas sampling as well as the newer noninvasive continuous real-time oxygen and carbon dioxide monitoring. These noninvasive monitoring methods are very close to becoming the standard of care for all pediatric anesthetic procedures, and many institutions now monitor in addition end-tidal concentrations of nitrous oxide, nitrogen, and the volatile anesthetic gases. These modalities may be monitored either by infrared gas analyzers or through mass spectrometry.

The currently used noninvasive methods for oxygen monitoring include the transcutaneous PO_2 measurement and the light absorbance oximetry methods. Transcutaneous PO_2 may be measured by placing a heated Clark electrode over the skin. In neonates or infants it will give a measurement close to the arterial PO_2 but not in children or adults. Its additional limitations include a marked fall of measurement with decreasing cardiac output, skin burns, and calibration requirements [18]. Noninvasive oximeters work by light absorbance (see Chapter 2). Hemoglobin and oxyhemoglobin absorb light at different wave lengths. The current generation of oximeters are easy to use and are rapidly becoming the standard of care in emergency departments, operating rooms, and critical care areas. Their limitations include poor signals with decreasing perfusion, light interference, and motion artifacts.

Infrared gas analyzers and mass spectrometers, as mentioned before, are now commonly used to monitor end-tidal carbon dioxide. They usually draw respiratory gases at a rate of 100 to 500 cc/minute and give real-time continuous display values. In pediatric patients the small tidal volumes and rapid respiratory rates may sometimes give values that have variable mixing of end-respiratory and fresh gas flows, thus reflecting a mixed respiratory value rather than a true end-tidal value. Also, conditions causing distorted ventilation-perfusion relationhips, such as bronchopulmonary dysplasia, may give erroneous values. However, a single arterial blood gas sample will quickly show the end-tidal to arterial gradient in that particular patient, making this modality quite predictable in any given situation.

In addition to monitoring ventilation and guiding ventilator therapy, end-tidal carbon dioxide monitors are useful for monitoring apnea and are excellent indicators of abrupt changes in cardiac output. A drop in the end-tidal carbon dioxide measurement over a very short period of time in the presence of constant ventilation is an instantaneous and accurate indicator of a decrease in cardiac output. An instantaneous drop to zero in this parameter is usually a potentially catastrophic respiratory event such as a kinked, obstructed, or misplaced endotracheal tube, airway disconnection, or ventilator malfunction. Thus these devices can be life saving. Because of their real-time continuous capability of trend monitoring of the patient's cardiac and respiratory status, these devices are extraordinarily valuable, and, like noninvasive light absorbance oximetry, they will shortly become the standard of care in respiratory monitoring in emergency departments and in critical care units.

Continuous noninvasive monitoring devices of all kinds are rapidly increasing in use and probably should be overused when in doubt because they do not exact a price in terms of patient morbidity or mortality. In many situations they may increase the quality of patient care even though this has been difficult to prove. The more traditional invasive monitoring methods are simply not as effective in many cases and do cause complications, probably more commonly than is reported in the literature. The invasive techniques will decline in use. Operating rooms and emergency departments that do not have the noninvasive monitors should start using them now.

NEONATAL CONSIDERATIONS

CIRCULATION

In the fetal circulation blood moves from the placenta to the inferior vena cava and then into the right atrium. It then crosses the patent foramen ovale into the left atrium and left ventricle and exits by way of the ascending aorta. Venous return from the central nervous system passes through the superior vena cava into the right atrium and right ventricle and then to the pulmonary arteries. The majority of the pulmonary arterial flow goes through the patent ductus arteriosus into the descending aorta. Only 5 percent of this blood flow goes to the fetal lung.

The fetal myocardium is poorly compliant and has an increased resting tension compared to that in the neonate, infant, or adult. It also generates less tension with any given stimulus [19].

The neonatal circulation is a transitional circulation lasting a variable period of time, usually only a matter of weeks. At the time of birth the placenta is removed, the umbilical cord is clamped, and the first breath is taken. This decreases cardiac output by approximately 40 percent [20]. The expansion of the lungs decreases pulmonary vascular resistance and increases pulmonary blood flow. The increasing PO_2 causes a functional closure of the patent ductus arteriosus. The increased pressure in the left atrium causes a functional closure of the foramen ovale.

Events occurring during the delicate and labile transitional period may prevent maturation and cause a regression to the fetal circulatory stage with its two main right-to-left shunts through the patent foramen ovale and the patent ductus arteriosus. The most common causes for regression to fetal circulation are hypoxemia and acidosis, because both lead to reflex pulmonary hypertension.

The transitional newborn myocardium has a limited ability to change its stroke volume. Fifty percent of the myocardium is connective tissue, and it has a decreased number of sarcomeres per gram of tissue [19, 20]. The neonatal cardiac output is about twice that of the adult in milliliters per kilogram.

The physiology of the transitional state changes rapidly during the first 24 hours. Changes then become more and more gradual, and the last transitional components are gone in 3 to 4 months [21]. Prematurity, illness, hypoxemia, and acidosis may prolong the transitional state or may cause a reversion back to the fetal circulatory state.

During the transitional circulatory period a high venous return is required to maintain adequate cardiac output, and dehydration is thus a greater risk than it is in the older individual [22]. The myocardial reserve is limited, and the cardiac output depends to a greater extent on heart rate. Because of the limited reserve and decreased ability to change stroke volume, bradycardia is poorly tolerated [23].

Halothane severely blunts the baroreceptors in the neonate [24]. During the transitional period the volatile anesthetic agents seem to cause a greater decrease in cardiac output, heart rate, and blood pressure than in older patients [25]. A number of newer studies dispute the older findings, however, and more work is needed in this area [26].

Normally, after 3 to 4 months the left ventricular and right ventricular weights, thickness, compliance, and electrocardiographic patterns have assumed relationships more like those of the adult heart (Table 8-11).

Table 8-11. Circulatory variables

| Age | Heart rate (beats/min) | Blood pressure (arterial) | | Oxygen consumption (ml/kg/min) |
		Systolic (mm Hg)	Diastolic (mm Hg)	
Preterm	150 ± 20	50 ± 3	30 ± 2	8 ± 1.4
Term	133 ± 18	67 ± 3	42 ± 4	6 ± 1.1
6 mo	120 ± 20	89 ± 29	60 ± 10	5 ± 0.9
12 mo	120 ± 20	96 ± 30	66 ± 25	5 ± 1.0
2 yr	105 ± 25	99 ± 25	64 ± 25	6 ± 1.2
3 yr	101 ± 15	100 ± 25	67 ± 23	6 ± 1.1
5 yr	90 ± 10	94 ± 14	55 ± 9	6 ± 1.1
12 yr	70 ± 17	109 ± 16	58 ± 9	3 ± 0.6
23 yr	77 ± 5	122 ± 30	75 ± 20	3 ± 0.6

Source: Modified from R. D. Miller (ed.), *Anesthesia* (2nd ed.). New York: Churchill Livingstone, 1986. With permission.

RESPIRATION

Surfactant is manufactured by type II pneumocytes and first appears in the lung tissue at 23 to 24 weeks of gestation. The severity of respiratory distress syndrome depends on the maturation of type II pneumocytes.

At birth, the lung expansion pulls pulmonary capillaries open, decreasing pulmonary vascular resistance and increasing pulmonary blood flow [27]. At this time there is a sharp increase in PO_2 and a decrease in PCO_2. The patent ductus arteriosus closes. The clamping of the umbilical vessels causes a sudden increase in systemic vascular resistance and a decrease in cardiac output. There is an increase in left ventricular afterload, an increase in left ventricular end-diastolic pressure, and a decrease in right ventricular afterload. The left atrial pressure now exceeds the right atrial pressure, and the foramen ovale functionally closes.

Ventilation-perfusion matching occurs in hours to days to an optimal degree [28]. Again, as mentioned before, hypoxemia or acidosis may increase pulmonary vascular resistance, open the foramen ovale, decrease the oxygen tension, and open the ductus arteriosus [29].

The first transpulmonary pressures may require negative intrapleural pressures of -60 to -80 mm Hg to expand the fluid-filled alveolae. However, the transpulmonary pressures are normal after 24 hours. Table 8-12 shows comparisons of some respiratory variables in the neonate and the adult.

The chest wall of the neonate has poor bellows function, the ribs are soft and cartilaginous, and the resting inspiratory flow rate is approximately 12 to 15 percent that of the adult. The specific compliance of the neonatal lung is the same as that of the adult. The closing volume in the newborn and

Table 8-12. Respiratory variables

	Neonate	Adult
Respiratory rate	40	15
Tidal volume (ml/kg)	7	7
Alveolar ventilation (ml/kg)	150	60
Oxygen consumption (ml/kg/min)	8	3
Functional residual capacity (ml/ kg)	30	35
Vital capacity (ml/kg)	35	70
FRC/VO$_2$	4	12
Resting inspiratory flow rates	3	24

young infant is greater than the functional respiratory capacity, thus contributing to an increased propensity for atelectasis and lower resting oxygen tensions.

During the initial transitional phases of respiration, the physiologic shunt is about three times that of the adult; thus the PO$_2$ in the newborn is 55 to 70 mm Hg [30]. Adult values are usually attained after 2 to 4 weeks, indicating complete functional closure of the foramen ovale and the ductus arteriosus.

RETINOPATHY OF PREMATURITY

Retrolental fibroplasia is now called retinopathy of prematurity. It was originally thought to be the result of hyperoxemia in small or preterm newborns. It has recently been shown to be a much more complicated process indeed, and is associated with much more than hyperoxemia alone. It is inversely related to gestational age and has been associated in various studies with hypoxemia, hypotension, hyperoxemia, vitamin E deficiency, hypercarbia, acidosis, sepsis, and prolonged hyperalimentation [31]. It usually occurs in the infant weighing less than 1250 gm. It does occur somewhat in the 1250- to 2500-gm weight group and is rarely reported in babies weighing more than 2500 gm, even in some who have never received supplemental oxygen. The retina does not mature until 44 weeks after conception, so theoretically every infant less than this age is susceptible. In spite of this, most cases have occurred in infants born less than 34 weeks after conception, and the great majority of these were less than 30 weeks old.

It seems appropriate to normalize the PO$_2$, PCO$_2$, pH, and blood pressure in most patients, and especially to avoid PO$_2$ values of greater than 70 or an oxygen saturation of more than 90 to 94 in all patients with susceptibility to retinopathy of prematurity. The emergency physician may not want to decrease the FiO$_2$ in a patient 38 to 40 weeks postconception who has just required resuscitation. However, it can be done safely with proper oximeter monitoring and should be considered rather than continuing with excessively high inspired oxygen levels. Additionally, it may be just as important to correct hypotension and acidosis quickly in these situations.

THERMOREGULATION

When placed in less than a neutral thermal environment, neonates try to keep their temperature normal by generating heat through metabolism of brown fat, crying, and moving. They do not shiver until several months of age. They may have a very high heat loss in cold environments because of a greater surface-to-volume ratio. This increases their already high metabolic rate, and, in trying to stay warm, they may exhaust glucose and calcium stores, setting the stage for hypoglycemia, hypocalcemia, and decreased systemic function. The transitional circulation may regress to fetal status with the ensuing fall in PO_2. Infants trying to compensate for cold surroundings need aggressive warming, extra glucose and calcium infusions, and frequent monitoring of temperature, glucose, and calcium levels.

Because of the additional systemic stresses involved, hypothermia, whether seen initially in the emergency department or later in the operating room, is especially dangerous to the newborn. Signs of hypoglycemia and hypocalcemia are masked by some drugs given in resuscitation efforts and by anesthesia. Additionally, many of the drugs we use (narcotics, relaxants, volatile anesthetics) interfere with temperature regulation. Operating rooms and emergency departments are cold, and cold preparation solutions make matters worse. Opening the chest and abdomen to air, infusing cold IV solutions and blood, and hyperventilation with dry gases accelerates the process.

In hypothermia there is an increase in arrhythmias, atelectasis, and aspiration. Anesthetic emergence is delayed. These patients should not be extubated postoperatively until they are normothermic.

Operating rooms and pediatric emergency areas should be warmed, and all gases should be warmed and humidified. Heating blankets are commonly used, and the head and extremities may be wrapped with plastic sheets or towels.

NEONATAL EMERGENCIES

Congenital Lobar Emphysema

In this process one lobe of the lung undergoes emphysematous expansion. It is usually an upper lobe, although occasionally it is the right middle lobe. The first symptoms are usually noted in the first 30 days of life. The neonate presents with dyspnea, wheezing, labored respirations, and cyanosis. Mediastinal shift and compression of the normal lung may produce severe respiratory distress.

Emergency bronchoscopy is indicated to exclude intraluminal obstruction, such as a mucous plug or a foreign body. Thoracotomy is then performed for lobectomy.

Airway and anesthetic management excludes nitrous oxide, which might further expand the emphysematous lobe. Spontaneous respiration is preferred because positive pressure breathing might produce a ball-valve mechanism, enlarging the emphysematous lobe even further. However, many of these patients are in severe respiratory distress and require careful controlled ventilation. A nasogastric tube is inserted to make sure the stomach is decompressed. Halothane is usually the volatile agent of choice. Intubation may be done with the patient awake or after an inhalation induction. Oxygen or oxygen-air mixtures may be used depending on the patient's postconceptual age, size, and degree of respiratory failure.

Congenital Diaphragmatic Hernia

The most common defect in this process is an incomplete closure of the pleuroperitoneal sinus, resulting in abdominal contents residing within the chest. Most commonly, small or large bowel or stomach is present. The defect is left sided in 75 to 90 percent of cases. It may occasionally be bilateral. It occurs once in every 2000 to 4000 births.

The onset and severity of symptoms depend on the quantity of the herniated viscera, its consistency, and the time of herniation. The herniation usually occurs early in development, and varying degrees of pulmonary hypoplasia are present. Significant bilateral hypoplasia may be present. The newborn may have a barrel chest, scaphoid abdomen, and decreased breath sounds on the affected side, as well as bowel sounds over the affected lung field. Severe respiratory distress may be present at birth.

Bag and mask ventilation has traditionally been discouraged because it may inflate the stomach, making the respiratory distress worse. Anesthetic considerations include intubation, avoidance of nitrous oxide, and careful monitoring and treatment of hypoxemia and acidosis. High ventilating pressures may produce lung barotrauma. Pneumothorax on the contralateral side is common and may be catastrophic.

Hypoxemia and acidosis are associated with persistence of the fetal circulatory state—i.e., with an open ductus arteriosus, a patent foramen ovale, and increased pulmonary vascular resistance, all making the hypoxemia worse. Pulmonary vasodilators such as priscoline or prostaglandin E are commonly used to treat the persistent fetal circulatory state.

Patients who continue to have severe respiratory failure while receiving maximum medical therapy may be candidates for extracorporeal membrane oxygenation (ECMO) for 10 to 14 days to provide time for lung growth and maturation.

In the high-risk group presenting with symptoms at birth some will respond to maximal therapy with a fall in pulmonary artery pressure and a postductal PO$_2$ greater than 60 for 12 to 24 hours. This is the so-called honeymoon period for these patients, and it is associated with a better prognosis. Patients whose pulmonary artery pressure is always greater than the systemic pressure and whose postductal PO$_2$ is always less than 60 are termed nonresponders and have a poorer prognosis [32].

Esophageal Atresia with Tracheoesophageal Fistula

This occurs once in every 2500 births. About one-third of these newborns weigh less than 2500 grams at birth. There are several types of esophageal defect, the most common consisting of a proximal esophageal atresia with the fistula extending from the distal trachea to the distal esophagus.

During fetal life, because these patients are unable to swallow amniotic fluid, polyhydramnios develops. After birth they cannot swallow their oral secretions. The diagnosis is easily made by inserting a nasogastric tube and taking an x-ray, thus demonstrating the coiled-up nasogastric tube just below the pharynx.

Infants with esophageal atresia aspirate both oral secretions and gastric contents, and their pulmonary status rapidly deteriorates. They become dehydrated due to inability to swallow oral secretions and feed. There is a high incidence of associated systemic anomalies including cardiovascular, gastrointestinal, musculoskeletal, and renal problems.

The approaches to therapy include primary repair and staged repair. Staged repair consists of a gastrostomy followed by several days of supportive care before the primary repair is done. It is usually done in patients who are premature or have associated respiratory distress syndrome (RDS), pneumonia, or associated systemic anomalies.

Airway management for the gastrostomy initially entails either an awake intubation followed by spontaneous respiration with nitrous oxide and halothane or an inhalation induction with halothane followed by intubation and the same kind of maintenance technique. Positive pressure ventilation may inflate the stomach and worsen the gastric reflux into the trachea. This in turn decreases ventilation by raising the intra-abdominal pressure and elevating the resting position of the diaphragms.

Because positive pressure is frequently necessary in these patients from the very start, some authorities recommend advancing the endotracheal tube past the fistula in order to prevent gastric distention during positive pressure ventilation. Others recommend bronchoscopic placement of a Foley catheter through the fistula to occlude the tract until repair can be carried out.

It is of note to emergency physicians that a significant number of these patients have residual long-term defects, including esophageal stricture, tracheomalacia, and gastroesophageal reflux. Eliciting the history of this anomaly may be very helpful in evaluating and diagnosing subsequent problems in these patients in the emergency department.

Omphalocele and Gastroschisis

A failure of the gut to return to the abdominal cavity at about the tenth week postconception results in an omphalocele, in which the abdominal contents lie outside the abdomen at birth. The contents are covered by a thin membrane. Omphalocele is associated with a high incidence of congenital heart disease and is also seen in various other syndromes.

Gastroschisis defects occur later in fetal life. In this condition there is no protective membrane covering the abdominal contents; the viscera are thus more prone to infection, and fluid loss is higher than in omphalocele.

Resuscitative and anesthetic management must consider associated defects and replace the large fluid deficits that sometimes occur. Extraordinary heat loss may occur from the exposed viscera.

SPECIFIC CLINICAL PROBLEMS

SURGERY ON THE YOUNG INFANT (1–3 MONTHS)

Hernia Repair

Two studies in 1984 reported a significant incidence of incarceration of inguinal hernias in small infants [33]. A certain percentage of these patients present with bowel obstruction. A gonad involved in an incarcerated hernia may be liable to infarction [34]. Irreducible hernias are associated with a higher incidence of other complications such as infection and bowel infarction. These data have made infant hernia surgery relatively urgent, the procedure generally being scheduled at the time of diagnosis regardless of age, weight, and associated conditions.

Hypertrophic Pyloric Stenosis

Patients with hypertrophic pyloric stenosis, usually males 2 to 6 weeks old, present with a history of days to weeks of varying amounts of projectile vomiting. They may have some weight loss after their initial weight gain. They have varying degrees of dehydration and loss of sodium, chloride, and hydrogen ion. Many need fluid resuscitation and electrolyte correction preoperatively. There is a large variation in the severity of dehydration present when the patient is seen in the emergency department. Even those infants who appear well hydrated invariably have some fluid deficit, and almost all are helped by an infusion of 10 ml/kg of normal saline or Ringer's lactate. Those infants with even the mildest signs or symptoms of dehydration may dramatically improve after an infusion of 20 ml/kg of normal saline or Ringer's lactate over 1 hour. Lethargic infants or those with a resting respiratory rate of less than 24 per minute may have the hypochloremic alkalosis seen with vomiting and may need electrolyte monitoring and appropriate adjustment over several hours.

Anesthesia considerations, in addition to fluid resuscitation, include emptying the stomach preoperatively. This may include gastric lavage if a barium study was done to make the diagnosis. Gastric lavage with warm normal saline or Ringer's lactate may be continued until the return contents are clear of the barium contrast material.

Induction may then proceed using a rapid sequence intravenous protocol with a barbiturate and muscle relaxant and cricoid pressure. Alternatively, an inhalation induction with nitrous oxide and halothane may be carried out. As with any induction, great care must be taken to avoid inadvertent stomach dilatation with its resultant potential for regurgitation and aspiration.

Maintenance techniques include inhalation alone or balanced anesthesia with relaxants and nitrous oxide.

Postoperatively, these infants may still have a metabolic alkalosis and may hypoventilate and retain carbon dioxide to compensate for this. For this reason extubation of these patients should be performed only after they are very awake and vigorous, and narcotic analgesics should be used with caution and in smaller than normal doses.

THE EX-PREMIE

Enormous advances in neonatology have increased the numbers of surviving premature infants. A significant number of these patients have systemic dysfunction including problems with the central nervous system, the lungs, and varying degrees of retinopathy of prematurity. Obviously, a number will present to the emergency department as infants. The most important problems are residual chronic obstructive pulmonary disease, apneas, and bradycardias.

In patients with bronchopulmonary dysplasia one may see abnormal blood gas values, abnormal resting flow rates, and an abnormal carbon dioxide response curve. These patients also have reactive airways and have an incidence of sudden infant death that is seven times normal [35]. They may have varying degrees of cor pulmonale and be on diuretic therapy. They may have more arrhythmias perioperatively than their normal counterparts.

A number of investigators have reported an increase in complications perioperatively in these patients. Steward reported an increase in the incidence of apnea, aspiration, and atelectasis in infants born prematurely who were undergoing hernia repair [36]. Liu reported a significant incidence of apnea during emergence from anesthesia in prematurely born infants with a history of idiopathic apneic episodes [37]. Because of these and other anecdotal reports and generalizations from them, prematurely born infants who are having surgery before they are 55 weeks post conception deserve special consideration [38]. They should not have surgery as outpatients and should be monitored postoperatively for 18 to 24 hours with apnea monitors and/or oximeters. They should be intubated for all but the shortest of procedures, and aspiration precautions should be taken during induction and emergence. These precautions may include a rapid sequence intravenous induction, cricoid pressure, preoperative gastric suctioning, and extubation only when alert, awake, and normothermic. Postoperative ventilation will be necessary in many major surgical procedures and even after minor procedures in some cases. Emergency physicians should use corresponding precautions for these patients after resuscitation.

When evaluating one of these infants in any stressed situation, the physician should remember the four As: apnea, aspiration, atelectasis, and arrhythmias, and react appropriately.

REFERENCES

1. Kunz, H., Michels, H., and Stickel, H. H. Differences in the binding of drugs to plasma proteins from newborn and adult man. *Europ. J. Clin. Pharmacol.* 11:469, 1977.
2. Borells, L. O., Jalling, B., and Kalberg, N. Clinical Pharmacology of Phenobarbital in the Neonatal Period. In P. L. Morselli (ed.), *Basic and Therapeutic Aspects of Perinatal Pharmacology.* New York: Raven Press, 1975.
3. Odell, G. B. Studies in kernicterus. I. The protein binding of bilirubin. *J. Clin. Invest.* 38:823, 1959.
4. Odell, G. B. Influence of binding on the toxicity of bilirubin. *Ann. N. Y. Acad. Sci.* 226:225, 1973.
5. Gregory, G. A. *Pediatric Anesthesia.* New York: Churchill Livingstone, 1983. P. 318.
6. Mangini, R. J. Clinically important cimetidine drug interactions. *Clin. Pharmacol.* 1:433, 1982.
7. Brandom, B. W., Brandom, R. B., and Cook, D. R. Uptake of halothane in infants. *Anesth. Analg.* 62:404, 1983.
8. Wark, H. J. Postoperative jaundice in children. *Anaesthesia* 38:237, 1983.
9. Gall, E. A. Report of the pathology panel. National Halothane study. *Anesthesiology* 29:233, 1968.
10. Berry, F. A. *Anesthetic Management of Routine and Difficult Pediatric Patients.* New York: Churchill Livingstone, 1986. P. 18.
11. Fisher, D. M., O'Keefe, C., Stanski, D. R., et al. Pharmacokinetics and dynamics of D-tubucurarine in infants, children, and adults. *Anesthesiology* 55:A391, 1981.
12. Cook, D. R., and Fischer, C. G. Neuromuscular blocking effects of succinylcholine in infants and children. *Anesthesiology* 42:662, 1975.
13. Ryan, J. F., Kagen, L. J., and Hyman, A. I. Myoglobinemia after a single dose of succinylcholine. *N. Engl. J. Med.* 285:824, 1971.
14. Zsigmond, E. K., Down, J., Jr. Plasma cholinesterase activity in infants and newborns. *Can. Anaesth. Soc. J.* 18:278, 1971.
15. Gardiner, M., Smith, M. L., Kagstrom, E., et al. Influence of blood glucose concentration on brain lactate accumulation during severe hypoxia and subsequent recovery of brain energy metabolism. *J. Cerebral Blood Flow Metab.* 2:429, 1982.
16. Smith, R. J., Keseg, D. P., Manley, L. K., et al. Intraosseus infusions by prehospital personnel in critically ill pediatric patients. *Ann. Emerg. Med.* 17:491, 1988.
17. Glaeser, P. W., and Losek, J. D. Emergency intraosseus infusions in children. *Am. J. Emerg. Med.* 4:34, 1986.
18. Tremper, K. K. Transcutaneous PO$_2$ measurement. *Can. Anaesth. Soc. J.* 31:664, 1984.

19. Friedman, W. F. The intrinsic properties of the developing heart. *Prog. Cardio-vasc. Dis.* 15:87, 1972.
20. Rudolph, A. M. *Congenital Diseases of the Heart.* Chicago: Year Book, 1974. Pp. 17–29.
21. Keen, E. H. The postnatal development of human cardiac ventricles. *J. Anaes.* 89:484, 1955.
22. Gilbert, R. D. Determinants of venous return in the fetal lamb. *Gynecol. Invest.* 8:233, 1977.
23. Guyton, A. C., and Sagawa, K. Compensations of cardiac output and other circulatory functions in areflexic dogs with large A-V fistulae. *Am. J. Physiol.* 200:1157, 1961.
24. Friesen, R. H., and Lichtor, J. L. Cardiovascular depression during halothane anesthesia in infants. A study of three induction techniques. *Anesth. Analg.* 61:42, 1982.
25. Lerman, J., Robinson, S., Willis, M. M., et al. Anesthetic requirements for halothane in young children 0–1 month and 1–6 months of age. *Anesthesiololgy* 59:421, 1983.
26. Gregory, G. A. The baro-responses of preterm infants during halothane anesthesia. *Can. Anaesth. Soc. J.* 29:105, 1982.
27. Rudolph, A. M. The changes in the circulation after birth. Their importance in congenital heart disease. *Circulation* 41:343, 1970.
28. Thibeault, D. W., Poblete, E., and Auld, P. A. M. Alveolar arterial O_2 and CO_2 differences and their relation to lung volume in the newborn. *Pediatrics* 41:574, 1968.
29. Rudolph, A. M., and Yuan, S. Response of the pulmonary vasculature to hypoxia and H^+ ion concentration changes. *J. Clin. Invest.* 45:399, 1966.
30. Lees, M. N., Way, R. C., and Ross, B. B. Ventilatory and respiratory gas transfer of infants with increased pulmonary blood flow. *Pediatrics* 40:259, 1967.
31. Shohat, M., Reisner, S. H., Kirkler, R., et al. Retinopathy of prematurity: Incidence and risk factors. *Pediatrics* 72:159, 1983.
32. Crone, R. K., et al. Survival of infants with CDH treated with perioperative anesthesia. *Anesthesiology* 63:3A–A481, 1985.
33. Rescorla, F. J., and Grosfeld, J. L. Inguinal hernia in the perinatal period and early infancy: Clinical considerations. *J. Pediatr. Surg.* 19:832, 1984.
34. Puri, P., Guiney, E. J., and O'Donnell, B. Inguinal hernia in infants: The fate of the testis following inguinal incarceration. *J. Pediatr. Surg.* 12:861, 1977.
35. Werthammer, J., Brown, E. R., Neff, R. K., et al. Sudden infant death syndrome in infants with bronchopulmonary dysplasia. *Pediatrics* 69:301, 1982.
36. Steward, D. J. Preterm infants are more prone to complications following minor surgery than are term infants. *Anesthesiology* 56:304, 1982.
37. Liu, L. M. P., Cote, C. J., Goudsouzian, N. G., et al. Life threatening apnea in infants recovering from anesthesia. *Anesthesiology* 59:506, 1983.
38. Berry, F. A. Anesthesia for premature nursery graduates. Children's Hospital, Los Angeles, Pediatric Anesthesia Conference, 1986.

9. Obstetric and Gynecologic Perspectives

Alan R. Snyder

The goals of this chapter are to discuss the anesthetic and medical needs of emergency department patients with obstetric or gynecologic problems. Review material is brief and is included in the discussions of particular patient problems. Many basic principles apply to different problems but are addressed only once to avoid repetition. For example, many of the considerations presented in the section on surgery in the pregnant patient apply to the pregnant patient who may present to the emergency department critically ill from trauma, hemorrhage, or eclampsia. In a desire to be practical, we have offered specific explanations or suggestions even though there are often a number of therapeutic options.

SURGERY IN THE PREGNANT PATIENT

Approximately 50,000 women per year in the United States undergo surgery while pregnant [1]. The two most common nonobstetric reasons for surgery during pregnancy are appendicitis and ovarian cysts. The primary considerations in providing preoperative care or anesthesia to the pregnant patient are the need to maximize both maternal safety and fetal safety.

To maximize maternal safety, a prior understanding of the physiologic alterations characteristic of pregnancy is desirable. Red cell volume increases during pregnancy (by approximately 20 percent), which is a smaller amount than the increase in plasma volume (approximately 40 percent). This accounts for the relative anemia of pregnancy [2]. As early as the first trimester, cardiac output in pregnant women increases about 40 percent above that of nonpregnant women, due in large part to increases in stroke volume (approximately 30 percent) and heart rate (approximately 15 percent).

Respiratory changes that occur during pregnancy are especially important to the emergency physician or anesthesiologist. The combination of increased minute ventilation and decreased functional residual capacity increases the rapidity with which alveolar concentrations of inhalational agents are altered. These factors, combined with the decreased minimum alveolar concentration (MAC) of inhalational anesthetics during pregnancy, increase the sensitivity of the pregnant patient to inhalational anesthetics. Additionally, increased capillary engorgement of the nasal and oral mucosa may make manipulation of the airway more difficult and hazardous [3].

Pregnant patients who become apneic during induction of general anesthesia are at a greater risk than nonpregnant patients for rapid decline in arterial oxygen concentration. This propensity for hypoxia also applies, of course, to the pregnant patient who presents to the emergency department in extremis for whatever reason. The primary factors that affect the speed of decline in PO_2 are the pregnant patient's decrease in functional residual capacity, which provides less oxygen reserve, increased use of oxygen, and increased alveolar-to-arterial oxygen gradient.

In addition to an increased sensitivity to inhalational anesthetics, the parturient usually requires a lower dose of local anesthetic in a spinal or epidural block to achieve the same degree of regional block. This is believed to be due in part to increased engorgement of the epidural veins, which decreases the available epidural or subarachnoid space. It is also believed that pregnancy causes increased sensitivity of the nerves to local anesthetics [3].

Pregnancy causes the following changes in the gastrointestinal system, necessitating the use of a cuffed endotracheal tube to reduce the risk of aspiration: First, the enlarged uterus displaces the pylorus upward and backward and consequently hinders gastric emptying. Second, the position of the stomach is altered, changing the angle of the gastroesophageal junction and predisposing the patient to gastric reflux. Third, the placenta produces the hormone gastrin, which stimulates gastric acid production and results in a lower gastric pH.

The principles involved in maximizing fetal safety can be considered in three categories: (1) avoiding teratogenic agents, (2) maximizing placental blood flow and oxygenation, and (3) avoiding premature labor.

To date, there are no studies that prove any anesthetic agent to be teratogenic when used during pregnancy. However, there are retrospective studies that suggest an association between the use of minor tranquilizers early in pregnancy and an increased incidence of congenital anomalies [4–6]. Despite the lack of definitive proof regarding their relative risk or safety, it may be advisable to avoid the use of minor tranquilizers during early pregnancy.

Placental blood flow and oxygenation are maximized by preventing maternal hypotension or hypoxia, and by avoiding excessive alterations in the maternal arterial carbon dioxide level. During the administration of a general anesthetic to a pregnant patient, it is desirable to maintain the inspired oxygen concentration at at least 50 percent. In addition, a pulse oximeter should be used.

Uterine displacement deserves special mention in connection with maximizing placental blood flow (Figs. 9-1 and 9-2). Maternal hypotension is more likely to occur in a pregnant patient placed in the supine position because the inferior vena cava is compressed, which decreases venous return to the heart. This decrease in preload results in decreased cardiac output and maternal hypotension. If maternal hypotension occurs, ephedrine (a nonselective synthetic noncatecholamine with both alpha- and beta-adrenergic properties [7]) in doses of 5 to 10 mg IV is the sympathomimetic of choice during pregnancy because it does not further decrease uterine blood flow. This action is in contrast to that of predominant alpha-agonists, which restore maternal blood pressure but may decrease uterine blood flow secondary to vasoconstriction [7]. Note, however, that maternal hypotension is not necessary for there to be decreased uterine blood flow. The nondisplaced gravid uterus may also compress the aorta and lower the perfusion pressure to the uterus without causing concomitant maternal symptoms.

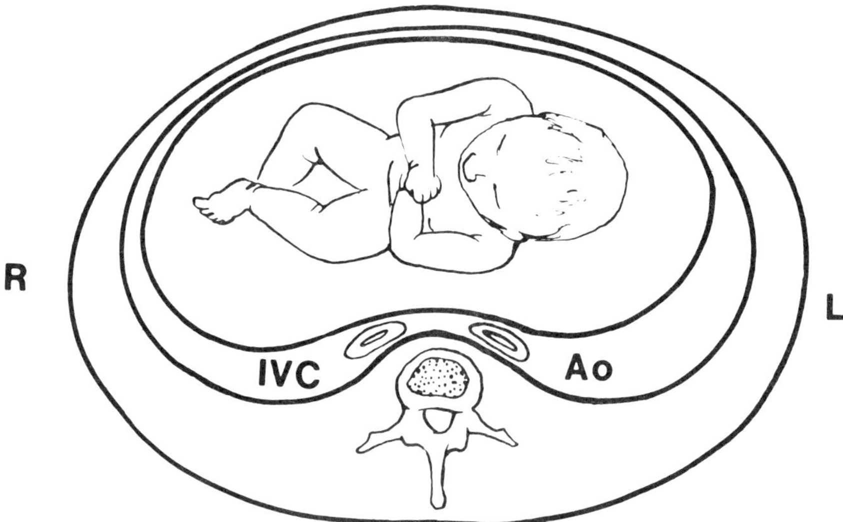

Fig. 9-1. Diagram demonstrating compression of both the inferior vena cava (IVC) and the abdominal aorta (Ao) when the parturient is supine. (From R. K. Stoelting and R. D. Miller [eds.], *Basics of Anesthesia.* New York: Churchill Livingstone, 1984. With permission.)

Avoiding premature labor is less a function of the type of anesthesia used than of the underlying pathology and the subsequent surgical procedure.

Specific recommendations have been made to help guide the delivery of anesthesia and surgery to the pregnant patient [8]. Elective surgery should be delayed until after delivery and maternal physiology has returned to normal. The possibility of pregnancy should be considered in all women of childbearing age.

When possible, it is preferable to avoid performing surgery in the first trimester of pregnancy. No anesthetic agent, whether premedicant, local, intravenous, or inhalational, has been proved to be teratogenic in humans. However, it is still prudent to minimize fetal exposure to medications, and a regional block is frequently recommended, especially in earlier gestations. A spinal block provides the lowest degree of fetal exposure to drugs. Precautions in the use of minor tranquilizers during early pregnancy have already been mentioned.

If surgery under general anesthesia is necessary, premedication with a nonparticulate oral antacid (e.g., sodium citrate, 30 ml PO) and a rapid sequence induction are frequently indicated. No specific technique of general anesthesia has been proved best during pregnancy. Special attention should be given to maintenance of a $PaCO_2$ normal for pregnancy (about 32 at term) as well as to adequate oxygenation. Left uterine displacement should be used during the second and third trimesters. Consideration should be given to monitoring fetal heart tones intraoperatively and monitoring for contractions postoperatively.

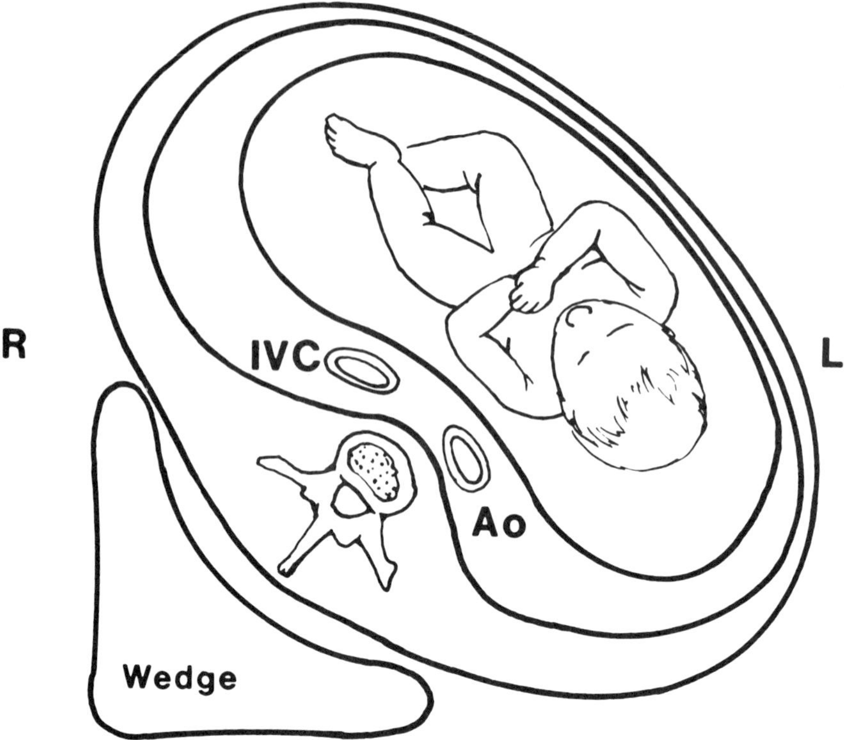

Fig. 9-2. Diagram demonstrating left uterine displacement by elevation of the parturient's right hip with a foam-rubber wedge. This position moves the gravid uterus off the inferior vena cava (IVC) and aorta (Ao). (From R. K. Stoelting and R. D. Miller [eds.], *Basics of Anesthesia.* New York: Churchill Livingstone, 1984. With permission.)

TRAUMA IN THE PREGNANT PATIENT

Trauma during pregnancy accounts for a significant percentage of nonobstetric deaths during pregnancy. The major causes of trauma during pregnancy are vehicular accidents, falls, and penetrating trauma [9]. Although evaluation and management of traumatized pregnant patients are similar to those of nonpregnant patients, some variations should be kept in mind in working with traumatized pregnant patients.

When placed supine, pregnant patients in their third trimester may manifest supine hypotensive syndrome secondary to aortocaval compression (see Figs. 9-1, 9-2). These patients should be placed in the left lateral position or at least have left uterine displacement. Left uterine displacement, however, should not take precedence over head and neck stabilization, when indicated, but once head and neck stabilization is achieved, left uterine displacement should be maintained.

Fetal well-being should be evaluated in conjunction with evaluation of the traumatized patient. Left uterine displacement and supplemental oxygen are appropriate to optimize fetal condition. Normal maternal responses to stress and trauma, such as vasoconstriction, may favor the mother while compromising the fetus.

Pregnancy may alter the presentation of or response to injury. Hypovolemia, slightly lower blood pressure, and a slightly higher pulse are normally present in pregnancy. Diagnosis of hypovolemia may be more difficult because the pregnant patient may be able to tolerate blood loss of up to 30 percent before clinical manifestations of hypovolemia appear [9]. Volume replacement is the preferred response to hypovolemia, and if necessary, ephedrine is preferable to alpha agents.

X-ray studies should be used selectively in pregnant patients, and the abdomen should be shielded when possible. Peritoneal lavage can still be effectively used in the pregnant patient, although the "open" technique (opening the peritoneum under direct vision) may be preferred.

CARDIOPULMONARY RESUSCITATION IN THE PREGNANT PATIENT

Cardiac arrest in the pregnant patient should be treated in the usual manner. Establishment of a secure airway, control of breathing, external cardiac massage, defibrillation if indicated, and use of medications are utilized as in the nonpregnant patient.

Normal $PaCO_2$ in a term pregnant patient is approximately 32 mm Hg, and an attempt should be made to maintain this level through ventilation. In addition, the pregnant uterus may make external cardiac compression less effective when the patient is supine, and hence left uterine displacement should be maintained if possible. However, in a pregnant patient in the third trimester undergoing cardiac arrest, it is difficult to perform effective cardiopulmonary resuscitation (CPR) with the patient in a lateral position, but it is also difficult to get effective perfusion with CPR with the patient in the supine position owing to aortocaval compression.

In this unfortunate situation, a perimortem cesarean section should be promptly considered to optimize chances for both the mother and the fetus [10, 11]. Even if the mother is not resuscitatable, a perimortem cesarean section should be considered if fetal heart tones are still present.

One possible technique for performing an emergency cesarean section would be as follows. While continuing ventilation and chest compressions on the mother, preparation of the abdomen can be performed by pouring povidone-iodine over the abdomen and then making a vertical midline incision from the pubic symphysis to the umbilicus. This incision can be carried down to the fascia. The fascial incision is extended with a pair of scissors. The peritoneum is entered from the upper portion of the incision to minimize the possibility of entering the bladder. The incision into the uterus can be done with either the "classic" vertical incision or a lower segment transverse incision depending on the experience of the operator. The infant is delivered from the uterus using upper abdominal pressure while guiding the infant out of the uterus. The cord is then doubly clamped and cut, and the infant is handed off for evaluation and any indicated resuscitation. The placenta is manually removed from the uterus, and the uterine incision is closed, usually with a running hemostatic closure. If uterine atony and subsequent blood loss are encountered, uterine massage may be utilized in addition to uterotonic agents. After securing hemostasis of the uterine incision, the peritoneum, fascia, and skin can be closed in a conventional manner.

ABNORMALITIES OF EARLY PREGNANCY

Abnormalities in early pregnancy frequently involve vaginal bleeding. Two common abnormalities are ectopic pregnancy and abortion.

Ectopic pregnancy is the abnormal implantation of a fertilized ovum, usually in the fallopian tube. Pain is the most common symptom of tubal pregnancy. Amenorrhea with or without atypical vaginal bleeding, lower abdominal pain, and an adnexal mass are the classic signs and symptoms of tubal pregnancy. Significant blood loss can accompany ectopic pregnancy, and the patient's clinical condition will dictate certain aspects of anesthetic management. In the emergency department, attention should be given to establishing good IV access, restoring blood volume, procuring appropriate laboratory tests, and symptomatic care as needed (e.g., oxygen by face mask and Trendelenburg positioning). If general anesthesia is necessary, ketamine is a good choice as an induction agent in the patient with acute blood loss.

Vaginal bleeding not associated with an ectopic pregnancy may also accompany one of the many different types of abortion. Threatened abortion is present in intrauterine pregnancies when vaginal bleeding occurs in the first 20 weeks. These pregnancies may go on to complete the abortion or may proceed to a viable gestation. Anesthetic care should be limited to close observation of the patient and avoidance of medications that are potentially harmful in early pregnancy. Abortions that are inevitable, incomplete, complete, or septic frequently are managed by performing a dilation and curettage. The same general principles of management apply as for ectopic pregnancies. If the bleeding is substantial and an operating room is not immediately available, it is possible to perform a dilation and curettage in the emergency department using a combination of intravenous sedation and a paracervical block.

A paracervical block is performed by injecting a local anesthetic into the fornix of the vagina lateral to the cervix in the area of Frankenhäuser's ganglion. This block can be accomplished by injecting 5 to 10 ml of 1% lidocaine lateral to the cervix at the 4 and 8 o'clock positions. This will provide anesthesia in the uterus, cervix, and upper vagina, although not in the area of the perineum.

Most experts advocate the use of Rh_o (D) immune globulin (RhoGAM) in Rh-negative women with abortions that have reached at least 8 weeks' gestation. The risk of the mother developing Rh sensitization far outweighs the risks associated with the administration of Rh_o (D) immune globulin when the fetal blood type is unknown.

A missed abortion is present when the uterus fails to expel the conceptus after it dies in utero. If the products of conception are maintained in utero for longer than 3 weeks after demise, development of a coagulation defect may occur. This is due to the absorption of thromboplastins released in the process of fetal autolysis. Patients suspected of having a missed abortion should have clotting studies done in connection with other laboratory work.

ANTEPARTUM AND POSTPARTUM HEMORRHAGE (BLEEDING IN LATE PREGNANCY)

Hemorrhage in late pregnancy, antepartum and postpartum, is a leading cause of maternal morbidity and mortality. The most common causes of serious bleeding in the third trimester are placenta previa and abruptio placentae. Uterine rupture is a less common event. The initial emergency management of antepartum hemorrhage is similar for all three types. Postpartum hemorrhage is typically caused by retained products of conception, uterine atony, or cervical or vaginal lacerations.

Placenta previa is the abnormally low implantation of the placenta in the uterus. This condition can lead to severe blood loss. The cardinal symptom of placenta previa is painless, bright red vaginal bleeding in the third trimester.

A vaginal examination should not be performed in the emergency department on a patient with third trimester bleeding. If placenta previa were present, a vaginal examination could precipitate a life-threatening hemorrhage. An ultrasound examination may help to locate the placenta. If a vaginal examination is desired for definitive diagnosis, it should only be performed in the operating room using a "double setup."

To prepare for a double setup, the emergency physician can be instrumental in organizing the notification and preparation of the operating team as well as ensuring the availability of blood and restoring the maternal volume. A central venous pressure line may be helpful in achieving normal maternal volume. At least one and preferably two large-bore intravenous lines should be in place. At least two units of crossmatched blood should be in the operating room. The patient should receive a nonparticulate antacid and a defasciculating dose of curare, preoxygenation should be done, and the abdomen should be prepped and draped with surgeons standing by prior to the vaginal examination. An assistant for the anesthesiologist should also be standing by to help apply cricoid pressure or assist with volume administration if a brisk hemorrhage occurs.

If a cesarean section is performed, ketamine is a good drug for use in induction of general anesthesia in patients with acute blood loss. It should be remembered that doses of ketamine in excess of 1 mg/kg are associated with increased uterine tone [12]. The infant delivered from a mother with bleeding placenta previa may be acidotic and hypovolemic.

Abruptio placentae is the separation of the normally implanted placenta from the uterus after the twentieth week of gestation but prior to delivery of the fetus. It can lead to severe blood loss or clotting abnormalities in the mother as well as fetal distress. It may be accompanied by dark vaginal bleeding, maternal hypovolemia, uterine irritability and tenderness, abdominal pain, and fetal distress.

The definitive management of abruptio placentae is emptying the uterus. If an emergency cesarean section is performed, ketamine is a good agent for induction of general anesthesia. Appropriate steps should be taken to treat blood loss or clotting abnormalities.

After the fetus and placenta are delivered, normal uterine tone may be more difficult to achieve than in a normal delivery. Intravenous (20 to 40 units/liter) or intramuscular (10 to 20 units IM) pitocin should be used to promote uterine tone, but it may not be sufficient. In those cases, intravenous or intramuscular methergine (0.2 to 0.3 mg) or intramuscular 15-methyl prostaglandin $F_{2\alpha}$ (250 mg) should be used immediately.

The major causes of postpartum hemorrhage are retained products of conception, uterine atony, and vaginal or cervical lacerations. Most episodes of early postpartum hemorrhage will occur in labor and delivery, but they may also occur initially in the emergency department in a recently delivered patient.

Retained products of conception frequently necessitate manual exploration of the inside of the uterus. If the patient cannot tolerate this examination or if the uterus is contracted around the retained fragments, a general anesthetic with endotracheal intubation may be required. Blood volume should promptly be restored toward normal. If uterine relaxation is required for exploration, the volatile agents (halothane, enflurane, and isoflurane) provide uterine relaxation, whereas ketamine increases uterine tone. After evacuation of the inside of the uterus, medication to augment uterine tone may be required.

Uterine atony is the most frequent cause of postpartum hemorrhage.

Emergency department management of this problem should include restoration of blood volume, symptomatic treatment, and both manual uterine massage and pharmacologic support to promote increased uterine tone.

The pharmacologic agents most often used to promote uterine tone are pitocin, methergine, and prostaglandin $F_{2\alpha}$ [13–15]. Oxytocin acts on the uterine smooth muscle, stimulating both the frequency and force of contractions. Dilute solutions of synthetic oxytocins (such as pitocin, 20 to 40 units/liter) exert minimal cardiovascular effects. However, bolus injections of pitocin may produce a decrease in the systolic and especially the diastolic blood pressures, tachycardia, and cardiac dysrhythmias. In high doses, an antidiuretic effect may occur [16].

Methergine in small doses also increases the frequency and force of contractions. In higher concentrations, contractions become more intense and prolonged, and there is an increase in resting tone between contractions. Effects on the cardiovascular system can include vasoconstriction or hypertension [16].

Intramuscular prostaglandin $F_{2\alpha}$ is also effective for increasing uterine tone. Nausea and vomiting may occur with its use. In asthmatic patients bronchospasm may occur [16].

If the above measures prove insufficient to control blood loss, surgical ligation of the internal iliac arteries or hysterectomy may become necessary.

Genital lacerations may be a cause of postpartum hemorrhage. These are usually apparent on close examination, and management consists of repair of the injuries and replacement of blood volume as well as general supportive measures.

OBSTETRIC EMERGENCIES

Premature rupture of membranes and premature labor are two related obstetric problems that may appear in the emergency department.

Premature rupture of membranes has variously been defined as rupture of membranes prior to term (term being 37 to 42 gestational weeks), or rupture of the membranes prior to the onset of labor, regardless of gestational age. Usually anesthetic care in the emergency room is minimal because these patients are generally referred to the obstetrician on call or to the labor and delivery department. Nevertheless, fetal heart tones should be at least briefly monitored in the emergency department. If possible, vaginal examinations should be avoided in patients with prematurely ruptured membranes because the greater the number of examinations, the greater the risk of subsequent infection.

Premature labor is the onset of labor prior to 37 weeks' gestation. If a tocolytic agent is used to treat premature labor, it is usually one of the beta-sympathomimetics (isoxsuprine, ritodrine, or terbutaline), although magnesium sulfate is also an effective tocolytic. The anesthetic implications of the use of magnesium are discussed below in the section on preeclampsia-eclampsia.

Numerous potential maternal side effects are associated with the use of beta-sympathomimetics that may interact with subsequent anesthetics. Maternal cardiovascular responses to beta-sympathomimetics can include tachycardia, cardiac dysrhythmias, hypotension due to decreased peripheral vascular resistance, and occasionally pulmonary edema. Additional maternal responses may include hyperglycemia, metabolic acidosis, and the shift of potassium intracellularly, manifested as hypokalemia [16]. Despite the presence of beta-sympathomimetic-induced hypokalemia, additional potassium has not been recommended as necessary.

Appropriate fetal monitoring in the emergency department may include an external tocometer for monitoring contractions, and an externally applied monitor to detect fetal heart tones (FHTs). Both the baseline of the FHTs and alterations from baseline, either accelerations or decelerations, are helpful in evaluating fetal condition. The normal baseline for FHTs is 110 to 160 beats per minute (bpm). Accelerations above baseline as well as variability in the baseline are usually indicative of fetal well-being. Decelerations can be classified into four categories:

1. Early decelerations (type I) (Fig. 9-3) mirror the contractions in onset, peak, and duration. This type of deceleration is believed to be a reflex vagal response secondary to fetal head compression. It is not a sign of fetal compromise.
2. Late decelerations (type II) (Fig. 9-4) occur after the onset of the contraction and last longer than the contraction. This type of deceleration is believed to be due to uteroplacental insufficiency and may indicate fetal distress. It is especially ominous if it is associated with fetal tachycardia and/or decreased variability.
3. Variable decelerations (type III) (Fig. 9-5) occur without any consistent relationship to the contractions. They are variable in onset, duration, and configuration. They are believed to be secondary to umbilical cord compression and are not necessarily associated with fetal distress.
4. Prolonged decelerations are decelerations in the fetal heart tones that last longer than 2 minutes. If this condition does not resolve, operative intervention should be anticipated.

PREECLAMPSIA-ECLAMPSIA

Preeclampsia is a syndrome that occurs after the twentieth week of gestation and is characterized by elevated blood pressure, generalized edema,

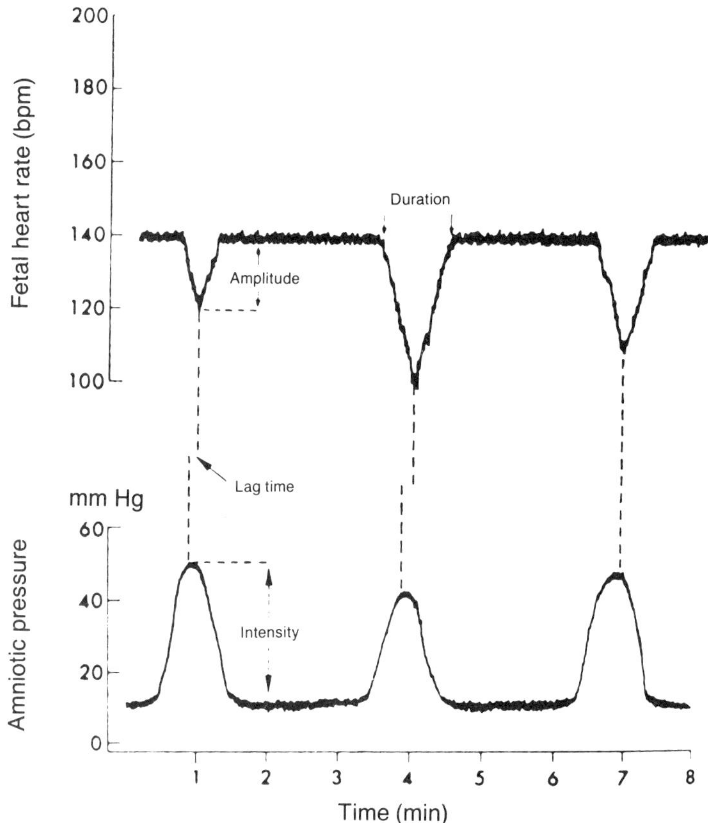

Fig. 9-3. Early decelerations of the fetal heart rate are characterized by a short lag time between the onset of the uterine contraction and the beginning of heart rate slowing. The maximum slowing of the fetal heart rate occurs at the peak intensity of the contraction. Fetal heart rate is back to normal by the time the contraction has ceased. The most likely explanation for this fetal heart rate slowing, which is generally considered benign, is vagal stimulation due to compression of the fetal head. (From S. M. Shnider. Diagnosis of Fetal Distress: Fetal Heart Rate. In S. M. Shnider [ed.], *Obstetrical Anesthesia: Current Concepts and Practice.* Baltimore: Williams & Wilkins, 1970. With permission.)

and proteinuria. For diagnosis, elevated blood pressure and at least one other sign or symptom is required. Elevation in blood pressure means an increase in the systolic blood pressure of at least 30 mm Hg (or to above 140 mm Hg), an increase in the diastolic blood pressure of at least 15 mm Hg (or to above 90 mm Hg), or an increase in the mean arterial pressure of at least 20 mm Hg (or to above 105 mm Hg). Severe preeclampsia exists if at least one of the following occurs: systolic blood pressure greater than

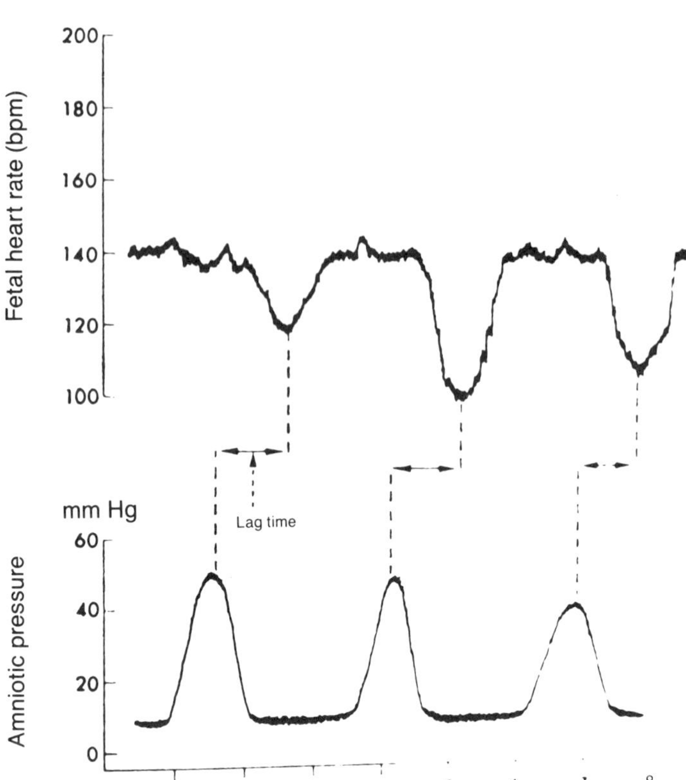

Fig. 9-4. Late decelerations of the fetal heart rate are characterized by a delay between the onset of the uterine contraction and the beginning of fetal heart rate slowing. The fetal heart rate does not return to normal until after the contraction has ceased. Late decelerations are ominous and indicate uteroplacental insufficiency. They mandate rapid correction of maternal hypotension and supplemental oxygen. If they are persistent, fetal scalp pH measurements and, if necessary, emergent cesarean section may be indicated. (From S. M. Shnider. Diagnosis of Fetal Distress: Fetal Heart Rate. In S. M. Shnider [ed.], *Obstetrical Anesthesia: Current Concepts and Practice.* Baltimore: Williams & Wilkins, 1970. With permission.)

160 mm Hg, diastolic blood pressure greater than 110 mm Hg, or mean arterial pressure greater than 120 mm Hg, proteinuria of greater than 5 gm/ 24 hours, headache or visual alterations, epigastric pain, pulmonary edema, or cyanosis. If seizures occur in addition to the preeclampsia, eclampsia is said to coexist.

Preclamptic patients are frequently intravascularly depleted, with low central venous pressures despite their generalized edema. The leading cause of maternal mortality incident to preeclampsia is intracranial hem-

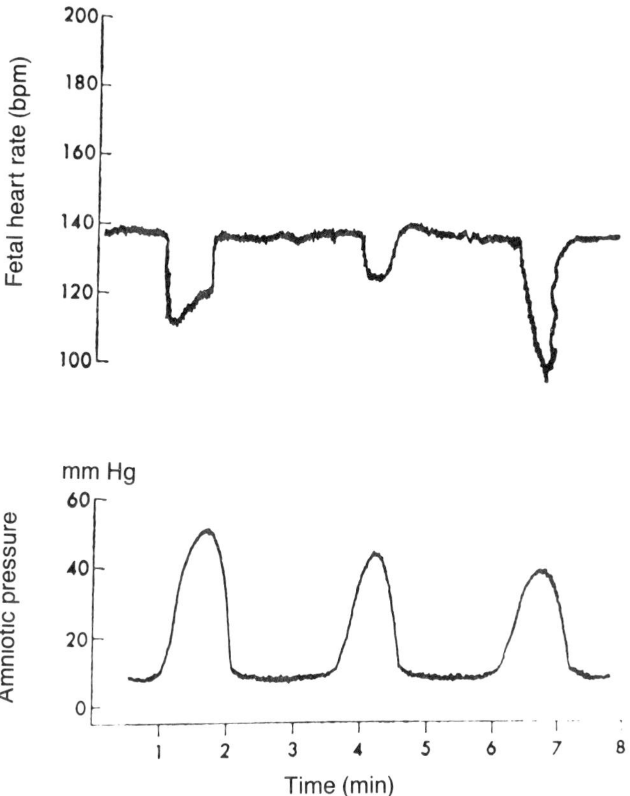

Fig. 9-5. Variable decelerations of fetal heart rate are characterized by varying magnitudes and time of onset of heart rate slowing. This pattern is usually benign but, if persistent, may reflect compression of the umbilical cord. (From S. M. Schnider. Diagnosis of Fetal Distress: Fetal Heart Rate. In S. M. Schnider [ed.], *Obstetrical Anesthesia: Current Concepts and Practice.* Baltimore: Williams & Wilkins, 1970. With permission.)

orrhage, and a careful neurologic examination is indicated in every patient with preeclampsia or eclampsia. A further potential complication of pre-eclampsia is the development of disseminated intravascular coagulation.

In eclampsia, the first priority is to control the seizures and ensure adequate oxygenation and ventilation. A number of medications have been suggested for immediate treatment of the seizures, including sodium thiopental 50 to 100 mg, diazepam 2.5 to 5 mg, or magnesium sulfate 2 to 6 gm intravenously. Occasionally it is necessary to apply cricoid pressure, give a muscle relaxant such as succinylcholine, and then intubate the patient. This may be required to control recurrent seizures, to protect the airway from aspiration, or to manage postictal respiratory depression. Further seizures are prevented by the administration of parenteral magnesium.

Following a seizure, maternal blood gases should be checked to assess the possible need for bicarbonate and the adequacy of ventilation and oxygenation. If cerebral edema is suspected, mannitol and possibly steroids should be considered. Care should be exercised in the use of mannitol if the urinary output is already low because of the risk of intravascular depletion.

Magnesium sulfate is used to prevent seizures in preeclamptic-eclamptic patients. It acts centrally to decrease the irritability of the central nervous system. It also acts at the neuromuscular junction to reduce the presynaptic release of acetylcholine, diminishing the sensitivity of the end plate to acetylcholine, and depressing the excitability of the muscle membrane. In light of its mechanisms of action, it is understandable that it would increase the sensitivity of the mother to both depolarizing and nondepolarizing muscle relaxants [17]. Therapeutic maternal blood levels of magnesium sulfate are approximately 4 to 8 meq/liter. Overdoses of magnesium sulfate are manifested first by abolition of deep tendon reflexes and then by onset of skeletal muscle weakness. Levels beyond this can lead to respiratory and then cardiac arrest. Magnesium also crosses the placenta. Intravenous calcium is an antidote to excessive levels of magnesium [18]. Magnesium is excreted renally, and care must be exercised in its administration to patients with impaired renal function or decreased urinary output.

The definitive treatment of preeclampsia-eclampsia is delivery of the fetus and placenta. In the interim, magnesium is frequently required, and antihypertensives may also be necessary.

The goal of antihypertensive therapy is not to bring the blood pressure down to the average range for a normal pregnancy but to maintain the diastolic pressure below 110 mm Hg. If the blood pressure is brought down too fast, there may be insufficient placental perfusion; accordingly, fetal heart tones need to be continuously monitored. Urinary output should also be followed.

Hydralazine is frequently the antihypertensive chosen to treat preeclamptic patients. It has a relatively rapid onset of action and tends to maintain or even improve renal blood flow.

For emergency treatment of a hypertensive crisis, intravenous trimethaphan, nitroprusside, or nitroglycerin provides a prompt response. Continued use of nitroprusside is discouraged, however, because cyanide can cross the placenta and potentially affect the fetus adversely.

As soon as possible, the patient should be transferred to the obstetric suite to await delivery and to allow continued monitoring of FHTs and maternal status.

In labor and delivery, there are a host of problems associated with delivery of anesthesia care to preeclamptic patients. Relative intravascular depletion requiring careful hydration must be balanced against an increased risk of development of pulmonary edema and congestive heart failure. Clotting studies must be checked prior to use of regional anesthesia. General anesthesia also has numerous potential pitfalls. Because magnesium potentiates skeletal muscle relaxants, caution should be exercised in using additional muscle relaxants after the intubating dose of succinylcholine has worn off because any further muscle relaxant may be difficult to reverse at the end of surgery. Precurarization is probably not necessary and is potentially hazardous in patients receiving magnesium. Generalized edema may also be present in the nasal and oral mucosa, making intubation both more difficult and more hazardous. Additionally, preeclamptic and eclamptic patients are especially sensitive to endogenous or exogenous catecholamines.

AMNIOTIC FLUID EMBOLISM

Amniotic fluid embolism is an obstetric emergency that occurs when amniotic fluid enters the maternal circulation, usually in association with a tumultuous labor. It is characterized by the sudden onset of respiratory distress, hypotension, and arterial hypoxemia and can quickly progress to include severe hemorrhage secondary to disseminated intravascular coagulation and uterine atony.

Once the amniotic fluid has entered the maternal circulation through a break in the membranes, a series of events occurs in the pulmonary vessels of the mother. Because of a combination of mechanical and vasospastic responses there is a sudden decrease in blood return to the left side of the heart, manifested as hypotension and a decrease in cardiac output; concomitantly, pulmonary hypertension and failure of the right side of the heart may occur. The resulting hypoxemia may be worsened by a ventilation-to-perfusion mismatch. This may be followed rapidly by severe hemorrhage secondary to coagulation defects and uterine atony.

Although the incidence of amniotic fluid embolism is rare, approximately 1 in 20,000 deliveries, the mortality associated with its occurrence is high, often quoted at approximately 80 percent [19]. Aggressive medical management is necessary if survival chances are to be improved.

The first step is to treat the respiratory distress and hypoxemia. This may require intubation and ventilation with 100% oxygen. The addition of positive end-expiratory pressure (PEEP) should be considered.

After establishing adequate ventilation and oxygenation, attention is focused on the circulatory system. If peripheral pulses are not palpable, cardiopulmonary resuscitation should be begun. Vasopressors and inotropes should be used as necessary. At least two large intravenous lines should be in place for administration of volume and medications.

The electrocardiogram should be monitored continuously, and central venous pressure and urinary output should be monitored as soon as possible. Arterial blood gases should be measured and full clotting studies done along with other indicated laboratory work.

Delivery of the fetus should be considered as soon as possible to maximize the chances of survival for both infant and mother. It is doubtful that even properly performed CPR will provide adequate uteroplacental perfusion in the term pregnant patient (see section on Cardiopulmonary Resuscitation in the Pregnant Patient). In addition, it is felt that once the uterus is empty and aortocaval compression is no longer present, resuscitation of the mother is more effective.

The administration of digoxin may be appropriate for the treatment of cardiac failure. Also, furosemide may be helpful in treating the pulmonary edema that frequently occurs as a result of amniotic fluid embolism. The use of 1- to 2-gm boluses of hydrocortisone also has been advocated.

After initial resuscitation and stabilization, attention should be directed toward restoring circulating blood volume and coagulation by administering blood to improve oxygen-carrying capacity and fresh frozen plasma, platelets, and possibly cryoprecipitate to correct clotting deficiencies.

REFERENCES

1. Levinson, G., and Shnider, S. M. Anesthesia for Surgery During Pregnancy. In S. M. Shnider and G. Levinson (eds.), *Anesthesia for Obstetrics* (2nd ed.). Baltimore: Williams & Wilkins, 1987. P. 188.
2. Campbell, C., and Ravindran, R. S. The Pregnant Patient. In R. K. Stoelting and S. F. Dierdorf (eds.), *Anesthesia and Co-existing Disease*. New York: Churchill Livingstone, 1983. Pp. 683–739.
3. Shnider, S. M., and Levinson, G. Obstetric Anesthesia. In R. D. Miller (ed.), *Anesthesia* (2nd ed.). New York: Churchill Livingstone, 1986. Pp. 1681–1728.
4. Milkovich, L., and Van den Berg, B. J. Effects of prenatal meprobamate and chlordiazepoxide on human embryonic and fetal development. *N. Engl. J. Med.* 291:1268–1271, 1974.
5. Saxen, I., and Saxen, L. Association between maternal intake of diazepam and oral clefts. *Lancet* 2:498, 1975.
6. Safra, M. J., and Oakley, G. P. Association between cleft lip with or without cleft palate and prenatal exposure to diazepam. *Lancet* 2:478–480, 1975.
7. Stoelting, R. K. Sympathomimetics. In R. K. Stoelting, *Pharmacology and Physiology in Anesthetic Practice*. Philadelphia: J. B. Lippincott, 1987. Pp. 251–268.
8. Levinson, G., and Shnider, S. M. Anesthesia for Surgery During Pregnancy. In S. M. Shnider and G. Levinson (eds.), *Anesthesia for Obstetrics* (2nd ed.). Baltimore: Williams & Wilkins, 1987. P. 201.
9. Hochbaum, S. R. Vaginal Bleeding. In P. Rosen (ed.), *Emergency Medicine* (2nd ed.). St. Louis: C. V. Mosby, 1988. Pp. 1605–1612.
10. Katz, V. L., Dotter, D. J., and Droegmuller, W. Perimortem cesarean delivery. *Obstet. Gynecol.* 68:571–576, 1986.
11. Marx, G. F. Cardiopulmonary resuscitation of late pregnant women. *Anesthesiology* 56:156, 1982.
12. Galloon, S. Ketamine for obstetric delivery. *Anesthesiology* 44:522–524, 1976.

13. Fredericksen, M. C. What place for ergot alkaloids in OB today? *Contemp. OB/ GYN* June 1988, 37–44.
14. Hayashi, R. H., Castillo, M. S., and Noah, M. L. Management of severe postpartum hemorrhage with a prostaglandin F2-alpha analogue. *Obstet. Gynecol.* 63:806–808, 1984.
15. Rall, T. W., and Scheifer, L. S. Oxytocin, Prostaglandins, Ergot Alkaloids and Other Drugs; Tocolytic Agents. In A. G. Gilman and L. S. Goodman (eds.), *The Pharmacologic Basis of Therapeutics* (7th ed.). New York: Macmillan, 1985. Pp. 926–945.
16. Stoelting, R. K. Hormones as Drugs. In R. K. Stoelting, *Pharmacology and Physiology in Anesthetic Practice.* Philadelphia: J. B. Lippincott, 1987. Pp. 394–413.
17. Ghomeim, N. M., and Long, J. P. The interaction between magnesium and other neuromuscular blocking agents. *Anesthesiology* 32:232–237, 1970.
18. Stoelting, R. K. Minerals. In R. K. Stoelting, *Pharmacology and Physiology in Anesthetic Practice.* Philadelphia: J. B. Lippincott, 1987. Pp. 394–413.
19. Morgan, M. Amniotic fluid embolism. *Anaesthesia* 34:20–32, 1979.

10. Gastrointestinal and Renal Considerations

Richard J. Unger

The emergency physician and anesthesiologist are often called on to treat patients with gastrointestinal and renal disorders. Not being wary of the patient with a full stomach can lead to disastrous pulmonary complications. Overvigorous iced saline gastric lavage can worsen hypothermia. Pharmacologic management of the patient with liver disease is challenging.

If the clinician is not vigilant, renal failure may develop in the trauma patient in the emergency department or during the perioperative period. Complications of chronic renal failure may be misunderstood. With these and other dilemmas in mind, this chapter has been written to elucidate some of the important aspects of renal and gastrointestinal disease for the emergency physician and anesthesiologist.

GASTROINTESTINAL DISORDERS

ASPIRATION PREVENTION AND PROPHYLAXIS

Aspiration of gastric contents may have disastrous consequences. The three most important factors that correlate with severity of aspiration are the presence of particulate matter, the volume of fluid aspirated (> 25 ml), and pH (< 2.5) [1]. Anything that decreases barrier pressure or lower esophageal sphincter (LES) tone or increases gastric volume or acidity will either make aspiration more likely or worsen the consequences of aspiration, respectively. Factors that increase gastric volume include recent ingestion of food (< 6 to 8 hours), bowel obstruction, pregnancy (> 20 weeks), or pain. Factors that lower pH include pregnancy, recent ingestion of food or alcohol, and certain drugs and endocrine disorders that lower gastric pH. Nasogastric tubes, hiatal hernia, scleroderma, airway trauma, and obesity all predispose to increased risk of aspiration by undermining the ability of the lower esophageal sphincter to function as a competent barrier. In addition, aging lowers LES pressures, the lithotomy position increases intragastric pressures, and trauma may interfere with the physiologic function of the lower esophageal sphincter [2].

The best way to prevent aspiration is to ensure that none of the aforementioned factors are present before intubation or before an anesthetic is administered. The presence of a cuffed endotracheal tube will prevent particulate aspiration but will not prevent small volumes of gastric fluid from leaking into the lungs around the cuff. Strategies exist to secure an endotracheal tube with some degree of safety. Awake intubation allows the clinician to insert the instrument in the airway while the patient's airway reflexes are still intact. These reflexes include the gag and cough reflex. Topical or regional anesthesia of the airway in combination with intravenous sedation are often used to facilitate awake intubation, but one must take care that the patient is not oversedated and has enough of a cough reflex present to prevent aspiration. Awake intubation can be accomplished blindly or with the aid of a standard laryngoscope or fiberoptic bronchoscope. Most patients tolerate awake nasotracheal intubation better than awake orotracheal intubation with a laryngoscope. The method used depends on the technical skill of the clinician and the clinical condition of the patient (see Chapter 2).

The other commonly used technique that provides rapid control of the airway is referred to as the rapid sequence induction (RSI) or "crash" induction, which depends on the aid of cricoid pressure. This technique consists of preoxygenation for 3 to 5 minutes, cricoid pressure and simultaneous administration of an anesthetic agent (sodium thiopental or ketamine), and a rapidly acting muscle relaxant (usually succinylcholine). The patient is preoxygenated for 3 to 5 minutes to allow complete washout of nitrogen, which allows the functional residual capacity (FRC) to serve as an oxygen reservoir while the airway is being secured. In healthy subjects with normal pulmonary gas exchange, FRC, and oxygen consumption, adequate preoxygenation will prevent oxygen desaturation for 8 to 10 minutes without ventilation. Patients who have impaired pulmonary gas exchange, low FRC, or high oxygen consumption have a lower margin of safety with preoxygenation.

Cricoid pressure (or the Sellick maneuver) is applied at the cricoid cartilage, not over the thyroid cartilage or the entire larynx (Fig. 10-1). The pressure should not be removed until proper position of the endotracheal tube has been confirmed [3]. Proper preoxygenation with continuous monitoring of oxygen saturation allows the airway to be controlled without the need of mask ventilation. Mask ventilation increases gastric pressures and volumes, which will further increase the likelihood of gastric aspiration. If mask ventilation is necessary, it should be done only while constant cricoid pressure is being maintained by an assistant (see Chapter 2) [4].

Certain drugs may help to prevent gastric aspiration and lessen sequelae from gastric aspiration. Metoclopramide (Reglan) is a dopamine antagonist that may be administered orally or parenterally. It increases LES tone and lowers pyloric and duodenal tone. It also enhances gastric and small bowel motility and, in addition, has central antinausea effects. Such a drug, which increases barrier pressure, decreases nausea, and lowers the chances of emesis, has obvious utility in both the emergency department and the opereating room. Ideally, the dose should be 10 mg PO 30 to 120 minutes before intubation or 10 mg IV 15 to 30 minutes before intubation in order to lower gastric volume and increase LES pressure optimally. The effect of the drug is quite rapid when given intravenously, and it may be efficacious if used emergently during preoxygenation. Side effects are unusual at these low doses and include dry mouth, sedation, facial edema, and extrapyramidal reactions. Extrapyramidal reactions are very rare and promptly respond to intravenous diphenylhydramine [5].

Antacids are used to increase gastric pH and thereby lower morbidity from aspiration of gastric contents. Nonparticulate antacids should be used because aluminum- and magnesium-containing antacids are themselves

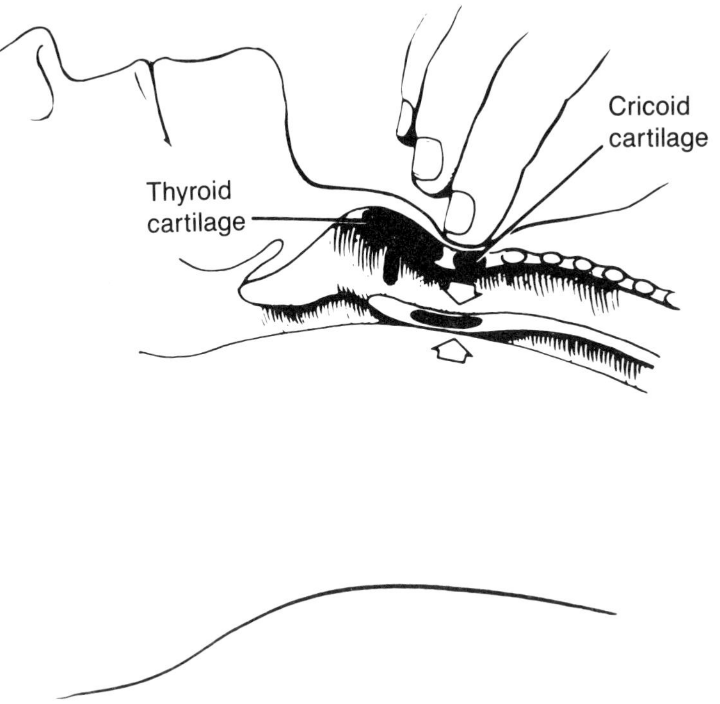

Fig. 10-1. Digital pressure on the cricoid cartilage (i.e., Sellick's maneuver) is demonstrated. Pressure on the thyroid cartilage, the "Adam's apple," is much less effective because only the cricoid ring has a cartilaginous posterior element. Cricoid pressure can block regurgitation but not active vomiting. (From W. Hamelberg and P. B. Bosomworth. *Aspiration Pneumonitis.* Springfield, Ill.: Thomas, 1968. With permission.)

harmful to the lung parenchyma [6]. Sodium citrate (Bicitra), 15 to 30 ml of 0.3 mol solution, will effectively raise gastric pH and should be administered before intubation, if possible, when the patient has an underlying hyperacidic condition such as pregnancy or Zollison-Ellinger syndrome. Antacids work quickly but have the decided disadvantage of increasing gastric volume [7, 8]. Their use in the emergency department is probably limited.

Histamine 2 (H_2) receptor blockers inhibit secretion of gastric acid mediated by way of histamine release. H_2 receptors are also present in the myocardium and central nervous system [9, 10]. H_2 blockers halt secretion of acid by the parietal cells but do nothing to empty the stomach or to neutralize the acid that is already present. H_2 blockers have no consistent effect on gastric volume [11].

Cimetidine (300 mg IV or PO) and ranitidine (50 mg IV, 150 mg PO) are available for both oral and parenteral use. High-risk patients should be treated with one dose the night before anesthesia and another dose the next morning 90 to 120 minutes before induction of anesthesia. If a more rapid effect is needed, as would be expected in the emergency department, or if the patient is unable to take oral medications, intravenous H_2 therapy should be used [12].

Cimetidine has a greater incidence of side effects than ranitidine because it penetrates cardiac and nervous tissue more readily. H_2 blockers may reduce heart rate and blood pressure, increase airway resistance, and cause agitation, confusion, and seizures [13]. Cimetidine can interfere with the metabolism of certain drugs such as lidocaine, propranolol, and diazepam through a reduction of hepatic blood flow and binding to cytochrome P_{450} enzymes [14]. Cimetidine may also interfere with the metabolism of inhalational anesthetic agents.

H_2 blockers are useful adjuncts in the high-risk patient (old, obese, hiatal hernia) scheduled for elective surgery. They have questionable utility in the patient who needs emergency surgery.

Once the airway has been secured with an endotracheal tube, the endotracheal tube should not be removed until the patient is awake enough to object to the tube and airway reflexes have returned.

BOWEL OBSTRUCTION

The patient with acute bowel obstruction poses one of the most difficult clinical dilemmas for the clinician. These patients have a great propensity for aspiration because of their large gastrointestinal volumes. Often an indwelling nasogastric tube is present, which may keep the gastroesophageal junction patent despite cricoid pressure. Furthermore, these patients tolerate a rapid sequence induction of anesthesia poorly because of their tenuous volume status [4].

Awake intubation is the safest way to secure these patients' airways, especially if there is *any question about the ease of endotracheal intubation.* These patients should be aggressively rehydrated, and this therapy should begin in the emergency department and be continued in the operating room. Often from 1 to 7 liters of warm crystalloid fluid will be needed, as will central venous pressure (CVP) or pulmonary artery (PA) pressure monitoring, arterial line placement, and placement of a Foley catheter. Close monitoring of electrolytes and blood gases often reveals acute hypokalemia and alkalosis. These metabolic problems may further complicate the management of these patients. Use of H_2 blockers may be helpful, but metoclopramide and antacids should probably be avoided in these patients, who do not have a patent gastrointestinal tract [5].

ACUTE GASTROINTESTINAL HEMORRHAGE

Considerations in the patient with gastrointestinal bleeding include monitoring of intravascular volume with CVP and/or PA catheters, assessment of the adequacy of oxygen-carrying capacity with noninvasive monitors and arterial catheters, and the availability of sufficient volumes of blood products. Monitoring of the adequacy of perfusion may be judged by mental status if the patient is awake and with urine output measurement if not. Adequate access to the circulation must be ensured with multiple large-bore IV catheters. Warming devices and rapid infusion devices may be necessary in the patient with rapid hemorrhage [4, 15, 16].

In the patient with upper gastrointestinal bleeding, iced lavage appears to be no more effective than room temperature saline lavage. Iced saline will aggravate the propensity of these patients toward hypothermia. Lavage serves the following purposes: (1) evaluation of the amount of bleeding, (2) determination as to whether the bleeding is ongoing, and (3) promotion of hemostasis. How lavage promotes hemostasis is scientifically unclear, but it has stood the clinical test of time. If after 3 to 10 liters of fluid have been used in lavage and the bleeding has not subsided, noradrenaline may be added to the lavage fluid to promote hemostasis [17]. The acute administration of antacids and H_2 blockers is of questionable value in the treatment of upper gastrointestinal bleeding. Vasopressin (0.1 to 0.4 units/minute IV) is often used in the treatment of acute upper gastrointestinal hemorrhage, but systemic use is probably no better than placebo [17]. Selective intra-arterial vasopressin with or without embolization is the best nonsurgical method of control of acute upper gastrointestinal hemorrhage [17].

LIVER FAILURE

Liver failure may be classified according to the course of illness: Acute liver disease stems from an acute insult in a patient with no previous history of liver disease. Acute liver failure is often a rapidly progressive illness, whereas chronic liver disease may be indolent because the body makes homeostatic adjustments to deranged liver function.

Acute liver disease is usually caused by viruses (hepatitis), poisons (acetaminophen, mushrooms), and hypoxic and/or metabolic insults, such as Wilson's disease or Reyes' syndrome.

The manifestations of acute liver failure are protean and include effects on the central nervous system (CNS) and on the coagulation, cardiovascular, pulmonary, metabolic, and gastrointestinal systems [18].

The CNS effects of liver failure are secondary to acute cerebral edema and to toxic metabolites such as ammonia and account for the "staging" of acute liver disease, which ranges from the awake, alert patient to the comatose or seizing patient [19].

Effects on the coagulation system from liver failure are secondary both to primary liver dysfunction and to the secondary consequences of liver failure. Primary liver dysfunction leads to a reduced production of coagulation factors, with factor VII levels the first to be affected owing to its short half-life. Secondary effects include the presence of fibrin degradation products (FDPs), which have an anticoagulant effect that is unmasked as the diseased liver fails to metabolize these products normally. Accumulation of these substances produces a clinical picture resembling that of disseminated intravascular coagulation. Malnutrition, increased platelet consumption, and hypersplenism all contribute to the profound thrombocytopenia that often accompanies acute liver failure.

Acute liver failure also produces profound vasodilation, which may lead to hypotension. This remains largely unexplained, but theories put forward to explain this phenomenon include failure of the liver to metabolize endotoxin, chronic entry of bacteria through the portal circulation, and mesenteric vasodilation and bleeding. Refractory hypotension is best treated with invasive monitoring, so that volume, ionotropic and vasoactive therapies can be customized on an individual basis.

Hypoxemia and hyperventilation often accompany acute liver failure. Hypoxemia is thought to be due to noncardiogenic pulmonary edema, pleural effusions, or increased intrapulmonary shunts. Hyperventilation is largely unexplained but is thought to be due to humoral factors related to impaired hepatic metabolic function.

Refractory hypoglycemia is seen in end-stage hepatic failure and is due to impaired gluconeogenesis and glycogenolysis. Hyponatremia and hypokalemia are also common. Liver failure increases the chances of aspiration of gastric contents by increasing intra-abdominal pressure, slowing gastric emptying, and lowering the gastroesophageal barrier pressure [20].

Chronic liver disease is classified according to criteria developed by Child that relates to chronic manifestations of liver disease, including jaundice, impaired protein anabolism, and ascites formation (Table 10-1). Child's classification system is useful because it allows the clinician to quantify roughly the amount of hepatocellular reserve remaining before end-stage liver failure develops. In addition to the manifestations mentioned above, chronic liver failure leads to more profound lowering of oncotic pressures, portal hypertension, and esophageal variceal bleeding and hepatorenal syndrome [20].

The patient with liver failure may present to the emergency department or operating room for treatment of several common complications of liver disease. The most common of these is acute gastrointestinal bleeding secondary to esophageal varices or other upper gastroduodenal sources. Often these patients require tracheal intubation to protect their airways and to allow diagnostic procedures to be done safely. Because of their bleeding diatheses, these patients should not be intubated nasally. In addition, such patients may have bleeding due to complications from hepatic transplantation, portosystemic venovenous shunts, or LeVeen (peritoneal venous) shunts.

There are many important anesthetic considerations in these patients. They have a high perioperative mortality due to the problems outlined above as well as risk from the concurrent medical problems that are often present. Hypoxia increases splanchnic arteriolar resistance, which decreases liver blood flow, exacerbates portal hypertension, and further compromises hepatic function. Respiratory acidosis or alkalosis will also decrease hepatic blood flow.

Table 10-1. Child's criteria for classification of liver dysfunction

Criteria	Class A	Class B	Class C
Bilirubin (mg/dl)	<2.0	2.0–3.0	>3.0
Albumin (gm/dl)	>3.5	3.0–3.5	<3.0
Ascites	None	Controlled	Severe
CNS symptoms	None	Mild	Advanced
Nutrition	Excellent	Good	Poor
Increase in prothrombin time (sec)	<2	2–3	3

The volume of distribution of drugs in patients with liver failure is often exaggerated, although drug metabolism is impaired. Pharmacologically, this fact implies that the loading dose of drugs may be supranormal but the maintenance doses often have to be reduced. Muscle relaxants should be carefully titrated with the aid of a neuromuscular stimulator so that their effect may be reversed when desired. Pancuronium and curare have a larger volume of distribution in patients with chronic liver disease, and therefore larger doses are required that last longer. Vecuronium largely depends on the liver for elimination, and doses should be carefully titrated. In the presence of end-stage liver disease, atracurium (metabolized via Hoffman elimination and ester-hydrolysis) may be the preferred muscle relaxant, although its tendency to release histamine may cause hypotension in the susceptible patient. Liver disease also decreases serum pseudocholinesterase levels because of decreased production. Succinylcholine may be safely used in these patients if moderate doses are administered [21].

Halothane lowers liver blood flow and should therefore be avoided in the patient with liver disease, although in this group halothane hepatitis is probably no more common. Isoflurane is considered by some to be the volatile anesthetic of choice in the patient with liver disease [20].

RENAL DISEASE

Patients with chronic and acute renal failure often present to the emergency department and operating suite, and these patients have special clinical problems.

ACUTE RENAL FAILURE

Acute oliguric renal failure is defined by a urine output of less than 20 ml/hour over 6 hours. There are many quantitative indices to help the clinician diagnose and treat the patient with oliguria, the most useful of which is the fractional excretion of sodium (Fe_{Na}).

$$Fe_{Na}\% = ([U_{Na}] \times [S_{Creatinine}]/[S_{Na}] \times [U_{Creatinine}]) \times 100$$

where U_{Na} = urine sodium concentration

$S_{Creatinine}$ = serum creatinine concentration

S_{Na} = serum sodium concentration

$U_{Creatinine}$ = urine creatinine concentration

The Fe_{Na} allows a rapid assessment of the etiology of oliguria using a spot urine and serum specimen. Acute renal failure (ARF) may be divided into three categories: prerenal, postrenal, and parenchymal-renal failure [22]. In the following section the use of Fe_{Na} in differentiating between the types of ARF will be examined.

Prerenal Azotemia

Prerenal azotemia, the most common type of acute renal failure, stems from an acute reduction in renal blood flow and an adaptive oliguria. The most common causes of prerenal azotemia are intravascular volume depletion secondary to hemorrhage, diuretics, gastrointestinal or surgical losses. Other causes of prerenal azotemia are cardiac insufficiency and renal arterial obstruction. The physical examination may reveal flat neck veins, orthostatic hypotension, and low cardiac filling pressures. Cardiogenic renal failure is diagnosed by decreased stroke volume despite adequate cardiac filling pressures. Laboratory study results that indicate the diagnosis include the Fe_{Na} value of less than 1 percent and a blood urea nitrogen (BUN)–creatinine ratio of greater than 10:1. (BUN is reabsorbed by the kidney with sodium and water.)

Management of patients with prerenal azotemia consists of therapy designed to correct diminished renal perfusion. The hypovolemic patient should be aggressively treated with fluid volume to prevent renal parenchymal damage. Invasive hemodynamic monitors should be used early to titrate therapy. Ionotropic agents and/or dopamine are used to optimize renal blood flow in the oliguric patient with a low Fe_{Na} despite adequate cardiac filling pressures [22].

Postrenal Azotemia

Postrenal azotemia accounts for 2 to 5 percent of all cases of ARF. Significant features in the history are anuria, history of nephrolithiasis, prostatic hypertrophy, previous radiation therapy, and/or trauma to the pelvis. Patients with anuric renal failure should have renal ultrasound examination to look for distended renal pelves. Such patients often have very high BUN-creatinine ratios. Work-up for these patients should be aggressive so that the obstruction can be corrected. Following decompression of the kidneys these patients often have a dramatic "postobstructive" diuresis that may require volume replacement [22].

Parenchymal Renal Failure

Parenchymal renal failure implies that there is some physiologic dysfunction secondary to injury to small blood vessels or glomeruli. Before this diagnosis can be made, prerenal and postrenal causes must be excluded. Parenchymal renal failure accounts for about 5 to 10 percent of all cases of ARF. Acute tubular necrosis (ATN) is the most common clinical cause of parenchymal renal failure, and prolonged ischemia to the kidney is the most common cause of ATN. This ischemia may be secondary to prolonged prerenal states, hypoxia, burns, sepsis, pancreatitis, obstetric disorders, or compromise of the major renal vessels. Commonly used drugs such as aminoglycosides, nonsteroidal anti-inflammatory agents, and radiocontrast dyes may also precipitate ATN [23]. Myoglobinuria secondary to muscular ischemia or trauma not only will cause ATN but may also cause renal tubular obstruction. Hemoglobinuria secondary to transfusion reactions or hemolysis may also cause ATN [24].

Diagnostic laboratory findings in these patients include Fe_{Na} of greater than 1 percent and a BUN-creatinine ratio of less than 10. The urinary sediment often shows red blood cell casts.

Treating patients with ATN is primarily supportive. When possible, the underlying cause should be reversed. If there is any question of prerenal oliguria a fluid challenge may be indicated. If the patient is oliguric, some experts recommend mannitol or furosemide to convert oliguric renal failure to nonoliguric renal failure [25]. Diuretics should be used with extreme caution because they may worsen renal ischemia and make the urine output a worthless barometer of renal function [25]. Additional vigilance with fluid and drug therapy is required in these patients.

CHRONIC RENAL FAILURE

There are some 12 million patients with chronic renal failure (CRF) in the United States. Many of these patients will eventually require dialysis or renal transplantation. Patients with CRF are often hospitalized and need surgery; such surgical procedures include vascular access, peritoneal dialysis access, renal transplantation, and surgery related to underlying disease or secondary to complications of CRF.

Renal insufficiency is well tolerated until the glomerular filtration rate (GFR) falls to less than 60 percent of normal. Patients with GRFs of approximately 50 percent of normal still have no electrolyte abnormalities or physical signs or symptoms of renal failure. Patients in whom 60 to 90 percent of nephrons are destroyed are classified as having "mild renal insufficiency." Clinical manifestations of mild renal insufficiency include anemia secondary to the loss of erythropoietin secretion and an elevation in the BUN and creatinine levels without overt symptoms of uremia. The patient with mild renal insufficiency has a decreased ability to concentrate the urine and to handle large free water loads.

When the GFR falls to less than 10 percent of normal, overt renal failure ensues [26]. These patients require dialysis or renal transplantation. CRF leads to multiple physiologic consequences, only some of which are dialysis responsive. The following section describes some of these problems.

1. *Anemia* (dialysis unresponsive). Anemia of chronic renal failure is secondary to impaired erythropoietin secretion and increased erythrocyte destruction. This anemia is remarkably well tolerated because of adaptive compensatory mechanisms. These include increased 2,3-diphosphoglyceric acid (DPG) concentrations in red blood cells and an increased cardiac output. The need for blood transfusion in these patients should be judged by their exercise tolerance, not by any arbitrary hemoglobin concentration. These patients also have lowered blood-gas partition coefficients, which may speed anesthetic induction.

2. *Hypertension* (dialysis unresponsive). Hypertension is one of the most frequent causes of CRF. In addition, most patients with CRF will develop hypertension secondary to a reduction in renal blood flow and increased renin secretion.

3. *Acidosis* (dialysis responsive). Acidosis is secondary to the kidney's inability to excrete organic and nonorganic acids. This is manifest by an increased serum ionic gap.

4. *Sodium imbalance* (dialysis responsive). When hyponatremia is present, total body sodium is paradoxically elevated because there is a relative excess of free water. Occasionally hyponatremia will be the initial indication for hemodialysis in the patient with CRF. If left untreated, hyponatremia can lead to altered mental status, coma, and seizures.

5. *Ca^{2+}, PO_4^{-2}, and Mg^+* abnormalities (dialysis unresponsive). Calcium, phosphorus, and magnesium balance is not responsive to dialysis, and therefore these patients are often treated with aluminum-containing antacids to control hyperphosphatemia. These patients may develop secondary hyperparathyroidism, mandating surgery.

6. *Hyperkalemia* (dialysis responsive). Hyperkalemia is the most common acute medical problem in the patient with CRF. Drugs, including penicillin V (Pen-Vee K), and fluids (lactated Ringer's) that contain potassium should be avoided in such patients.

7. *Central nervous system abnormalities* (dialysis responsive). CNS manifestations of uremia may range from malaise, fatigue, and intellectual impairment to seizures, coma, and death. These manifestations are thought to be due to toxic metabolites that are not excreted by the kidney.

8. *Peripheral nervous system abnormalities* (dialysis responsive). Peripheral neuropathies are common with CRF; dialytic therapy may improve

this condition. Patients with CRF have decreased sensation in the extremities as well as chronic itching and burning sensations.

9. *Autonomic neuropathies* (dialysis unresponsive). Postural hypotension (autonomic insufficiency) is seen in these patients and is often manifest by an inability to tolerate fluid shifts during dialysis and surgery and an increased sensitivity to anesthetic agents.

10. *Gastrointestinal abnormalities* (dialysis responsive). Uremic patients have a variety of gastrointestinal symptoms that are common and nonspecific: nausea, vomiting, and anorexia. Less common but more troublesome are chronic hiccups and gastrointestinal bleeding.

11. *Immune system defects* (dialysis unresponsive). Humoral and cellular immunity is impaired in patients with CRF. The exact mechanism of immunodeficiency is unclear. It results, however, in frequent infections with unusual organisms. Because of the need for frequent blood transfusions, these patients have an extraordinarily high incidence of hepatitis B and presumably human immunodeficiency virus (HIV) infection. Therefore, it is prudent to use the same careful precautions one would use to prevent all blood and body fluid contact.

12. *Platelet function defects* (dialysis responsive). Platelet function is impaired in patients with CRF for multiple reasons. They have low platelet counts secondary to consumption from hemodialysis tubing and membrane contact. Qualitative function is impaired because of decreased platelet factor III and decreased platelet aggregation in response to adenosine diphosphate (ADP). Platelet function is measured clinically with the bleeding time. Treatment of platelet dysfunction emergently is accomplished with platelets or desmopressin (DDAVP).

13. *Decreased protein binding.* Normal protein binding sites may be bound by circulating metabolic products, which will exaggerate the effects of certain drugs, notably barbiturates and benzodiazepines.

14. *Decreased pseudocholinesterase levels.* These patients have decreased pseudocholinesterase levels, but this is usually of little clinical significance. Succinylcholine can be used safely in these patients, even in the presence of mild hyperkalemia.

Considering all the complications secondary to CRF, it is easy to understand why these patients have frequent emergency department visits and an increased perioperative morbidity. Judicious management of these patients should include compulsive attention to volume status because they have an inability to handle excess sodium and water. The clinician should have a low threshold for the use of invasive hemodynamic monitors to optimize fluid therapy. Preoperative dialysis has been shown to reduce perioperative morbidity, presumably by reducing fluid and potassium loads [27].

Patients with CRF have unpredictable drug responses because of their electrolyte abnormalities and their inability to excrete certain drugs. High Ca^{2+} and low K^+ levels will increase the sensitivity of the neuromuscular junction to nondepolarizing muscle relaxants. Likewise, cardiotonic drugs may have unusual effects because of abnormal intracellular and extracellular electrolyte concentrations. Because of the inability of CRF patients to excrete certain drugs, it is best to avoid volatile anesthetics that are metabolized such as ethrane or halothane. Gallamine and dimethyl tubocurarine iodide (Metubine iodide) rely on renal excretion for elimination and should also be avoided. Atracurium and vecuronium retain their predictable half-lives in the setting of CRF [26].

Another phenomenon seen in these patients is rebound heparinization. This is thought to be due to release of stored heparin. Rebound heparinization can be especially dangerous in the immediate postdialysis period. The partial thromboplastin time (PTT) will be elevated in these circumstances, and the coagulopathy will respond promptly to protamine administration.

Positioning injuries are more common in these patients because their nerves are already damaged from their uremic states and because they often have arteriovenous fistulas that may be damaged by incorrect positioning.

If no platelet dysfunction or coagulopathy is present, regional anesthesia is attractive in these patients with multisystem disease. Normocapnia should be maintained. Any change in PCO_2 will not only change the concentration of K^+ and H^+ but will also impair oxygen delivery by shifting the oxyhemoglobin dissociation curve. Patients with CRF represent a challenge to the clinician. However, an increased understanding of the pathophysiology of CRF will ideally assist in the management of these patients [26].

REFERENCES

1. James, C. F., Modell, J. H., Gibbs, C. P., et al. Pulmonary effects of volume and pH in the rat. *Anesth. Analg.* 63:665–668, 1984.
2. Stoelting, R. K. Liver and Gastrointestinal Tract. In R. K. Stoelting. *Pharmacology and Physiology in Anesthetic Practice.* Philadelphia: Lippincott, 1987. Pp. 788–791.
3. Sellick, B. A. Cricoid pressure to control regurgitation of stomach contents during induction of anesthesia. *Lancet* 2:404, 1961.
4. Weiskopf, R. B., and Fairley, H. B. Anesthesia for major trauma. *Surg. Clin. North Am.* 62:31, 1982.
5. Schulze-Delrieu, K. Drug therapy: Metoclopramide. *N. Engl. J. Med.* 305:28–33, 1981.
6. Gibbs, C. P., Schwartz, D. J., Wynee, J. W., et al. Antacid aspiration in the dog. *Anesthesiology* 51:38–85, 1979.
7. Viegas, O. J., Ravindran, R. S., and Shumacker, C. A. Gastric fluid pH in patients receiving sodium citrate. *Anesth. Analg.* 60:521–523, 1981.
8. Gibbs, C. P., Spohr, L., and Schmidt, D. The effectiveness of sodium citrate as an antacid. *Anesthesiology* 57:44–46, 1982.
9. Ginsberg, R., Bristow, M. R., Stinson, E. B., et al. Histamine receptors in the human heart. *Life Sci.* 26:2245–2249, 1980.

10. Mogelnicki, S., Waller, J., and Finlayson, D. Physostigmine reversal of cimetidine-induced mental confusion. *J.A.M.A.* 241:826–827, 1979.
11. Coombs, D. W., Hooper, D., and Colton, T. Acid aspiration prophylaxis by use of preoperative oral administration of cimetidine. *Anesthesiology* 51:352–356, 1979.
12. Stoelting, R. K. Histamine and Histamine Receptor Antagonists. In R. K. Stoelting. *Pharmacology and Physiology in Anesthetic Practice.* Philadelphia: Lippincott, 1987. Pp. 378–381.
13. McGuigan, J. E. A consideration of the adverse effects of cimetidine. *Gastroenterology* 80:181–192, 1981.
14. Feely, J., Wilkinson, G. R., and Wood, A. J. Reduction of liver blood flow and propranolol metabolism by cimetidine. *N. Engl. J. Med.* 304:692–695, 1981.
15. Boyan, C. P., and Howland, W. S. Blood temperature: A critical factor in massive transfusion. *Anesthesiology* 22:559, 1961.
16. Schiller, K. F. R., and Coltton, P. B. Acute upper gastrointestinal hemorrhage. *Clin. Gastroenterol.* 7:595, 1978.
17. Eckstein, M. R., Kelemouridis, V., Athanasoulis, C. A., et al. Gastric bleeding: Therapy with intra-arterial vasopressin and transcatheter embolization. *Radiology* 152:643–646, 1984.
18. Christensen, E., Bremmelgaard, A., Bahnsen, M., et al. Prediction of fatality in fulminant hepatic failure. *Scand. J. Gastroenterol.* 19:90–96, 1984.
19. Van Dyke, R. W., Scharschmidt, B. F. Hepatic Encephalopathy and Hepatic Failure. In D. Watts (ed.), *Gastrointestinal Disease.* Los Altos: Lange Medical, 1984.
20. Merritt, W. T. Liver Disease. In M. C. Rogers (ed.), *Current Practice in Anesthesiology.* Philadelphia: B.C. Decker, 1988. Pp. 31–36.
21. Williams, R. L. Drug administration in hepatic disease. *N. Engl. J. Med.* 309:1616–1622, 1983.
22. Schrier, R. W., and Conger, J. D. Acute Renal Failure: Pathogenesis, Diagnosis and Management. In R. W. Schrier (ed.), *Renal and Electrolyte Disorders* (3rd ed.). Boston: Little, Brown, 1986. Pp. 423–460.
23. Anderson, R. J., Linas, S. L., Berns, A. S., et al. Non-oliguric acute renal failure. *N. Engl. J. Med.* 296:1134, 1977.
24. Gabow, P. A., Kaehny, W. P., and Kelleher, S. P. The spectrum of rhabdomyolysis. *Medicine* 61:125, 1982.
25. Eneas, J. F., Schoenfeld, P. Y., and Humphreys, M. H. The effect of infusion of mannitol-sodium bicarbonate on the clinical course of myoglobinuria. *Arch. Intern. Med.* 139:801, 1979.
26. Burke, G. R., and Gulyassy, P. F. Surgery in the patient with renal disease and related electrolyte disorders. *Med. Clin. North Am.* 63:1191, 1979.
27. Alfrey, A. C. Chronic Renal Failure: Manifestations and Pathogenesis. In R. W. Schrier (ed.), *Renal and Electrolyte Disorders* (3rd ed.). Boston: Little, Brown, 1986. Pp. 461–494.

11. Infectious Disease Considerations

Marie Csete Prager

CENTRAL VENOUS CATHETER–RELATED INFECTIONS

All indwelling catheters, regardless of site or technique of insertion, can cause local or systemic infection. Sterile insertion technique by emergency physicians and anesthesiologists is the most important defense against these lethal infections.

Serious infectious sequelae are most common with percutaneously placed central venous lines. Three types of infections have been described in this setting. The first is clear-cut catheter-related sepsis. The clinical definition of catheter-related sepsis is a septic syndrome during which the same micro-organism is cultured from both the catheter tip and any blood culture obtained within 48 hours before or after catheter removal. The definition implies the absence of other infectious sources.

A second infection of concern is clinical catheter-related sepsis (or non-bacteremic catheter-related sepsis) during which the patient manifests a septic picture and the catheter, when cultured, is infected. In addition, the patient improves within 2 days of catheter removal. Blood cultures, however, have not been drawn (for whatever reason) or blood cultures are sterile. This syndrome is accepted as catheter-related sepsis because catheters are thought to seed the blood stream only intermittently, and timing of blood cultures may not correlate with the bacteremic episodes.

The third infection is simple catheter infection without an associated septic picture (in other words, catheter-related sepsis in the making). About half of all central line infections are local. The degree or severity of catheter infection has been prospectively shown to be positively associated with bacteremia. Over the years various culturing techniques have been used to assess the severity of catheter infection, but the current standard is the semiquantitative technique (Maki technique) [1].

For this culturing technique, the catheter is removed as cleanly as possible. If the skin insertion site appears infected, a skin culture is first obtained. The area surrounding the insertion site is then cleaned with povidone-iodine (Betadine) or a similar solution. The operator wears mask and sterile gloves and uses a sterile instrument to keep the skin away from the catheter as it is withdrawn. This same technique is mandatory in the emergency department if catheterized patients present with fever during a home course of antibiotics or intravenous nutrition. Approximately 5 cm of the distal catheter tip is sterilely clipped and placed in a culture tube. If this procedure is done at night, the tube may be stored in a refrigerator and sent for culturing in the morning.

In the laboratory, the catheter is rolled four or five times over a blood agar plate and then incubated at 37°C. The catheter segment is considered to be significantly colonized if it results in the growth of more than 15 colonies per agar plate.

One convincing study of the utility of this technique was done by Cooper and Hopkins at the Massachusetts General Hospital [2]. A total of 330 catheters were cultured for suspected catheter-related infection. Of those catheters that were positive for colonization by the semiquantitative technique, 34 percent were associated with bacteremia. Of those catheters that did not yield significant growth, none were associated with bacteremia.

Another culturing technique cited in the literature is a pour-plate method, using blood drawn back from the central line. This practice carries a theoretical risk of increasing the likelihood of infection, since there is a strong correlation between central line violations (including blood drawing) and the development of infections. Yet another technique is comparative quantitative culturing of central venous and peripheral venous specimens. A fivefold difference in bacterial concentrations between central and venous blood was found to be significant in one study [3].

The reported incidence of central catheter-related sepsis varies from about 4 to 10 percent of catheters placed. Representative studies are cited in Table 11-1 [2, 4–10]. From this literature, no hard data are available on mortality from catheter-related infections. Morbidity from antibiotic therapy and repeated cannulation of central veins is also a significant but unquantitated phenomenon.

The most common pathogens are *Staphylococcus epidermidis* and *S. aureus.* Production of a glycoprotein slime by *S. epidermidis* enhances the adherence of the bacteria to plastic catheters and may decrease the efficacy of antibiotics. In patients who receive total parenteral nutrition through a central venous line, *Candida albicans* is a common pathogen.

In the older literature, an assumption was made that the source of bacterial seeding of central catheters was the blood stream. That assumption has been discarded, and most catheter-related infections are thought to derive from skin, with direct extension along the catheter. Several investigators have looked at the relationship between simultaneous skin and catheter cultures and have demonstrated some correlation. Unfortunately, however, skin cultures are not sensitive enough to dictate therapy, and definitive di-

Table 11-1. Incidence of catheter-related sepsis

Study	Use of catheter	CRS rate (%)
Ryan [4], 1974	TPN	7.0
Bjornson [5], 1982	TPN	7.0
Snydman [6], 1982	TPN	5.0
Pettigrew [7], 1985	TPN	3.3
Sitzmann [8], 1985	TPN	5.7
Cooper [2], 1985	Mixed	12.5 colonized
Bozetti [9], 1985	No TPN	7.6
Brun-Buisson [10], 1987	No TPN	10.8

agnoses require catheter removal. When removed central or peripheral intravenous catheters are Gram stained and examined at 1000 × power (a technique that, in experienced hands, is more sensitive than semiquantitative culturing) [2], organisms are found concentrated on the external surface of the catheter. (One can speculate that this location is due to direct extension from the skin rather than infusion-related colonization.)

Clearly, prevention of skin-to-catheter infection is in the hands of the physician. Strict aseptic technique is the rule for insertion of all central venous lines regardless of site (internal jugular, external jugular, subclavian, antecubital, or femoral). Ideally, the physician scrubs before dressing in head covering, mask, gown, and surgical gloves. The patient's skin is prepared with povidone-iodine or a similar surgical antiseptic, and sterile towels are used to isolate the field. Central lines placed without sterile technique in an emergency situation should be identified as such in the chart by the physician who placed them and subsequently removed, cultured, and replaced in sterile fashion when the patient's condition allows.

There is a positive correlation between the number of attempts to insert a central line and the subsequent incidence of infection. A typical scenario is one in which one physician makes many attempts before a second physician enters the field. By the time a second person attempts line placement, the field barriers are wet or torn and all needles in the central line kit are bloodied. In order to minimize the incidence of catheter-related infections the entire sterile procedure should be redone and fresh equipment used.

Aseptic dressing technique is also important. In general, dressings are easier to maintain on the flat surface of the subclavian area than on the lateral neck where there is more movement. Internal jugular veins may thus be more likely to become infected than subclavian lines. Nutritional support teams generally prefer a subclavian approach for alimentation lines for this reason. On a flat surface, a transparent adhesive plastic dressing (e.g., Tegaderm) can be safely maintained between dressing changes (every day or every 2 days). Because these types of dressings usually do not adhere to lateral neck sites for long periods of time, occlusive-type dressings are generally preferred.

Percutaneously placed catheters are generally reported to cause a higher rate of catheter-related infections than catheters tunneled under the skin. Tunneled catheters, it should be noted, are usually placed in the operating room. A few series show similar rates of infection between the two catheter types; with careful insertion techniques, the percutaneous route can be as safe as the tunneled route. The type of plastic may also have an influence on the rate of infection. In animals antibiotic bonding of catheters has shown promise in preventing catheter-related infections [11]. In most, though not all, series there is a direct correlation between the length of time the catheter is in place and the rate of infection. The time interval between "routine" central venous line changes is a matter of local practice and varies considerably among institutions (anywhere from 3 days to 2 weeks).

A related controversy concerns changing a central catheter over a guidewire. Several investigations [5–7] have concluded that, from a bacteriologic viewpoint, changing catheters over wires is safe practice with less morbidity than that associated with fresh needle sticks. When such studies are viewed as a whole, it is clear that there is a small but significant transfer of infection to the new catheter. Therefore, most clinicians agree that patients who appear toxic or septic are not candidates for a change of catheter over a guidewire.

Treatment of catheter-related infection is usually initiated before culture results are available. In most patients, vancomycin and an aminoglycoside provide suitable empiric coverage pending culture results. In neutropenic patients antipseudomonal coverage is added (such as mezlocillin, ticarcillin). The current conservative standard therapy also includes removal of the catheter and reinsertion at a new site by sterile technique. Some groups have reported successful therapy with catheters remaining in place [3], but this practice should be reserved for patients who are uncompromised by their infection.

PULMONARY ARTERIAL LINE INFECTIONS

Endocarditis is a particular concern in patients who have indwelling pulmonary arterial lines. From both animal models and numerous human autopsy studies [12, 13] it is clear that the incidence of right-sided endocardial lesions is high (3.4—75 percent) in this setting. Infected endocardial lesions develop at the sites of catheter-induced damage; again, this is documented in both animal and human autopsy studies.

Because pulmonary arterial lines often migrate and must be repositioned, sheaths have been designed to maintain a sterile external portion of catheter, giving physicians a "safe" area of catheter to manipulate. Many studies have demonstrated that the catheters under the sheaths are commonly contaminated [14, 15]. This contamination has not, however, readily led to catheter-related infection. Nonetheless, the pulmonary arterial line sheath is not a cause for complacency; sterile dressing changes are required routinely, and the line should be violated as little as possible. Fluids used to measure cardiac outputs are also a potential source of contamination.

ARTERIAL LINE INFECTIONS

Serious infections due to arterial catheters are less common than infections from central venous catheters. (High flows through arterial lines may afford some protection against infections.) In one large series of compromised patients, however, serious infectious sequelae were seen in 4 percent of patients with arterial lines [16]. The lower incidence of infectious problems occurs in spite of a high incidence of partial or complete arterial occlusion (about 25 percent for radial lines) [17]. Radial arteries are most commonly used for cannulation because of the hand's collateral circulation and because of easy access. In some institutions, axillary and femoral arteries are used successfully for chronic arterial cannulation. In one series the reported rate of catheter-related sepsis from axillary arterial lines was 2.2 percent [18], despite the difficulties inherent in maintaining sterile conditions in the axilla.

Proper placement of an arterial line implies a sterile technique. The skin is prepared with povidone-iodine, and the operator wears sterile gloves and mask. Full sterile gowning is generally not performed unless the patient is severely immunocompromised.

All fluids connected to arterial or venous lines are potential sources of contamination. This includes transducers and manometers. All tubing should be changed every 3 days; all fluid bags or bottles should be changed daily.

PERIPHERAL INTRAVENOUS LINE INFECTIONS

Peripheral venous lines are easily contaminated by skin micro-organisms, yet many physicians make little effort to decontaminate the skin before inserting a venous catheter. Often a small alcohol wipe is the only precaution. With this technique, the incidence of infection is high, especially after 72 hours of continuous cannulation. Fortunately, serious consequences are minimized by daily inspection of the site and by routine line changes every 72 hours. At the first sign of inflammation or purulence the catheter should be removed. Septic phlebitis is a serious sequelae that requires surgical intervention.

Strict sterile technique for peripheral lines should be observed in patients who are immunocompromised, in patients at risk for bacterial endocarditis, and in patients with grafts or prostheses. If endocarditis is a particular concern, scalp vein needles are recommended instead of plastic catheters.

Intravenous tubing can be safely changed every 72 hours [19]. Direct contamination from intravenous fluids is rare, though certain bacteria grow readily at room temperature in standard electrolyte solutions.

In one recent study the type of dressing applied to a peripheral intravenous line was found to have no particular bearing on the rate of catheter-related infection. The dressing should be inspected daily and changed if it is wet or no longer adherent.

HEPATITIS

HEPATITIS A

Hepatitis A is usually transmitted by the fecal-oral route, and has an incubation period of about 28 days. Risk factors include contact with children attending day care centers and foreign travel. Homosexual men and IV drug abusers also have increased risk of hepatitis A. Contact with a hepatitis A patient is certainly a major risk factor.

Traditionally hepatitis A outbreaks were not considered a major nosocomial problem because adult patients generally do not present themselves until jaundice is apparent. By this stage in the disease viral shedding via the gut is diminished or absent. Nonetheless, several in-hospital outbreaks of hepatitis A have been reported. The best prevention is careful hand washing between patients and gloving if there is contact with feces. For exposed health care workers or patients, immune serum globulin given within 2 weeks of exposure is effective in preventing clinical disease.

Most causes of hepatitis A resolve over weeks, and a chronic carrier state has not been reported. A few patients may be symptomatic for as long as a year with cholestatic variant [20]. These patients are not infectious. Rarely hepatitis A causes an acute fulminant hepatic failure that may be fatal.

Confirmatory diagnosis of the acute disease is made by demonstrating elevated titers of IgM antihepatitis A virus (IgM anti-HAV). These antibody titers usually peak within 4 weeks of clinical illness and disappear by 3 to 6 months. (IgG antibody persists indefinitely and is an indicator of immunity.)

Post-transfusion hepatitis A is extremely rare, probably because active viremia is so short-lived [21].

HEPATITIS B

Hepatitis B is now the most frequently reported type of hepatitis in the United States [22]. The disease is usually transmitted by percutaneous inoculation with hepatitis B–containing blood or serum (therefore IV drug abusers are at risk) or is acquired from a sexual partner. The incubation period is about 6 to 24 weeks. Hepatitis B can be transfusion acquired, although most cases of transfusion-related hepatitis are attributable to non-A, non-B virus. The symptoms of acute hepatitis are not unique to the viral type. Generally, patients experience fatigue, decreased appetite, nausea, vomiting, and right upper quadrant discomfort with a low-grade fever. Patients with hepatitis B are more likely to exhibit extrahepatic manifestations such as rash or arthralgia, but these signs are not virus specific. Many patients experience seroconversion without evidence of clinical illness.

The serologic diagnosis of acute hepatitis B is established if the patient has a positive hepatitis B surface antigen (HBsAg) and IgM-specific antibody to hepatitis B core antigen (IgM-specific anti-HBc). The presence of a positive HBsAg and high titers of total anti-HBc is characteristic of either acute or chronic infection. Hepatitis Be antigenemia (HBeAg) is a marker of active viremia. Unfortunately, not all patients with acute disease have demonstrable HBsAg. Other markers may also be difficult to detect.

In patients with hepatitis B in whom the acute disease is resolved (and no chronic hepatitis develops), HBsAg antigenemia disappears within 6 months. HBeAg is demonstrable in these uncomplicated patients for an even shorter time. At about 6 months, these patients will develop antibody to the surface antigen (anti-HBs). Anti-HBc (IgG) will be sustained. Antibody to surface antigen is generally considered evidence of prior infection or immunization, and therefore of immunity.

Patients who develop chronic hepatitis B continue to have elevated HBsAg levels and high titers of IgG anti-HBc. In these patients HBeAg is a particularly useful marker of infectivity, while anti-HBe positivity indicates that the patient is not likely to be infectious. Health care workers who are carriers of HBsAg should not have patient contact during the acute stage of disease. Health care workers who are discovered to be HBsAg positive but have no acute illness are allowed to have normal patient contact, provided they use appropriate precautions (gloves and mask, depending on the nature of the contact). These are the same precautions used to protect the physician from patient-acquired hepatitis. Some institutions use HBeAg testing to determine whether or not patient contact is appropriate, but this is not our policy.

Patients with chronic hepatitis should be referred to a gastroenterologist. These patients are followed with serial liver function tests, serologies, and liver biopsy. Patients with more severe chronic active hepatitis are generally given a trial of steroids. These patients are at risk for cirrhosis. Patients with milder chronic persistent hepatitis do not require steroid therapy.

Anesthesiologists and emergency physicians are clearly at increased risk of hepatitis B and its chronic sequelae because of exposure to blood products and secretions. In one multicenter study, 12.7 percent of anesthesia residents were seropositive for hepatitis B [23]. As in other studies, years in anesthesia practice were positively correlated with seropositivity, and anesthesia faculty had a 23.3 percent seropositive rate [23].

Anesthesia and emergency personnel should immunize themselves against hepatitis B. A safe, effective vaccine is available, and the great majority of health care workers are protected by the vaccine for at least 5 years. After three doses of vaccine, anti-HBs levels are used as a marker of protection. Routine screening after vaccination is not a uniform practice but should be considered in patients who are re-exposed and have an unknown antibody status, or in patients who may be poor responders (such as the obese) [24]. Additional vaccine doses may benefit some hyporesponders or nonresponders to the original vaccine series [25].

In addition, gloves should be used when handling blood products (despite an epidemiologic survey that demonstrated that gloves were of no benefit in oral surgery) [26], and contaminated needles should be discarded promptly, without bending, manipulating, or capping. Certainly such precautions are mandatory when handling products known to be infected, but our current standard is to practice gloving and careful needle disposal in all settings in which there is contact with bodily fluids.

Hepatitis delta virus infection is a particularly virulent cotraveller of hepatitis B. This defective virus requires hepatitis B virus in order to replicate. Hepatitis delta virus infection may be acquired at the same time as hepatitis B or may be superimposed on hepatitis B infections. The combination of hepatitis delta and hepatitis B carries a considerably poorer prognosis than hepatitis B alone.

NON-A, NON-B HEPATITIS

Non-A, non-B hepatitis is generally a post-transfusion phenomenon with an incubation period of about 3 to 18 weeks. The risk of developing hepatitis after transfusion is approximately 2 to 4 percent. The risk of icteric disease is about 1 percent. Approximately 80 percent of post-transfusion hepatitis cases are caused by non-A, non-B virus(es). There are no commercially available markers of non-A, non-B hepatitis, although recent reports indicate that this situation may soon change. Currently, non-A, non-B hepatitis is a diagnosis of exclusion. Elevated serum alanine aminotransferase levels (persisting over weeks) are necessary for diagnosis, and the patient must have negative serologic findings for acute hepatitis A and B, cytomegalovirus, herpesvirus, and Epstein-Barr virus. Unfortunately, approximately 20 percent of patients with this form of hepatitis will develop a chronic carrier state.

ACUTE FULMINANT HEPATITIS

The majority of patients with acute hepatitis of any cause do not require hospitalization. In most patients, therapeutic interventions are not needed. Occasionally patients require pharmacologic intervention for pruritus or vomiting. In addition, patients with acute hepatitis require serial liver function measurements until the disease has resolved.

A few patients with viral hepatitis, however, present with a picture of acute fulminant hepatic failure characterized by encephalopathy developing within 2 months of the onset of symptoms. These patients may have profound hepatocellular damage with coagulopathy and hypoglycemia. Encephalopathy may progress to frank hepatic coma, with elevated intracranial pressure (and cerebral edema on CT scan). In addition, these patients are at risk of developing acute renal failure (hepatorenal syndrome). Survival with medical management is about 20 to 30 percent.

All three types of hepatitis virus can cause acute fulminant hepatic failure. In addition, toxic causes should be sought (*Amanita* mushroom poisoning, acetaminophen overdose). A pulmonary artery line is useful in the management of these patients, especially if renal failure is superimposed. Patients may have enormous cardiac outputs in this setting.

Encephalopathic patients require intubation for airway protection. If coagulation parameters are not normal, nasal intubation is not recommended. Fresh frozen plasma (and vitamin K) may be required in large volumes to keep the prothrombin time (PT) in reasonable range. Clear communication with the blood bank is mandatory. Cryoprecipitate may be required to keep fibrinogen in reasonable range (for example, above 150 mg/dl). Acute thrombocytopenia may also be a complicating factor, and platelet transfusion may be necessary. Patients are often febrile because of hepatic necrosis but surveillance cultures are necessary to rule out intercurrent infections.

In a few centers hepatic encephalopathy has improved after either charcoal hemoperfusion [27] or postdilution hemofiltration [28]. It is not clear whether these techniques have an effect on elevated intracranial pressures, but there is preliminary evidence to suggest a beneficial effect [29].

Elevated intracranial pressure (ICP) in these patients has been treated successfully with mannitol in some cases. Hyperventilation is a useful tool, and we have recently used barbiturate coma successfully in three patients with acute fulminant hepatic failure and elevated intracranial pressures. Monitoring the intracranial pressure may be complicated by intracranial bleeding in patients with profound coaguloathy and is still a controversial issue. In some centers epidural catheters have been used for ICP monitoring with success. Steroids have had variable effect.

While the patient is being stabilized, communication should be established with a center that has the capacity to perform liver transplantation. In several small series, emergency liver transplantation yielded better survival rates than medical therapy alone [30, 31]. In addition, such centers are valuable resources for stabilizing patients with this complicated disease.

ACQUIRED IMMUNODEFICIENCY SYNDROME (AIDS)

AIDS is a complex disorder characterized by the appearance of either opportunistic infection or malignancy in the setting of seropositivity for antibody to HIV (human immunodeficiency virus). Neurologic disorders may also be a presentation of AIDS. The virus is transmitted by contact with contaminated blood products or by sexual contact. Intravenous drug users who share needles are at high risk of contracting AIDS. Homosexual men who do not use condoms are at high risk of contracting AIDS. Neonatal AIDS is also a serious problem, resulting from blood-borne transmission of virus from mother to fetus.

A detailed description of the immunologic defect in AIDS is beyond the scope of this chapter. Simply stated, HIV is trophic for T lymphocytes and for monocyte-macrophage cells. Abnormalities in the numbers of T-cell populations are associated with deficient recognition of antigen [32]. B-lymphocyte function is not spared either and may be severely impaired [33]. Virus can also bind directly to cells in the central nervous system.

The AIDS virus can involve any organ system. Infections are a common presentation. Hematologic disorders such as circulating coagulation inhibitors [34] and thrombocytopenia [35] have been described. Enteropathy [36] and malabsorption [37] as well as biliary tract obstruction [38] are associated with HIV infection. Various renal abnormalities have been observed in AIDS patients [39], and adrenal insufficiency [40] may also occur. Polymyositis associated with AIDS [41] may herald the syndrome. The list above is only partial but is an indication of the many problems encountered in HIV-positive patients. Physicians must maintain a high degree of suspicion of AIDS in patients at high risk for disease simply because the patient's presentation is so variable.

Probably the single most common emergency department presentation in this disease is infection. Skin lesions should be sought, and, in consultation with an infectious disease specialist, scrapings should be sent for appropriate examination and culture. Pneumonias are an important problem in AIDS patients. Emergency physicians may be called on to gather culture information before starting antibiotic therapy. Again consultation with the hospital laboratory is important to ensure that correct media are used for culturing and that cultures are stored properly.

The most common pulmonary infection is *Pneumocystis carinii,* often heralded by dyspnea and hypoxemia. Induced sputum samples may yield the diagnosis, but patients may require bronchoscopy (for washings or biopsy) in order to make the diagnosis.

Other common pathogens include cytomegalovirus, *Mycobacterium avium-intracellulare* and *M. tuberculosis, Cryptococcus,* and *Toxoplasma gondii* [42]. Various other bacterial, viral, parasitic, and fungal infections have developed in these immunosuppressed patients. Multiple infections are common. Pulmonary infiltrates may be nonspecific (no infectious agent identified) or due to malignancy.

Atypical pneumonia may alert the practitioner to the possibility of AIDS. However, it is our current practice to treat all emergency patients as potential carriers. Gloves and eye protection are worn whenever contact with body fluids or secretions is anticipated. Gowns are used if gross spills are anticipated. On equipment, bleach or sodium hypochlorite (0.5 to 1% solution) quickly inactivates HIV [43]. In one study from Baltimore, 3 percent of 203 critically ill or injured patients in an emergency department were seropositive for HIV antibody [44]. In the same study 16 percent of trauma patients (for whom significant blood contact can be anticipated) were seropositive. In California, HIV antibody assays cannot be done without the express permission of the patient. Physicians must be aware of such regulations in their own hospital and state.

Fortunately, transmission of HIV from patient to health care worker is a rare event. Following needlestick exposure from a seropositive patient the chance of acquiring HIV seropositivity is less than 1 percent. If such exposure is documented or suspected, the exposed health care worker should be tested for HIV antibody at the time of exposure, at 6 weeks, and at 3, 6, and 12 months after exposure. In addition, the health care worker should contact the Centers for Disease Control [45], where such exposures are recorded and followed. Exposed health care workers should also be tested for hepatitis B (see discussion above). Asymptomatic HIV antibody-positive health care workers may continue normal patient contact, using gloves and mask when appropriate.

REFERENCES

1. Maki, D. G., Weise, C. E., and Sarafin, H. W. A semiquantitative culture method for identifying intravenous-catheter-related infection. *N. Engl. J. Med.* 296:1305, 1977.
2. Cooper, G. L., and Hopkins, C. C. Rapid diagnosis of intravascular catheter-associated infection by direct Gram staining of catheter segments. *N. Engl. J. Med.* 312:1142, 1985.
3. Flynn, P. M., Shenep, J. L., Stokes, D. C., et al. In situ management of confirmed central venous catheter-related bacteremia. *Pediatr. Infect. Dis. J.* 6:729, 1987.
4. Ryan, J. A., Jr., Abel, R. M., Abbott, W. M., et al. Catheter complications in total parenteral nutrition. *N. Engl. J. Med.* 290:757, 1974.
5. Bjornson, H. S., Colley, R., Bower, R. H., et al. Association between micro-organism growth at the catheter insertion site and colonization of the catheter in patients receiving total parenteral nutrition. *Surgery* 92:720, 1982.
6. Snydman, D. R., Murray, S. A., Kornfeld, S. J., et al. Total parenteral nutrition-related infections. Prospective epidemiologic study using semiquantitative methods. *Am. J. Med.* 73:695, 1982.
7. Pettigrew, R. A., Lang, S. D. R., Haydock, D. A., et al. Catheter-related sepsis in patients on intravenous nutrition: A prospective study of quantitative catheter cultures and guidewire changes for suspected sepsis. *Br. J. Surg.* 72:52, 1985.
8. Sitzmann, J. V., Townsend, T. R., Siler, M. C., et al. Septic and technical complications of central venous catheterization: A prospective study of 200 consecutive patients. *Ann. Surg.* 202:766, 1985.
9. Bozetti, F. Central venous catheter sepsis: The experience of the Instituto Nazionale Tumori of Milan. *Acta Anaesth. Scand.* S81:53, 1985.
10. Brun-Buisson, C., Abrouk, F., Legrand, P., et al. Diagnosis of central venous catheter-related sepsis: Critical level of quantitative tip cultures. *Arch. Intern. Med.* 147:873, 1987.
11. Trooskin, S. Z., Harvey, R. A., and Greco, R. S. Prevention of catheter sepsis by antibiotic bonding. *Surg. Forum* 34:132, 1983.
12. Ducatman, B. S., McMichan, J. C., and Edwards, W. D. Catheter-related lesions of the right side of the heart. *J.A.M.A.* 253:791, 1985.

13. Becker, R. C., Martin, R. G., and Underwood, D. A. Right-sided endocardial lesions and flow-directed pulmonary artery. *Cleveland Clin. J. Med.* 54:384–388, 1987.

14. Murray, M. J., Wignes, M., and McMichan, J. C. Assessment of sterility of pulmonary arterial catheter sheaths. *Anesth. Analg.* 65:1218, 1986.

15. Hudson-Civetta, J. A., Civetta, J. M., Martinez, O. V., et al. Risk and detection of pulmonary artery catheter-related infection in septic surgical patients. *Crit. Care Med.* 15:29, 1987.

16. Band, J. D., and Maki, D. G. Infections caused by arterial catheters used for hemodynamic monitoring. *Am. J. Med.* 67:735, 1979.

17. Slogoff, S., Keats, A. S., and Arlund, C. On the safety of radial artery cannulation. *Anesthesiology* 59:42, 1983.

18. Gurman, G. M., and Kriemerman, S. Cannulation of big arteries in critically ill patients. *Crit. Care Med.* 13:217, 1985.

19. Snydmann, D. R., Donnelly-Reidy, M., Perry, L. K., et al. Intravenous tubing containing burettes can be safely changed at 72 hour intervals. *Infect. Control* 8:113, 1987.

20. Gordon, S. C., Reddy, K. R., Schiff, L., et al. Prolonged intrahepatic cholestasis secondary to acute hepatitis A. *Ann. Intern. Med.* 101:635, 1984.

21. Hollinger, F. B., Khan, N. C., Oefinger, P. E., et al. Posttransfusion hepatitis type A. *J.A.M.A.* 250:2313, 1983.

22. Centers for Disease Control, Department of Health and Human Services: Update on Hepatitis B prevention. Recommendations of the Immunization Practices Advisory Committee. *Ann. Intern. Med.* 107:353, 1987.

23. Berry, A. J., Isaacsom, I. J., Kane, M. A., et al. A multicenter study of the epidemiology of hepatitis B in anesthesia residents. *Anesth. Analg.* 64:672, 1985.

24. Weber, D. J., Rutala, W. A., Samsa, G. P., et al. Obesity as a predictor of poor antibody response to hepatitis B plasma vaccine. *J.A.M.A.* 254:3187, 1985.

25. Craven, D. E., Awdeh, Z. L., Kunches, L. M., et al. Nonresponsiveness to hepatitis B vaccine in health care workers. *Ann. Intern. Med.* 105:356, 1986.

26. Reingold, A. L., Kane, M. A., and Hightower, A. W. Failure of gloves and other protective devices to prevent transmission of hepatitis B virus to oral surgeons. *J.A.M.A.* 259:2558, 1988.

27. Gimson, A. E. S., Braude, S., Mellon, P. J., et al. Earlier charcoal haemoperfusion in fulminant hepatic failure. *Lancet* 2:681, 1982.

28. Rakela, J., Kurtz, S. B., McCarthy, J. T., et al. Postdilution hemofiltration in the management of acute hepatic failure: A pilot study. *Mayo Clin. Proc.* 63:113, 1988.

29. Pappas, S. C. Fulminant hepatic failure and the need for artificial liver support (Editorial). *Mayo Clin. Proc.* 63:198, 1988.

30. Bismuth, H., Samuel, D., Gugenheim, J., et al. Emergency liver transplantation for fulminant hepatitis. *Ann. Intern. Med.* 107:337, 1987.

31. Brems, J. J., Hiatt, J. R., Ramming, K. P., et al. Fulminant hepatic failure: The role of liver transplantation as primary therapy. *Am. J. Surg.* 154:137, 1987.

32. Seligmann, M., Chess, L., Fahey, J. L., et al. AIDS—An immunologic reevaluation. *N. Engl. J. Med.* 311:1286, 1984.

33. Pahwa, S. G., Quilop, M. T. J., Lange, M., et al. Defective B-lymphocyte function in homosexual men in relation to the acquired immunodeficiency syndrome. *Ann. Intern. Med.* 101:757, 1984.

34. Cohen, A. J., Philips, T. M., Kessler, C. M. Circulating coagulation inhibitors in the acquired immunodeficiency syndrome. *Ann. Intern. Med.* 104:175, 1986.

35. Pollak, A. N., Janinis, J., and Green, D. Successful intravenous immune globulin therapy for human immunodeficiency virus-associated thrombocytopenia. *Arch. Intern. Med.* 148:695, 1988.

36. Kotler, D. P., Gaetz, H. P., Lange, M., et al. Enteropathy associated with the acquired immunodeficiency syndrome. *Ann. Intern. Med.* 101:421, 1984.
37. Gillin, J. S., Shike, M., Alcock, N., et al. Malabsorption and mucosal abnormalities of the small intestine in the acquired immunodeficiency syndrome. *Ann. Intern. Med.* 102:619, 1985.
38. Margulis, S. J., Honig, C. L., Soave, R., et al. Biliary tract obstruction in the acquired immunodeficiency syndrome. *Ann. Intern. Med.* 105:207, 1986.
39. Rao, T. K. S., Friedman, E. A., and Nicastri, A. D. The types of renal disease in the acquired immunodeficiency syndrome. *N. Engl. J. Med.* 316:1062, 1987.
40. Greene, L. W., Cole, W., Greene, J. B., et al. Adrenal insufficiency as a complication of the acquired immunodeficiency syndrome. *Ann. Intern. Med.* 101:497, 1984.
41. Dalakas, M. C., Pezeshkpour, G. H., Gravell, M., et al. Polymyositis associated with AIDS retrovirus. *J.A.M.A.* 256:2381, 1986.
42. Fishman, J. An approach to pulmonary infection in AIDS. *Hosp. Pract.* April 15, 1988, pp. 196–204.
43. Spire, B., Barre-Sinoussi, F., Montagnier, L., et al. Inactivation of lymphadenopathy associated virus by chemical disinfectants. *Lancet* 2:899, 1984.
44. Baker, J. L., Kelen, G. D., Sivertson, K. T., et al. Unsuspected human immunodeficiency virus in critically ill emergency patients. *J.A.M.A.* 257:2609, 1987.
45. Centers for Disease Control. Summary: Recommendations for preventing transmission of infection with HTLV-III/LAV in the workplace. *Morbid. Mortal. Wkly. Report* 34:681, 1985.

12. Trauma Management

Glenn S. Vanstrum

OVERVIEW

TRAUMA REGIONALIZATION

History

The roots of organized trauma care may be found in military conflict. Such care has evolved from the Roman legions, who were the first to designate war injury hospitals, to Larrey's use of horse-driven field ambulances in Napoleon's army, to the battalion aid stations of the World Wars [1]. The real models for modern civilian trauma care are found in the Korean and Vietnam conflicts, where injured U.S. soldiers were transported from the field to mobile army surgical hospitals (MASH) in the former war and directly to the surgical hospitals in the latter. Average time from injury to definitive treatment was 81 minutes in one Vietnam study [1].

Unfortunately, the civilian sector was tardy in adapting the military's rapid transport and specialized treatment of trauma victims. The civilian sector was spurred, however, by the landmark paper presented by West, Trunkey, and Lim in 1979, in which they showed that preventable deaths in 1974 were markedly lowered in one California county (San Francisco) that had regionalized trauma care compared to another California urban county (Orange) that did not have trauma centers and simply had triage of injured patients to the "nearest facility" [2]. Orange County subsequently established trauma regionalization, in which dedicated trauma physicians and hospitals treated severely injured patients who were rapidly transported past "nearest facilities" directly to the trauma centers. Careful evaluation by an autopsy method [3] revealed marked reduction in preventable deaths in the new program. Similar positive results were seen in San Diego County after regionalization [4].

Although further reduction in mortality in the civilian sector has been achieved by improvements in prehospital care [5, 6], trauma remains the number one cause of death in individuals under 40 years of age, with one of every eight hospital beds occupied by a trauma patient [7]. Thus it has enormous societal implications. Unfortunately, preventive measures, ultimately the most cost-effective means of reducing mortality, such as handgun control and seat belt and motorcycle helmet laws, are often embroiled in political controversy in this country (see Chapter 15). Although it certainly can play a major role in prevention, it is ultimately up to the medical profession to render acute care when prevention fails. Anesthesiologists and emergency physicians are central players in this field of health care.

SPECIALIST INTERACTION

Trauma care is an odd business at times. Peak volume comes after 6 P.M., often after midnight. Financial reimbursement for those in private practice is uncertain, especially in caring for patients with penetrating trauma [8]. Physicians and other health care personnel who are involved in trauma resuscitation are at increased risk for hepatitis and human immunosuppressive virus infections, both because of the patient population and because of the generally chaotic atmosphere and need for multiple invasive procedures. Stress is high, especially when multiple victims require treatment. Why then do physicians join a trauma team?

In trauma resuscitation, emergency physicians and anesthesiologists have an opportunity to utilize fully their many diagnostic and procedural skills. There is a sense of pride in working in a hospital that can effectively handle major trauma. Finally, there is the realization that, even though many times one is up all night with yet another drunken motorcyclist who failed to wear his helmet, or yet another phencyclidine dealer shot when his drug deal went sour, the next patient might well be a loved one who made a mistake on the freeway, or a child who got adventurous and fell too far.

Unfortunately, while many hospitals have eagerly sought trauma center designation, hoping to gain favorable publicity and prestige, they often realize later the great expense involved in treating the many indigent patients who so often seem to get into traumatic situations. Without funding from governmental sources, concern has been voiced that trauma centers will not survive [9].

On a specialist level, trauma center designation may mean changes in roles. The presence of an in-house trauma surgeon who assumes command of the resuscitation effort does leave the emergency physician with an uncertain role at times. Except in teaching hospitals, it is unusual for trauma anesthesiologists to be in-house, and thus emergency physicians, who routinely handle cardiac arrests, often become the local in-house airway expert. Of course, in a multiply injured patient, all three physicians can and do optimally work as a team simultaneously, with, for example, one intubating, one starting and maintaining lines, and one placing chest tubes.

In community hospitals that receive trauma but are not designated trauma centers, the role of the emergency physician becomes even more central, because surgical and anesthesiologic back-up are often less prompt. Although the trauma census may be lower in such a hospital, this is not always the case.

Teaching hospitals, of course, have their own complex specialist interactions. Usually specialist back-up at the resident level is omnipresent, although the huge patient census one often finds in large inner city teaching hospitals can leave inexperienced (and weary!) residents with complex problems.

TRAUMA AIRWAY MANAGEMENT

BLUNT TRAUMA

Cervical Spine Protection

As discussed in Chapter 2, protection of the injured or potentially injured neck is a paramount consideration in trauma airway management. There are four major options. First, one may judge that a patient is ventilating adequately spontaneously and may only need supplemental oxygen or perhaps a nasal trumpet, jaw thrust, or other modality to clear the upper airway. One must be ever vigilant in this case for subtle deterioration in ventilation and oxygenation. Often the patient with multiple rib fractures will do quite well initially but later tire and show increasing flail movement (Fig. 12-1) and less air exchange. Generally, the tendency is to wait too long, and if there is swelling of an injured tongue or nasopharynx, late intubation may become technically more difficult. If a patient has had major trauma, particularly chest trauma, and intubation is postponed, constant physician observation of the airway is advised. Trouble often occurs in the radiology suite with an unattended patient.

Second, there is nasotracheal intubation with cervical spine traction or immobilization. This is a favorite technique of many physicians, and when it works, it works well. Often, however, a stuporous, semicomatose patient will suddenly become agitated as the tube is passed, shake the head and neck violently, or vomit. Many of these patients eventually develop severe sinus infections later in the intensive care unit (ICU), often with nosocomial organisms that are difficult to treat (see Chapters 2 and 11).

A third option is orotracheal intubation with in-line axial traction. If the patient is not comatose, this often requires the use of muscle relaxants, which can be dangerous in the hands of the unwary or inexperienced physician. Direct laryngoscopy is a terrific stimulus, often of greater magnitude than skin incision for operation. Especially in the patient with increased intracranial pressure, the common hyperdynamic response to this stimulus can be disastrous and may require the use of potent and potentially dangerous agents such as sodium thiopental. Finally, the efficacy of the in-line traction is still controversial. It will be discussed below.

The final option is surgical cricothyroidotomy. This also can have deleterious results, including bleeding, failure, or delayed tracheal abnormalities (see Chapter 2). Optimally, the cervical spine should be immobilized adequately for this procedure as well, and it becomes technically more difficult when the neck is maintained in the neutral (as opposed to the hyperextended) position.

Of the various options, then, none is ideal. One must remember, however, that the *airway always has priority.* No matter which airway option is followed, however, the phrases "adequate immobilization" and "in-line trac-

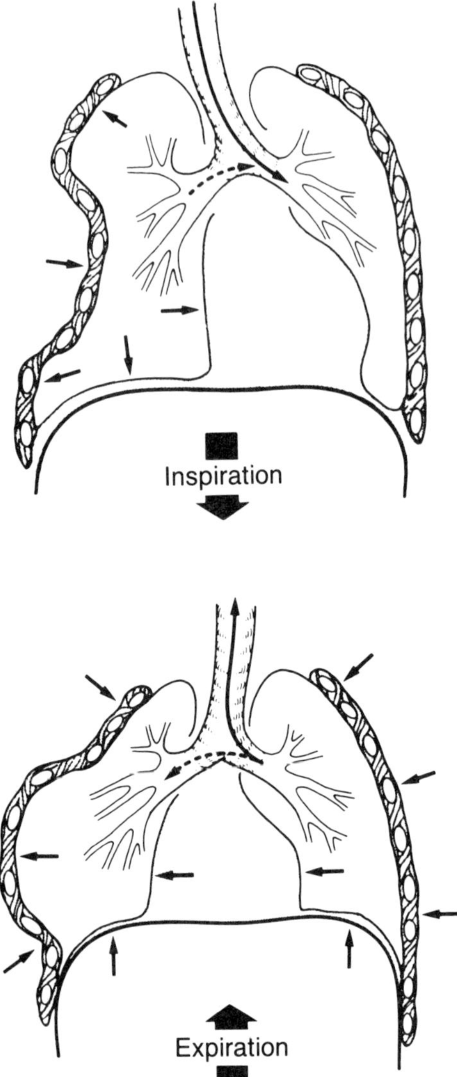

Fig. 12-1. Diagram of flail chest (amount of flail is exaggerated for illustration). As a patient tires, smaller and smaller ventilatory excursions occur as less and less muscular splinting is available. This leads to increasing V/Q mismatch and worsening blood gas tensions. Definitive therapy is institution of positive pressure ventilation after endotracheal intubation. (From W. G. Baxt. *Trauma: The First Hour.* Norwalk, Conn: Appleton-Century-Crofts, 1985. With permission.)

tion" are pertinent. Unfortunately, the literature does not abound with research investigating these modalities. Aprahamian and others presented an interesting work in 1984 in which they created C5–6 instability surgically in a cadaver model [10]. They severed essentially all interspinous ligaments, both anterior and posterior, subjected the cadaver to various airway maneuvers, and examined the resultant changes radiographically. Although one must note critically that the maneuvers could be performed quite differently by different individuals, they concluded that oral airway placement, head tilt, and nasal trumpet placement were relatively safe, and that chin lift, jaw thrust, and nasal or oral intubation all produced marked radiographic changes, such as widening of the disk space, narrowing of the disk space, or subluxation.

In examining this model, one must realize that in a similar clinical injury, say, a flexion-rotation injury with both anterior and posterior disruption, widening of the disk space, which would no doubt accompany in-line cervical traction, would be much less deleterious to the spinal cord than subluxation, which was noted during positioning for nasal tracheal intubation. Unfortunately, the authors did not examine the effect of in-line traction.

A second interesting study was performed on normal volunteers by Majernick and others [11]. They also used radiographic documentation of cervical spine movement and demonstrated that significantly less movement occurred during orotracheal intubation in which in-line traction was present than when a semirigid (Philadelphia) collar was in place. Podolsky also documented the lack of efficacy of soft and Philadelphia collars as a means of immobilization [12] and found that the best protection was afforded by use of laterally placed sandbags on either side of the patient's head and neck, with adhesive tape placed over the forehead onto the bags and secured down to a backboard.

A totally different experimental model was used by Magnaes in Norway [13]. He measured pressure on the cervical spinal cord during endotracheal intubation in patients with cervical spondylosis. This condition mimics injuries of the lower cervical spine. He showed marked diminution of cervical spinous pressures during orotracheal intubation in which anterior longitudinal traction was present. The traction tongs were placed midway between the auditory canal and the orbit, some 3 to 5 cm anterior to the usual position recommended for Gardner Wells tong placement [14]. He substantiated the resultant extension by citing the work of Brieg [15], who showed that some extension of the neck relaxes the spinal cord. Thus, slight extension with traction serves to both relax the cord and stabilize the spine.

Bivins et al. presented a differing study in which they examined the effect of intubation with in-line traction on four deceased trauma victims with unstable neck fractures [16]. Although their study had no control group, and although they did not quantitate in any way the amount of force used by the laryngoscopist, their results indicated that considerable motion occurred. A recommendation in an editorial accompanying this study was made to use only cricothyroidotomy or nasal intubation in patients with suspected neck fractures [17]. The extrapolation of Bivins' cadaver work to the live patient was criticized by Dronen and Syverud [18], who argue for more clinically applicable research before making a blanket endorsement of nasotracheal intubation. Condemnation of axial traction is in disagreement with neurosurgical [19, 20] and orthopedic [21] tradition, in which traction has been used universally and successfully in treating unstable cervical spine fractures. This tradition is substantiated in the anesthesia literature, where, for example, Grande et al. reported on the use of manual in-line axial traction for the intubation of 3000 trauma patients without change in spinal cord function [22].

This issue is related to the controversy about the need for surgical intervention in a patient with possible cervical fracture. Although the Advanced Trauma Life Support (ATLS) course sponsored by the American College of Surgeons (ACS) initially advocated rapid cricothyroidotomy strongly, the ACS has modified their position and now recommend initial in-line axial traction and endotracheal intubation [23]. Most anesthesiologists are wary of cricothyroidotomy due to concerns about the considerable morbidity associated with the procedure, which includes tracheal stenosis, bleeding, infection, and pneumothorax [24] but also because it is common in their experience to intubate easily and successfully, by the oral route, known cervical fracture patients for spinal fusion procedures. This author agrees with Stewart [25] that airway management in the setting of cervical spine injury can often best be performed with axial traction and gentle oral endotracheal intubation.

In conclusion, airway management in the setting of cervical spine injury is uniformly risky. There is substantiation in the literature that in-line traction is efficacious in stabilizing the spine and reducing spinal cord pressure, although more study in this area is needed. The most unstable injuries involve flexion and rotation [26], and if any movement from neutral is to be tolerated, slight extension is best. The author prefers neutral in-line traction, the use of muscle relaxants if necessary, an appropriate dose of sodium thiopental or narcotics (withheld if the patient is hypovolemic), and orotracheal intubation. It is recognized that other modalities, such as conservative treatment, nasotracheal intubation, and cricothyroidotomy, have their place in alternative settings.

The appropriate muscle relaxant for emergent intubation in a trauma patient is the subject of much discussion. The advantages of succinylcholine, the depolarizing agent, are rapid onset after a dose of 1 to 1.5 mg/kg IV (30- to 45-second intubation conditions) and rapid offset in the event intubation is impossible (5 minutes, which is, of course, long enough to cause possible anoxic brain damage if hypoxia is extreme and bag ventilation impossible). Disadvantages include vagally induced bradycardias or even asystole, fasciculations, which can increase gastric pressure and lead to large increases in serum potassium, and the fact that succinylcholine is a trigger agent for malignant hyperthermia. Advantages of a nondepolarizing agent such as vecuronium include the virtual lack of hemodynamic side effects and the presence of good intubating conditions after a dose of 0.1 mg/kg IV [27]. The major disadvantage of this agent is the prolonged period of paralysis it induces (20 to 30 minutes), This author prefers the latter drug, although others may prefer succinylcholine. Either drug can be potentially lethal or life saving.

PENETRATING TRAUMA

Airway management in patients with penetrating trauma is, for the most part, straightforward. There are, however, several pitfalls for the unwary physician. Knife or gunshot wounds can damage the cervical spine and cord, or a person can fall after such a wound is inflicted and damage the neck. Although such injuries are rare, cervical spine protection in a nonresponsive patient is always essential.

Penetrating trauma that results in pericardial tamponade presents another special instance. Venous filling to the heart is restricted and must be maximized prior to surgical intervention. Rapid and decisive thoracotomy is indicated once the diagnosis is made, but in patients who are still conscious and alert, some would perform pericardiocentesis, leave a catheter in the pericardium, and transfer the patient to the operating room. Whether in the operating room or the emergency department, the patient must be intubated prior to incision. One must not allow a prolonged period after intubation with institution of positive pressure ventilation before release of the tamponade. The negative inspiratory force of spontaneous respiration augments what little venous return these patients have, and to substitute positive respiration in its place will lead to arrest rapidly.

Thus, patients who have tamponade in cardiac arrest have little need for decision making. Intubate and incise. The alert and seemingly stable patient with a blood pressure of 80 mm Hg, however, requires surgical preparation, a rapid sequence induction (one set of options would be: cricoid pressure, preoxygenation, IV ketamine 1 mg/kg (see Chapters 5 and 15 for a more complete discussion of this drug), and IV succinylcholine 1.5 mg/kg, wait 45 seconds, intubate), and a stat lateral thoracotomy incision. No delay in preparing sternal saws, looking for rib retractors, or any other wasting of seconds will be tolerated.

One other special circumstance in airway control in patients with penetrating trauma deserves attention. This is penetration of the unilateral pulmonary great vessels with intrabronchial bleeding. In this dire circumstance the use of the double-lumen endobronchial tube is necessary (Figs. 12-2 and 12-3). Isolation of the hemorrhage may preserve the noninvolved lung

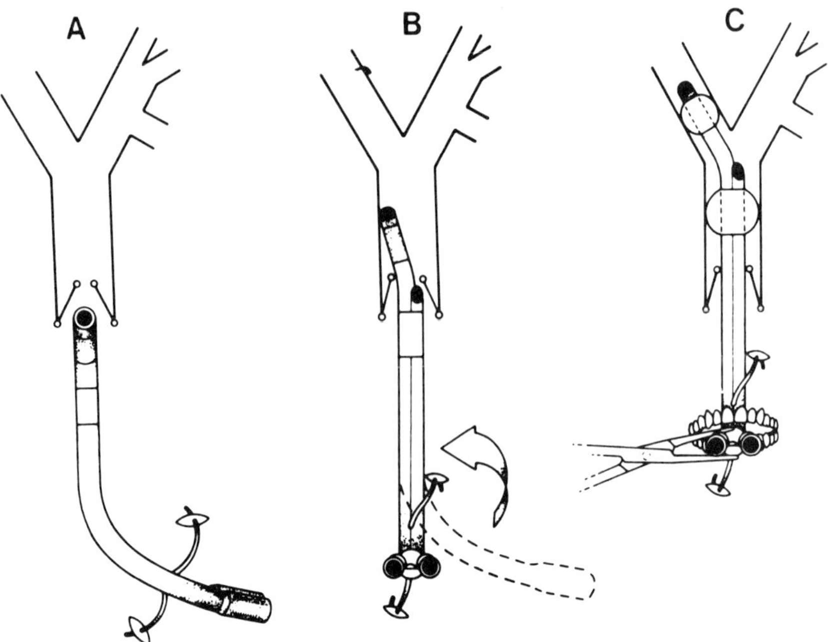

Fig. 12-2. Placement of the double lumen tube. This tube allows isolated ventilation of an individual lung and can protect a lung from hemorrhage or contamination from lung abscess; it can also provide excellent surgical exposure. Accurate placement can be difficult and requires substantial operating room training on elective patients. Fiberoptic bronchoscopy may be needed to confirm placement. It can be a lifesaving technique.

Passage of the left Robertshaw tube is shown. *A.* The distal curvature should be anterior initially as the tube tip passes througoh the glottis, and the proximal curve should be to the right and parallel to the floor. *B.* After the distal tube tip passes the vocal cords, the entire tube should be rotated 90 degrees to the left so that the proximal curvature is now concave anteriorly and the distal curvature is to the left and parallel to the floor. *C.* The tube should be advanced until the common molding or parting of the individual lumen is at or near the teeth, or until moderate resistance to further passage is encountered. (From J. L. Benumof and D. D. Alfery. Anesthesia for Thoracic Surgery. In R. D. Miller [ed.]. *Anesthesia* [2nd ed.]. New York: Churchill Livingstone, 1986. With permission.)

and thus be lifesaving. Use of these tubes is not simple or straightforward and is best done by someone with training in their use during less emergent circumstances.

INTRAVENOUS RESUSCITATION

Timely and adequate volume replacement is the cornerstone of trauma resuscitation. Adequate infusion of warm crystalloids and blood products is

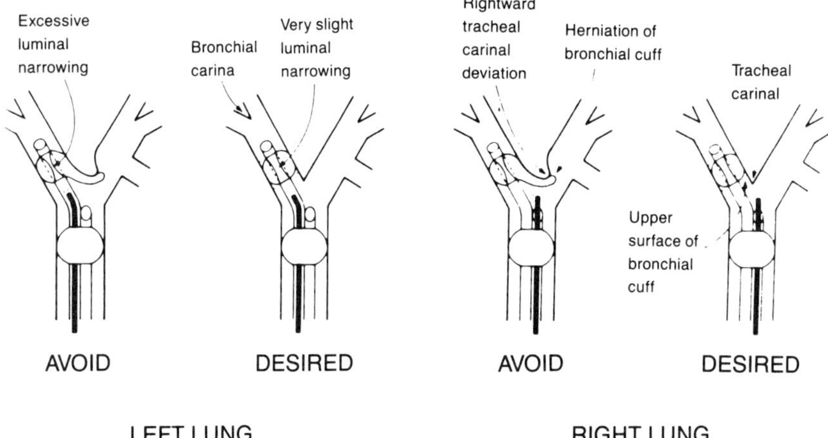

Fig. 12-3. Use of the fiberoptic bronchoscope to determine position of the double lumen tube. When the bronchoscope is passed down the right side, the tracheal carina should be apparent, and the upper surface of the endobronchial cuff should just be visible. When the bronchoscope is passed down the left side, the bronchial carina should be seen past a very slight luminal narrowing. (From J. L. Benumof and D. D. Alfery. Anesthesia for Thoracic Surgery. In R. D. Miller [ed.]. *Anesthesia* [2nd ed.]. New York: Churchill Livingstone, 1986. With permission.)

essential to shock resuscitation. The ACS has published useful guidelines correlating percent of blood volume loss with physical and laboratory findings [23]. When in doubt, however, *give volume.* Complications from volume therapy in adequately monitored trauma patients are rare and easily treated, while morbidity from inadequate replenishment is great. Even isolated head-injured patients at times need large amounts of volume, since, for example, the injured scalp can bleed prodigiously.

PLACEMENT OF PERIPHERAL LINES

Large-Bore Peripheral Lines

The placement of 14- and 16-gauge intravenous lines may be mundane, but in hypothermic, volume-depleted trauma patients vasoconstriction makes the procedure anything but routine. Some tricks include hanging the arm in a dependent position prior to tourniquet placement and warming the arm locally if time permits (and using volume warmers subsequently to keep the patient warm!). One can also use a reverse Esmarch technique by wrapping an Esmarch bandage in a proximal to distal direction to distend the distal extremity veins [28]. Good technique also includes, besides the obvious sterile preparation, the making of a skin hole with another needle prior to insertion of the catheter-needle assembly. Veins can be remarkably tough, and one wants the needle sharp and not dulled by the skin nor occluded with a skin plug. A slight popping motion, in addition to traction maintained with the other hand to immobilize the vessel, is also helpful in penetrating the venous wall. A syringe may be attached to the catheter if penetration of the back wall of the vein occurs. One then gently aspirates as one withdraws, and on getting blood return, advances the catheter with a gentle twisting motion.

In performing any kind of surgical procedure, it is wise to use only the delicate and coordinated muscles of the fingers, not coarse wrist motions or, even worse, motion of the more proximal joints. In watching others perform procedures, one might be amazed at how often they use such coarse musculature for fine coordinated tasks. Critical, detached, and objective self-observation is a much harder skill to develop but will do even more toward improving technique and aiding patients.

Alternate sites (other than antecubital and arm veins) for large-bore peripheral lines are limited to the external jugular (EJ) veins, although sometimes it is possible to cannulate the greater saphenous vein. The head-down or Trendelenburg table position is a prerequisite for EJ placement, and the attached syringe-aspiration technique mentioned above is often helpful. Catheterization of these veins requires rotation of the head, which may obstruct venous drainage from the brain, a consideration that limits its efficacy in head trauma (ICP can increase) and spinal trauma (spinal cord immobilization is violated). The head-down position is also very deleterious for adequate respiratory mechanics.

Controversy exists about the need for placement of large-bore intravenous lines in the field. The average time for such placement has been documented at 8 to 12 minutes [29, 30]. Lewis has developed a computer model incorporating fluid flow rate, transport time, and bleeding rates [26]. His conclusion is that if transport time from scene to definitive care is less than 15 to 20 minutes, initiating IV therapy is not warranted for any type of bleeding. If transport time is greater than 30 minutes, IV therapy is warranted, according to Dr. Lewis.

Others, however, disagree. Pons and associates at Denver General demonstrated increased blood pressure as a result of on-the-scene fluid therapy [31]. Their paramedics, who participate in an intensely supervised and didactic program, spent an average of 10 minutes total on the scene of 203 gunshot or stab wound victims. This included, in addition to intravenous line placement, assessment and base station communication, airway manipulations, and pneumatic antishock garment placement as well. Other studies support their view that prehospital resuscitation is valuable [32, 33]. While the controversy rages, one point is best remembered: Whether an IV line is placed in the field or the ED in the heat of a trauma resuscitation, it should probably be discontinued after 24 hours because of increased risk of infection.

Intraosseous Infusion

Because of the difficulty of establishing intravenous access in pediatric patients in the under 3-year-old age group, the technique of intraosseous infusion has been shown to speed vascular access in patients with cardiac arrest [34]. It involves placement of a large-bore needle, usually a bone marrow biopsy needle, into the marrow of a long bone, usually the anterior tibia, where confirmation of placement is achieved by bone marrow aspiration [35]. Not only will volume loads given in this manner be rapidly absorbed systemically, but also drugs may be infused as well [35]. Contraindications include local infection, fracture, and chronic bony disease.

Venous Cutdown

Because of the wide use of central venous lines and the increased rate of infection with any emergent cutdown technique, this procedure has fallen from favor. One can, however, place an intravenous line with the Luer-lok connector removed directly into the greater saphenous vein by cutdown, and this can be a useful fluid line in a major resuscitation effort. To perform this, one should apply a povidone-iodine splash preparation, make a 2-cm incision just anterior to the medial malleolus, dissect bluntly in a longitudinal fashion to expose the vein, and pass two 2–0 silk ties proximally and distally under the vein. The author recommends placing these ties under traction with mosquito clamps rather than unnecessarily tying the distal tie. One then makes a nick in the isolated vein segment, widens the opening with a clamp, and passes the sterile intravenous tubing or pediatric feeding tube into the lumen. At this point one may tie the silks around the tubing.

Other sites for cutdown include the antecubital fossa, the proximal saphenous vein, and the axillary vein at the deltopectoral groove. The second choice is useful in pediatric trauma (see Chapter 8).

PLACEMENT OF CENTRAL LINES

Indications, Complications, and Sites

Absolute indications for central venous access are less common than would be expected in young trauma patients. Short, large-bore peripheral lines (especially 12- or 14-gauge) function better for volume resuscitation than the usual 6-inch 16-gauge central venous pressure (CVP) catheter. While it is helpful to know the central venous pressure in cases of suspected tension pneumothorax or pericardial tamponade, these diagnoses may be made by noninvasive means (chest radiograph or cardiac echocardiography) or by needle aspiration, which is a treatment as well as a diagnostic method. Nevertheless, knowledge of increased CVP is helpful in making certain clinical decisions, e.g., whether to perform pericardiocentesis in a slightly hypotensive victim with a normal chest radiograph. CVP as a guide to volume replacement is approximate, at best, especially in patients with coronary disease, in which knowledge of left-sided filling pressures for effective volume replacement is prerequisite (see Chapter 3). Still, other parameters that may be used to follow volume status can be misleading, and the CVP is often a helpful piece of data that is related to many organ systems. Is the drop in urine output prerenal, secondary to renal injury, or due to postrenal obstruction or trauma? Is the patient stuporous due to hypovolemia or head injury? Finally, it is often important to have venous access for vasotonic drips, the ability to aspirate blood samples and venous gases easily, and a conduit through which large volume introducers may be passed or through which pulmonary artery catheters may be inserted. Thus, although not always a first priority, CVP access is frequently useful.

Sites for CVP lines are well known and include the brachial, femoral, subclavian, supraclavicular, and internal jugular veins. The brachial vein is difficult to thread consistently toward the right atrium but is relatively safe. The femoral approach carries no risk of pneumothorax and does not require the head-down position for insertion but is located in an area of the body where absolute bacterial counts are high. If the inferior vena cava is disrupted, femoral resuscitation is useless. The subclavian approach requires the head-down position for insertion (with concomitant deleterious effects on ventilation), has a 5 to 10 percent risk of pneumothorax [36] and subjects the catheter to kinking from compression by the first rib and clavicle. The supraclavicular approach, in which the needle is inserted at an angle that bisects the clavicle and the clavicular head of the sternocleidomastoid muscle, also has a high risk of pneumothorax and requires the head-down position.

Finally, the internal jugular (IJ) approach, although it has a somewhat lesser risk of pneumothorax in skilled hands, carries the risk of carotid artery puncture, and although this is usually compressible, it can lead to trachea-compressing hematoma or cerebrovascular neurologic damage. Inadvertent passage of the commonly used 8 Fr introducer through the carotid may necessitate surgical repair. It is difficult to place an IJ catheter when movement of the neck is contraindicated; thus, placement of such a line requires cervical spine clearance. One should be leary of rotating the head in an unconscious, head-injured patient who has only had a normal lateral cervical spine radiograph. Fractures of the odontoid can at times be noted only on the open-mouth odontoid view. Vascular compression in the neck due to hematoma or positioning, which can lead to impedance of venous return and elevated ICP, is a good reason to approach the IJ position with reserve in patients with neurologic trauma.

Other, more general complications of CVP lines are legion and include air embolism, thromboembolism, and later infection. The many risks and benefits must be constantly weighed for each unique clinical situation. Usually, however, with careful technique (see below) these important adjuncts can be placed safely.

Technique and Equipment

The Seldinger technique has become established as the safest and best manner of inserting central lines. It involves, as a standard approach, location of the vein with a long, thin-walled 18-gauge needle, followed by placement of a 0.032-inch guidewire into the vein. The presence of atrial or ventricular aberrant contractions verifies the location of the guidewire in the right side of the heart; their absence neither confirms nor rejects the location. One then makes a skin nick around the wire with a No. 11 blade and passes the catheter or dilator over the wire into the vein with a twisting motion.

Prior to use of the 18-gauge needle it is helpful to use a 22-gauge, 1½-inch needle to locate the vein, especially if one of the internal jugular approaches is used. It is also helpful to pass the 18-gauge needle a millimeter or two into the vein after blood flashes in the syringe. If the guidewire does not thread easily, even with rotation, one must reposition the needle. It is best to apply pressure to the site whenever the needle is removed after an unsuccessful attempt to prevent hematoma formation. Once this occurs the site is usually no longer usable.

In patients who are anticoagulated or in pediatric patients, one may want to use one of the various "micro" size thin-walled needle and guidewire kits that are now on the market. One must be cautious in withdrawing such a guidewire from these needles after an unsuccessful attempt because the wires are so thin that they may be sheared easily.

Prevention of pneumothorax is important in these patients. Obviously, if an existing pneumothorax has been treated with a tube thoracostomy, that is the side that should be considered for a subclavian line. If the patient is awake and coughs with a needle stick, suspect iatrogenic pneumothorax. Prolonged general anesthesia and positive pressure ventilation in a patient with an undiagnosed pneumothorax can convert a simple pneumothorax to the tension variety. Similarly, use of nitrous oxide in the setting of trauma is unwise because it can diffuse rapidly into the pneumothorax and increase its size (see Chapter 5).

Perforation of the superior vena cava or the right atrium can result in life-threatening pericardial tamponade if a CVP catheter is located within the pericardial reflection [37, 38]. Such a disastrous complication has an incidence of from 0.25 to 1.4 percent of CVP lines placed [38]. Positioning of the tip of the catheter, which is often assumed to be adequate if it is in the right atrium or the superior vena cava, may need to be more distal to the heart in light of these reports, probably near the sternal notch on chest radiograph. Such a catastrophic complication of central venous line placement occurred within 24 hours in 36 percent of 49 cases found in Karnauchow's literature review [37] and should be kept in mind in any cardiac arrest occurring in an individual who has such a line in place.

The choice of the femoral CVP line is all too often neglected when it may be the safest route. These lines should, however, be changed to another site later in the ICU to prevent infection. At times the femoral artery may be cannulated during an arrest situation. If no vasoactive drips are given through this line, it may be considered just as effective for volume administration as a venous line (arterial lines are discussed below).

FLUID RESUSCITATION

Mobilization of Interstitial Fluid and the Hematocrit

Although the hematocrit may remain unchanged for several hours after major hemorrhage in which there is no fluid replacement with crystalloid, in young, previously healthy trauma patients spontaneous fluid mobilization from the interstitium after major hemorrhage can be extremely rapid. Some of the earliest work on this phenomenon was done by Francis Moore, who performed phlebotomy in medical students and measured their hematocrits [39]. He calculated, for a two-unit or 1000-ml phlebotomy, that the rate of fluid mobilization was about 200 ml/hr. This author has seen, in a 20-year-old male who had had a stab wound to the chest 30 minutes previously and a 2000-ml hemothorax (without fluid resuscitation), a hematocrit of 22 on the initial CVP line aspiration sample. This is not to say that modern street warriors are somehow physiologically superior to Harvard medical students but that there is a large amount of variability in fluid mobilization. The hematocrit or hemoglobin level is nevertheless very valuable and should be followed serially as an indicator of occult bleeding.

From work in rheology spurred by cardiac surgery, the balance between viscosity and oxygen-carrying capacity is probably optimized at a hematocrit value of 25 to 30. This value is lower in hypothermic states because viscosity is raised and oxygen needs are diminished with hypothermia. In children this value may be altered (see Chapter 8).

Crystalloid vs Colloid. There is still controversy about the use of such crystalloid solutions as Ringer's lactate or normal saline as opposed to colloid solutions such as 5% albumin (hydroxyethyl starch and dextran solutions inhibit platelet function and should be avoided in trauma patients). The classic view in support of crystalloid is that the deficit of interstitial fluid caused by hemorrhagic shock must be replaced by a similar fluid, i.e., a crystalloid, for optimal survival [40]. Although several well-designed studies have shown that there is no real difference in pulmonary function or hemodynamic parameters with either type of solution [41, 42], Dawson has criticized these studies [43], pointing out that both included the use of whole blood, which must be viewed as a colloid. He recommends the use of colloid if packed red cells are used (see section on type O blood below) because it increases the speed of resuscitation and improves hemodynamic indices.

Gammage has done a thorough and dispassionate review of the subject [44]. He acknowledges that there is increased peripheral edema with crystalloid resuscitation and cites some theoretic evidence that this may hinder wound healing and nutrient transport. On the other hand, he notes that albumin costs are far from negligible, with 30 percent of some pharmacy budgets spent on colloid. He concludes, and this author thinks wisely so, that extreme positions in this controversy are unwarranted, that close monitoring of filling pressures is advised, that routine use of colloid in fluid resuscitation is unreasonable, but that it is just as unreasonable to refuse categorically the use of colloid. Whatever philosophy is followed, it seems clear that the primary danger in fluid resuscitation of patients with major trauma is inadequate volume and blood resuscitation or the infusion of hypothermic solutions.

Hypothermia and Fluid Warming. Trauma patients are at increased risk for hypothermia because of prehospital exposure associated with prolonged extrication, necessary exposure in the resuscitation area for diagnosis and treatment, and difficulties associated with the administration of chilled blood and cool resuscitation fluids. The dangers of hypothermia are many. As mentioned above, blood viscosity increases dramatically as blood temperature drops, leading to microcirculatory sludging and impairment of oxygen distribution to energy-starved tissue. At temperatures below 31°C, spontaneous ventricular fibrillation is possible. One of the most common sequelae of hypothermia is its contribution to coagulopathy [45]. Enzymes in homeothermic mammals such as *Homo sapiens* malfunction at abnormal temperatures, and the coagulation system enzymes are no exception.

Consideration for rewarming must be considered at all phases of trauma resuscitation. Paramedics should carry warmed crystalloid solutions. In the ED resuscitation area fluid warmers should be used for all administered fluids. Once a patient has had primary and secondary surveys and treatment has begun in the ED, blankets should be provided as soon as possible. When severe hypothermia exists, active rewarming by nasogastric or peritoneal lavage may be considered. In the operating room, where definitive care may take 12 or more hours, heated, humidified ventilation should be available as well as the above-mentioned modalities. Pure hypothermia without associated trauma has been treated with heparinization and cardiopulmonary bypass (see Chapter 4).

Hyperthermia. This disorder is less rarely involved in trauma but should be searched for and treated just as scrupulously as hypothermia. Volume replenishment and external cooling measures are especially important in neurologic trauma (see Chapter 13). Callaham has written an excellent review of the gamut of heat illness. He recommends use of a combination of evaporation and cooling packs to the neck, groin, and axilla for hyperthermia [46].

Malignant hyperthermia is a genetic disorder that may have fatal symptoms usually triggered by use of such agents as succinylcholine, halothane, or other volatile anesthetic agents. Rarely, it may appear in the ED in susceptible persons under stress without a history of anesthesia or in a more chronic form in patients taking neuroleptics such as haloperidol or the phenothiazines [47]. It is often first noted by unexplained tachycardia or other dysrhythmia, and the diagnosis may be confirmed by demonstrating marked metabolic acidosis by arterial blood gas measurement. Temperature elevation, often extreme, may be a late event. Treatment includes IV dantrolene, a phenytoin relative that prevents excessive calcium release from the sarcoplasmic reticulum, in a starting dose of 3 mg/kg.

Pressure Devices. Two types of pressure devices can be used in trauma resuscitation. The first is the inflatable bag for rapid blood and fluid infusion. This increases fluid flows dramatically when filled to 300 mm Hg and frees one's hands from manually pumping fluids for other tasks. Its use should be routine in all EDs and ORs.

The second pressure device, somewhat more controversial, squeezes the patient and has been called MAST (military antishock trousers) and PASG (pneumatic antishock garment). Initially, this device was thought to "autotransfuse" a patient by compressing blood in the venous capacitance system. Work by Bivens [48] and Gaffney [49] refuted this, showing that an elevation in systemic vascular resistance (SVR) resulted instead. Neither of these investigators used a hypovolemic model, however, and Bellamy and colleagues, in a swine shock model, found little change in SVR but increases in cardiac output and aortic pressure instead [50]. Whatever the hemodynamic effects, these garments provide excellent temporizing treatment for blood loss from pelvic and lower extremity fractures. They should not be left inflated for prolonged periods of time, however, because compartment syndrome, sometimes requiring amputation, is a known complication [51]. Removal, best done in the OR, involves deflation of the abdominal section first. If adequate vital signs are maintained, each leg can then be deflated sequentially.

Other Devices for Massive Fluid Loading

Conventional resuscitation for hypovolemic patients generally leads to several large-bore peripheral intravenous lines, an arterial line, perhaps a CVP line as well, Foley catheter, nasogastric and endotracheal tubes, chest tubes, and so on. Transporting such patients is inevitably necessary, whether to the OR, CT scanning area, or ICU. Not only does the plethora of lines tend to become tangled into a mess of plastic spaghetti, but the patients are often unstable and need things done rapidly and correctly through all those lines and tubes. To alleviate this problem, many have advocated a single combined fluid system to simplify at least the intravenous therapy aspect. Some have recommended the use of 8 and 9 Fr CVP introducers, introduced by means of a Seldinger-technique guidewire with a dilator/introducer [52]. Such lines deliver flow rates with 200 mm Hg of pressure of 540 ml/min and 566 ml/min, respectively, compared with 484 ml/min for a 2-inch 14-gauge peripheral catheter [52]. These introducers are not to be confused with the side-arm ports provided on other large introducers. For example, it has been shown that the flow characteristics from such a side port are similar to those from a 20-gauge, 5.1-cm length catheter [53].

More recently, Iserson and associates have developed a 14-Fr introducer, through which crystalloid and blood products are infused at rates of from 28 to 41 liters/hr [54]. They surmounted rewarming problems by combining warmed crystalloid solutions with the chilled blood products. Other devices that have active rewarming units and flow rates of 30 liters/hr have also been introduced to the market (e.g., Level 1 fluid warmer, manufactured by Level 1 Technologies, Plymouth, MA). Any active trauma center should consider having available some kind of rapid infusion device, because giving multiple warmed units of blood and factors in a very short time through several lines is labor intensive, inefficient, and often chaotic.

AUTOTRANSFUSION

There is no better volume replacement for shed blood than a patient's own warm blood. Especially in cases of hemothorax and cardiac bleeding, in which there is little chance of bowel flora contamination, reinfusion of shed blood can be lifesaving. There are several autotransfusion devices on the market. The simplest is the Sorenson or Pleurovac autotransfusion system, in which blood is collected from (usually) chest tube drainage directly into special bags containing citrate anticoagulant. Blood is collected at less than − 40 cm of suction to avoid traumatic hemolysis and is directed into a disposable liner held in a reusable outer shell. Efforts to minimize blood-air interface are recommended [55]. Acid citrate dextrose anticoagulant is added, preferably so that it is mixed with blood before it reaches the liner, in a 1:7 ratio [55]. Two 170-μm filters are supplied to remove aggregates and particulate matter prior to reinfusion, but some would recommend the addition of a 20- or 40-μm micropore filter as well [56, 57]. This system is relatively simple to use and inexpensive. Because they do not remove platelets and labile clotting factors, the Sorenson and similar Pleurovac autotransfusion devices require anticoagulation and have been implicated in the complication of disseminated intravascular coagulation (DIC) [58]. Blood shed into the thoracic cavity does form fibrin, however, and, except in cases of massive major vessel bleeding, in which brisk bleeding prevents fibrin formation, anticoagulant is not needed, only filtering [59].

Another system, one that has fallen from popularity, is the Bentley autotransfusion device. It utilizes a roller-head pump similar to those used on cardiopulmonary bypass pumps, although 100 percent occlusion at the roller pump head is used to provide negative suction pressure. It requires systemic anticoagulation (an extremely negative feature in patients with multiple trauma) and has been associated with air embolism [57, 58].

A final category of autotransfusion device utilizes the cell-washing technique. Blood is aspirated from the surgical field or chest cavity, anticoagulant (usually heparin) is added, and the resultant blood is washed and centrifuged to produce concentrated red blood cells from which debris, anticoagulant, platelets (which are usually degranulated and of little value to the patient), and white blood cells (usually vacuolated) are all removed. These systems, produced by Haemonetics Corp. (Cell-Saver) and IBM (Cell Processor), require operation by a skilled technician, usually a cardiopulmonary bypass perfusionist. Thus labor and equipment expense is their major drawback. They have not been associated with DIC, although the washed cells must often be supplemented with transfused platelets and plasma for depleted factors [58].

Recently, Timberlake and McSwain reported on the use of cell-washing autotransfusion for patients with penetrating thoracoabdominal trauma and enteric-contaminated blood [60]. Although most washed specimens had positive cultures and 3 of 11 patients developed infections in spite of broad-spectrum antibiotic coverage, there were no cases of intra-abdominal sepsis, and all 11 patients lived and were discharged. Thus the proscription against using enteric-contaminated blood may deserve further study.

In the emergency department setting, systems such as the Sorenson device are recommended by some [61] owing to their simplicity and inexpensive attributes. Cell-washing techniques are probably superior in many regards, however, and if one's hospital has a high enough volume of trauma cases and adequately trained personnel, these systems are worth considering. Certainly their use in any operating room that performs vascular and cardiac surgery should be commonplace.

BLOOD PRODUCTS

Preservatives

Citrate phosphate dextrose (CPD) is the most common anticoagulant-preservative used today. It provides 70 percent red cell survival 24 hours post-infusion for 28 days of storage at 1° to 6°C, although federal regulations deem it outdated at 21 days. Adenine is also added to form CPDA-1. This prolongs storage from 21 to 35 days. The citrate component binds calcium and thus prevents clotting. It can cause serum calcium deficiency during rapid massive transfusion, although the body can usually mobilize the ion rapidly from bony storage sites. Such "citrate toxicity" can be diagnosed clinically by the presence of hypotension accompanied by widening of the QT interval on the ECG. Administration of IV calcium chloride can be gratifying under these circumstances. Because Ringer's lactate (RL) contains 3 meq/liter of calcium, there is a theoretical objection to using this fluid in conjunction with CPD stored blood, and using normal saline instead. This author has noted an increased need to change macropore filters due to clotting after the infusion of several units of blood diluted with Ringer's lactate. No clinical advantage to RL over normal saline has been shown conclusively; thus, the use of normal saline is recommended with blood transfusion.

During storage of blood, glycolysis is slowed by cooling but still occurs, aided by the dextrose additive. Lactate and hydrogen ions are produced, although buffering from the CPD does occur. 2,3-Diphosphoglyceric acid (2,3-DPG) levels progressively fall with a concomitant left shift of the oxyhemoglobin curve and increased hemoglobin affinity for oxygen, and there has been much speculation and controversy about whether or not clinically important organ hypoxia results from this or not. Miller and Brizica have reviewed this topic, and although they acknowledge that more definitive work remains to be done in this field, they do recommend the avoidance of excessive bicarbonate administration, the use of blood that is 1 week old or less for patients who cannot increase cardiac output, and the use of frozen red cells if possible [62].

Frozen red cells, processed in glycerol, can be stored for years and still have adequate survival rates after a somewhat complicated thawing and glycerol-washing process. Advantages of this technique include the fact that rare blood types can be stocked, 2,3-DPG levels are maintained, and fibrin and leukocyte aggregates and antigens are low owing to the washing process [62, 63]. The preparation of such cells does take some time, which precludes their use for early trauma resuscitation.

Component vs. Whole Blood

Although many physicians still prefer whole blood, there are good reasons for using components as needed. First, this allows better distribution of a precious resource. Second, the advantages of whole blood are questionable. The major coagulation defect associated with massive transfusion is thrombocytopenia [62], yet platelet counts in CPD blood fall to 10 percent in only 24 hours. Factors V and VIII, supplied in whole blood or fresh frozen plasma, are rarely a cause of coagulopathy [64]. Thus it may make more sense to use packed red cells, crystalloid, and fresh platelets as needed, even for patients with major trauma. Patients with major trauma probably need a platelet count of greater than 100,000 cells/mm^3. The use of O-negative packed cells for emergency transfusion when time for crossmatch is not available is recommended over O-negative whole blood because the discarded serum often contains antibodies to the A and B major antigens.

The excessive use of fresh frozen plasma (FFP) has been condemned because benefits are questionable and risks of infectious disease contamination are great. A recent National Institutes of Health (NIH) conference issued a list of indications for the use of FFP [64]. This list includes replacement of documented factor deficiency, rapid reversal of warfarin (vitamin K administration requires several days to take effect), and antithrombin III deficiency (the cause of failure of heparin to anticoagulate). FFP is needed for massive transfusion when levels of factors V and VIII are less than 25 percent [62]. In cases of DIC, in which platelets and clotting factors are both massively consumed, one must replace platelets and FFP as needed until the underlying cause of the DIC is remedied.

In spite of the purported advantages of component therapy, criteria for use of FFP and platelets are still unclear in the setting of massive transfusion and DIC, and hence some believe the pendulum is swinging back toward the use of fresh whole blood [65]. More research in this area is obviously needed.

Religious Considerations—Jehovah's Witnesses

The legal aspects of this topic are discussed in Chapter 14. Emergency resuscitation physicians should have a thorough knowledge of the legal guidelines (which, unfortunately, are not as clear as they could be). Many persons of this sect, who refuse blood transfusion, will accept the use of the autotransfusion devices mentioned above, especially if "continuity with the patient" is preserved. Emergent need for blood in minors or pregnant patients can be satisfied after court order (see Chapter 14).

Micro and Macro Filtration

Standard intravenous blood administration sets carry an in-line 170-μm filter, which removes clot and debris associated with stored blood products. Since 1970, when Moseley and Doty [66] demonstrated that some of this material is not removed by such "macro" filtration, there has been controversy about the need for additional "micro" filtration, such as that provided by the many 20- or 40-μm filters now on the market. They also demonstrated that "older" blood has more clot and debris than fresh blood, and that macropore filters are less and less efficient as more units are transfused through them [66].

Pulmonary dysfunction after shock and transfusion therapy, seen clinically as hypoxemia due to shunt and ventilation-perfusion abnormalities associated with the adult respiratory distress syndrome (ARDS), has been related to the effects of granulocytes on the pulmonary microvasculature [67] and to large, fibrin-granulocyte-platelet aggregates that form in blood stored for 10 days [62]. Platelet aggregates do not begin to form until the second to fifth day of storage, yet this author has commonly seen transient hypoxemia after fresh platelet transfusion. This may well be due to vasoactive amine release [68], for which filtration will obviously be of little efficacy. A study by Durtschi and coworkers was unable to show any difference in pulmonary function in patients who received massive transfusion through micro filters compared with those who had the benefit of standard macro filtration [69]. In this study, interestingly, 40-μm filters were found to remove only 12 percent of the aggregates in the first unit of transfused blood and actually to add aggregates in later units. More work needs to be done in this area, but pending new research to the contrary it would seem that the major drawback of the slowing of transfusion caused by micro filtration outweighs any real or imagined advantages given by such devices. Pulmonary platelet sequestration is increased by low flow states [70], and thus rapid volume restoration, already of prime importance, takes on new emphasis in relation to pulmonary function and prevention of coagulopathy. All transfusions should, however, be given with the standard 170-μm filtration [71], which has little effect on infusion rate.

Complications of Transfusion

Transfusion reactions are generally classified as hemolytic, allergic or febrile, and delayed. The former are usually caused by an error in ABO antigen, type, and crossmatch. Hemoglobinuria may be the only sign of a hemolytic reaction in a patient who is severely traumatized and undergoing resuscitation. Prompt treatment consisting of transfusion cessation, fluids, mannitol, furosemide, and alkalinization of the urine may prevent renal damage due to hemoglobinuria. Delayed hemolytic reactions are generally less severe and are caused by incompatibility in the lesser antigens, such as the Rh or Kidd systems. Febrile reactions are common, and the major concern is to rule out hemolytic reaction, which may be done by demonstrating the absence of free hemoglobin or by performance of a direct antiglobin test [62]. Allergic reactions, unless they are of the anaphylactic variety associated with a rare IgA deficiency, are generally mild and are treatable with antihistamines.

Infectious diseases can be and are transferred by transfusion. Human immunodeficiency virus and viral hepatitis are of prime concern, but other diseases such as malaria, cytomegalovirus, and syphilis have been transmitted (see Chapter 11).

Use of Type-Specific and Universal Donor Blood

Most of the progress in this area has been made on the battlefield. Extensive use of group O transfusion was first done at the Anzio beachhead in April, 1944 [72], and transfusion reactions were noted in patients receiving blood with high anti-A and anti-B titers. High-titer group O blood was subsequently identified and not used. Another problem of universal donor blood was identified during the Korean War—that of multiple transfusions with group O blood causing subsequent hemolysis of the patient's usual type-specific cells given later, lysis caused by antibodies still circulating from the group O blood [73]. Because of this problem, Crosby recommended that a period of 2 weeks should transpire after a large transfusion of group O blood before group-specific blood is given [74].

The use of type-specific blood (blood matched according to ABO group and Rh group only) and universal donor blood in Vietnam demonstrated the relative safety of these techniques. During a 10-month period, 230,323 units were transfused [74]. Only 24 hemolytic reactions were observed (0.01 percent), and all but one involved type-specific transfusions and administrative error. As the war progressed, greater and greater percentages of universal donor blood were given, a reflection of concern with these hemolytic reactions. Clusters of these reactions appeared and were associated with chaotic mass casualty situations.

The current consensus among civilian medical authorities in the United States is to take the 5 or 10 minutes required to use type-specific blood for an emergency situation. There is still lingering doubt about detection of dangerous high-titer universal donor blood. Barnes has studied this topic extensively and disagrees [72]. He feels that there is greater risk of administrative error in using type-specific blood, especially in chaotic situations with multiple patients, and that one or two units of O-negative packed red cells should be given immediately because packed cells have a low risk of causing antibody problems. Although packed cells are difficult to give rapidly as such, they may be easily diluted with normal saline for rapid transfusion. One can then switch to type-specific blood without problems.

Lefebre and coworkers reported on the use of 537 units of O-negative packed cells in 133 trauma patients and had no clinical complications [75]. They did find that 10 of 116 patients showed positive results on direct antiglobin tests, seven of these ten having received more than eight units of type O blood. Thus, if large amounts (greater than four to eight units) of O blood are given, it is advisable to continue with universal donor blood until direct antiglobin tests are negative.

Pulmonary Complications

As alluded to above in the discussion on filters, pulmonary deterioration can occur as a direct result of massive transfusion. In this author's experience, this complication is related most closely to the need for transfusion of platelets and FFP, especially the former. After a protracted resuscitation in a patient with coagulopathy, in which scores of units of factors are often required during 12 to 24 hours, not to mention multiple autotransfusions of shed blood and red cell transfusions, the lungs commonly develop the usual stigmata of the adult respiratory distress syndrome (ARDS). Compliance drops, intra-alveolar filling occurs, and hypoxia, even with toxic inspired oxygen concentrations, is common. Maximal use of positive end-expiratory pressure (PEEP) and careful pulmonary toilet and antibiotic use

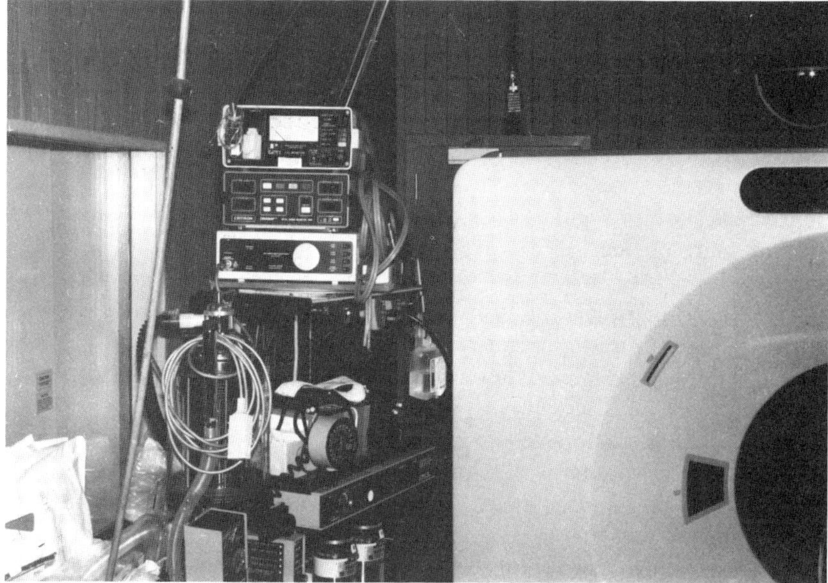

Fig. 12-4. Computed tomography monitoring and anesthetic apparatus. Note the tier of three monitors mounted on a swivel above the anesthesia machine. This arrangement permits observation of monitors from control room (*far left*) or while positioning patient in scan apparatus (*far right*). Stacked from top down are an end-tidal CO_2 monitor, automatic blood pressure device, and oxygen saturation monitor. (Courtesy of Sharp Memorial Hospital, San Diego, California.)

are the only therapeutic options that are efficacious in this setting (see Chapter 3). If right heart failure develops, infusion of prostaglandin E (PGE) may dilate the pulmonary vasculature without marked systemic effects. Differential vasoconstriction can be achieved systemically during thorocotomy, if and when PGE causes hypotension, by administering phenylephrine via a left atrial line (see Chapter 4).

MONITORING

PULMONARY STATUS

Effective monitoring of the pulmonary system is discussed in Chapters 2 and 3. It is only important to repeat here that at the present time, oxygen saturation monitoring and end-tidal CO_2 monitoring are fast becoming state-of-the-art procedures and will probably be considered the standard of care in all emergency departments and operating rooms shortly. Their use in computed tomography suites is also invaluable and should be considered in any trauma center (Fig. 12-4).

BLOOD PRESSURE

The condition of trauma patients, like cardiac patients, can deteriorate rapidly and unexpectedly. It is essential in a patient with major trauma to maintain constant vigilance of arterial pressure by either repeated (every 3 to 5 minutes) occlusive cuff measurements or second-to-second pressure monitoring by arterial line. The former may be done by hand, which is labor intensive and often irregularly performed. There are a number of automatic blood pressure devices on the market, most of which work by the oscillometric method [76], but some work by the auscultatory method or by Doppler detection of wall motion. These devices are rapidly becoming the standard of care in trauma resuscitation areas and operating rooms. Unfortunately, at lower pressures they function less effectively and even in the best of circumstances they give only intermittent information.

Arterial catheterization and transducer pressure monitoring is the gold standard of blood pressure measurement. Rapid institution of such monitoring in the ED is essential in critically ill trauma patients. Most transducers use variable resistance by means of a Wheatstone bridge to convert the fluid wave pressure changes through distortion of wires or semiconductor elements to an electronic signal that can be displayed on an oscillograph. Sites for arterial cannulization in trauma patients include the radial, brachial, femoral, and axillary approaches. Usually the radial artery is preferred because the ulnar artery usually provides collateral circulation should occlusion later occur. This may happen in 20 to 50 percent of patients [77, 78], although serious results of this are rare (Fig. 12-5). Embolization of thrombi released from the catheter can produce occlusion of the digital artery and loss of part of a digit [79]. A 20-gauge catheter is preferred at this site.

Brachial and femoral artery catheters are also useful in trauma patients. Prys-Roberts strongly defends the former [79], especially in comparison with the radial site, but he emphasizes the need to use short, small catheters (18- or 20-gauge) and to avoid cutdown. Others are distrustful of this site because it is an "end" artery. The femoral site is ideal for a patient with hypotension or a patient in extremis. Generally the Seldinger technique is preferred, and a 12- to 15-cm 18-gauge catheter is used. If a patient has no palpable pulse, one can still usually find the artery if effective chest compressions are instituted, midway between the pubic tubercle and the iliac crest. Although thorough sterile preparation should precede any cannulation, this site is especially prone to infection and should always be prepared with povidone-iodine solution.

Technique for successful percutaneous cannulation includes sterile preparation, liberal use of local anesthetic both for pain and to decrease vasospasm, and placement of a skin hole with another needle. One then enters the artery using the finger muscles to direct the needle in a 45-degree angle. Once blood return occurs, it is helpful to lower the needle so that it is almost parallel to the skin and advance it a bit more. If one can advance the

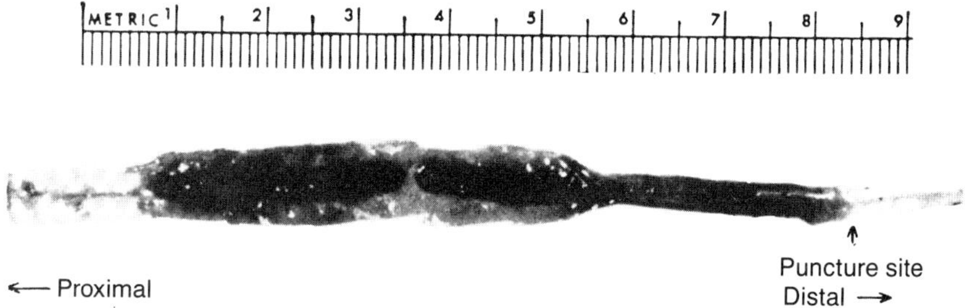

Fig. 12-5. Postmortem specimen of a 22-day-old partially organized radial-artery thrombus that developed 28 hours after cannulation. The thrombus extends proximally from the site of arterial puncture. Such thrombi occurred in 40 of 105 cannulations studied prospectively [77]. Of the 20 patients who were followed with radial artery thrombi, all subsequently had recanalization, and no major ischemic complications were noted. (From R. F. Bedford and H. Wollman. Complications of percutaneous radial-artery cannulation: An objective prospective study in man. *Anesthesiology* 38:228–236, 1973. With permission.)

needle enough to ensure that the outer cannula is inside the vessel (usually 2 mm), one can slide the catheter into the vessel. If, however, the needle penetrates the back wall of the artery, simply remove the needle and slowly withdraw the catheter until vigorous blood return is noted and then advance the catheter with a gentle, twisting motion.

Arterial line placement can be messy, and in this day of fatal infectious disease this is of more than aesthetic concern. Some advocate placing pressure tubing and syringe or a similar sysstem on the catheter prior to cannulation to avoid splatter of blood. Such a system is cumbersome and makes determination of entry into the vessel more difficult. Although strict sterile technique is a must, latex gloves do diminish sensation and, if the arterial pulse is faint, can lower rates of success. One can, while keeping one hand sterile, palpate the artery above the sterile puncture site, transfix the artery with the other gloved and sterile hand, and then glove both hands prior to threading the catheter. This technique lacks style but is effective. When using the Seldinger technique, one must prepare, drape, and glove in the usual sterile fashion. This guidewire technique is messy but usually effective, although it is possible to create a false lumen and dissect the artery with the guidewire.

Once the cannula is placed, one connects the shortest possible length of pressure tubing feasible to the transducer to minimize harmonic accentuation of systolic pressure. Aspiration before flushing is important to remove air bubbles. Retrograde flow does occur with arterial flushing, and one can thus drive air bubbles to the cerebral or coronary circulation with careless, vigorous arterial line flushing. Suture or secure taping of the line should always be done carefully.

Once the arterial line is connected to a properly zeroed transducer, one can derive a great deal of information from the pulse tracing. Heart rate, an estimate of myocardial contractility from the slope of the upstroke, resistance and compliance from the slope of the downstroke, and the effect of cardiac dysrhythmia on hemodynamics can all be appreciated in addition to blood pressure [79]. A marked decrease in beat-to-beat pressure with positive pressure ventilation is a sign of hypovolemia. Should the pressure damp suddenly or lower to dangerous levels, it is always important to examine the patient and the pressure monitoring system carefully before jumping to the conclusion that the patient is in extremis and needs radical therapy. This author has seen an epinephrine bolus cause needless prolonged hypertension in a patient who had a kinked arterial line and a normal blood pressure earlier.

Although it is known that infection rates are higher in cutdown cannulations, this is still a worthwhile technique to use when percutaneous cannulation is difficult or impossible and femoral cannulation is not an available alternative. Useful instruments for a cutdown tray include a small self-retaining retractor, several clamps, a scalpel, preparation materials, sponges, and silk 2–0 ties. The technique is similar to the one described above for venous cutdown. After a careful preparation, one makes a lateral incision, usually at the radial artery site, and uses a mosquito clamp to dissect bluntly parallel to the artery. Sharp dissection and lateral dissection at right angles to the artery will surely lead to complications. One then passes the ties under the artery and places the artery under tension by clamping the ties to the drape distally and proximally. Again, one should not tie off the distal tie but simply provide tension with a mosquito clamp. Good surgical technique dictates penetrating the skin distal to the incision with the catheter/needle assembly. One penetrates the artery under direct vision, places the catheter, connects the pressure tubing, removes the ties, sutures the catheter to the skin, and closes the wound with a nonabsorbable, nonbraided suture such as Prolene. A skilled practitioner can reliably place an arterial line in this fashion in 5 minutes, even in a patient with extreme hypotension. This is often preferable to spending 20 minutes sticking a patient in all four limbs ("four-postering"), creating multiple hematomas and needle puncture sites, and possibly failing anyway.

VENOUS PRESSURE MONITORING

Techniques and indications for CVP monitoring are discussed above, and pulmonary artery catheter monitoring is discussed in Chapter 4. Suffice it to say here that although the great majority of young penetrating trauma victims rarely benefit initially from pulmonary artery (PA) catheter monitoring or even from CVP pressure monitoring, for that matter, many elderly blunt trauma patients do need a PA catheter for the accurate estimation of filling pressures and for determination of vascular resistances. Often a motor vehicle accident results as a direct corollary of a medical problem, such as cardiac-induced syncope or a cerebral vascular event. Such invasive monitoring can shed important light on the therapy of such difficult patients.

PATIENT TRANSFER

BACK MECHANICS AND PRESERVATION

Whether one works in the field, the emergency department, or the operating room, it seems constantly necessary to move patients from one place to another. Such work is dangerous to the well-being of a vertebral spine only recently required by evolution to assume the vertical position. More simply put, if one's back is a source of agony, work becomes impossible. If one cannot work, one's patients suffer. There are two cornerstones of prevention of back injury, which all medical personnel must appreciate. The first relates to knowledge of sound lifting mechanics. The second is related to the need for optimal specific physical conditioning to prevent injury.

The act of lifting requires adherence to four laws. First, keep the axial skeleton in a vertical position—i.e., do not bend the back while lifting. Up and down lifting motion is provided by the legs, not the back. Second, avoid loads that are at a lateral distance to the axial skeleton—i.e., keep weight close to one's body, not at arm's length. Laterally distanced loads apply force unevenly to the spinal column and predispose to the shifting of disks. Third, avoid rotation while bearing a load. Rotation also predisposes to uneven force applied to the spinal column. Fourth, tighten the abdominal musculature while lifting. This acts as an internal brace and relieves the load on the spinal muscles and ligaments.

Proper conditioning is closely related to the fourth point above. A soft, protuberant abdomen is the precursor to lumbar laminectomy surgery. Daily abdominal exercises and tightening of the abdomen while lifting, paradoxical as they may seem, are the key to prevention of back injury.

TRANSFER MODES

Ground Vehicle

Modern ambulances are usually staffed by nonphysician paramedics or emergency medical technicians, sometimes with physician contact by radio. Care in the field can be quite sophisticated with this arrangement, although as transfer times become shorter, the "scoop and run" philosophy becomes more cogent. In the United States, such vehicles today usually have equipment for airway maintenance, splinting, and volume administration. Except in a few areas, where paramedics use nitrous oxide for certain medical patients, oxygen is the only gas provided. Morphine is the usual analgesic agent used. During a recent trip to the Soviet Union, the author was surprised to find that not only do anesthesiologists (or emergency physicians/anesthesiologists, or "reanimatologists," as they are called) staff ambulances, but also many vehicles contain small anesthesia machines that can provide oxygen, nitrous oxide, and methoxyflurane (rarely used in the United States because of renal toxicity). The use of nitrous oxide in patients who may have a pneumothorax is contraindicated because it tends to expand such an air collection rapidly; still, such a prehospital system is interesting. Other European trauma systems, especially in France and Germany, also provide physicians as part of field resuscitation.

Helicopter Transfer

Since the Korean War helicopters have played an important role in casualty transfer and improved rapid resuscitation of trauma patients. Recent work by Baxt and coworkers has clearly demonstrated that helicopters can significantly improve survival in civilian trauma [80, 81]. Such improved survival is expensive, however, and the price paid is not only financial. A number of medical helicopters have crashed with fatal outcomes, and the tendency to use wartime criteria for flights in inclement weather may be responsible. Careful criteria in regard to patient selection is a first step in reducing these costs [82]. The Federal Aviation Administration is currently preparing guidelines that should help to prevent such problems, but at the time of this writing they are not yet available (personal communication, William Baxt, M.D., Life Flight, UCSD) (Fig. 12-6).

Intrahospital Transfer

Often neglected as a source of danger, transfers of critically ill patients between departments should be regarded as extremely hazardous. Use of oxygen and ECG monitoring has become standard, but physician attendance is just as important. It may not be safe for critically ill, intubated patients to be sent to the CT scan area without a physician (preferably an anesthesiologist or an emergency physician) in attendance. Because it is often difficult for the ED physician to leave a busy ED, an anesthesiologist should be recruited for such a role. As will be discussed below, in trauma the first priority of an anesthesiologist is resuscitation and preservation of homeostasis, and only then the administration of anesthesia and analgesia. Thus the European term of *reanimatologist* (used for both ED physicians and anesthesiologists) may be more appropriate.

General guidelines for intrahospital patient transfer must include disconnecting endotracheal tubes just before bed-to-bed transfer and prompt reconnection after transfer. A backboard should be used with the patient's forehead taped down securely to prevent cervical spine injury. Most CT

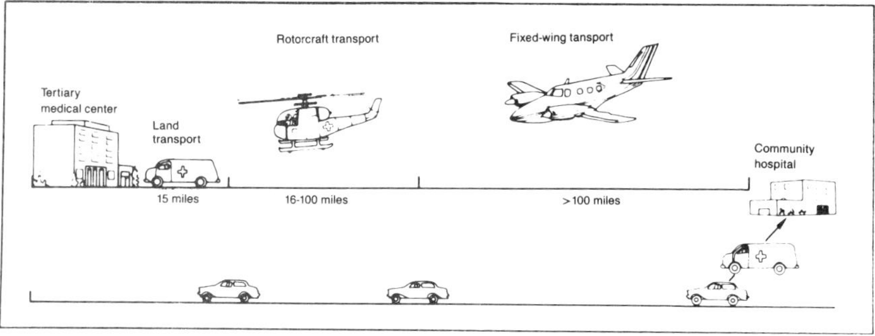

Fig. 12-6. Proposed scheme for rapid transport of patients. Helicopter transport is used by 36 percent of hospitals represented by physicians who answered questionnaire in Chapter 1. (From W. G. Baxt. *Trauma: The First Hour.* Norwalk, Conn: Appleton-Century-Crofts, 1985. With permission.)

scanning equipment has a means of scanning such a patient without any manipulation of the neck. This often requires removing the usual head restraint present on such devices. If there is no backboard, the individual responsible for the patient's head must not be required to assume any other body weight because first, the head is very heavy, and second, assuming its weight during transfer without any cervical spine movement requires full attention. Optimal monitoring in the CT scan area includes oxygen saturation and end-tidal CO_2 monitoring, especially if hyperventilation is necessary.

Organization of intravenous lines and arterial lines is essential during patient transfer. It is facilitated by making sure connections are tight initially (most tubing requires a push-and-twist motion), by providing adequate extensions for IV tubing initially (only arterial lines should be short, see above), and by securing lines at the skin thoroughly (arterial lines and CVP lines sutured and IV lines taped). Use of IVAC-type devices are to be avoided, if possible, when transfers are anticipated. Blood warmers are usually bulky but are an essential part of continuing therapy in trauma patients.

EMERGENCY OPERATION IN THE EMERGENCY DEPARTMENT

GENERAL CONSIDERATIONS

Of the various functions of an anesthesiologist, i.e., provision of analgesia, amnesia, hypnosis, muscle relaxation, and maintenance of homeostasis, in patients with major trauma the last item overshadows the others. Thus, as stated before, resuscitation must occur before drugs that ease pain, prevent memory, and induce sleep can be given. Most such drugs cause some degree of vasodilatation and hypotension and must be withheld initially. Even ketamine, which usually increases blood pressure and heart rate by catecholamine release, may cause hypotension in a patient in extremis who is catecholamine depleted (see Chapter 5). Thus there is a high incidence of awareness among surviving trauma patients during initial resuscitation. Bogetz and Katz at the University of California, San Francisco reported on two groups of major trauma patients, one group of 37 who were stable enough to receive some anesthesia, and another group of 14 who were severely injured and did not receive anesthesia per se during intubation or for 20 or more minutes during operation [83]. Eleven percent of the first group and 43 percent of the second had recall of surgery, and several considered this memory their worst hospital experience. The authors concluded that identification of aware patients was impossible and that postoperative discussion of the problem was beneficial in minimizing psychiatric sequelae. Others have commented that the giving of sufficient drugs to obliterate all awareness would expose many patients to dangerously deep levels of anesthesia, and that pain per se has not been the usual problem, only awareness [84]. Thus, one's first responsibility is to keep the patient alive. To quote Dr. Gilbert Kinyon, current secretary of the American Society of Anesthesiologists (ASA), "You can kill a patient with kindness" (personal communication).

Below are discussed surgical and anesthetic aspects of the three operations most commonly performed in the emergency department. The reader should bear in mind that these procedures are not to be undertaken by any physician or in the absence of an unprepared ED team. The potential for iatrogenic injury runs high, and physicians who undertake these procedures require adequate training and previous clinical experience. Simon and Brenner have presented much more detailed discussions of the procedural aspects discussed below [85], and the reader is encouraged to consult their work or one of many excellent surgical textbooks dealing with these procedures. There are considerable risks of transmission of infectious diseases during these often chaotic procedures, and all personnel must wear gloves and avoid contact with needles, scalpels, and splattering blood.

TUBE THORACOSTOMY

Surgical Technique

Placement of a tube to drain air or blood from the thorax can be life saving. If the patient is awake and stable one prepares and gives an adequate local anesthetic (see below). A 3-cm incision is then made over the fourth or fifth rib at the anterior axillary line. (Chest tubes are rarely placed for pneumothorax between the first and second ribs at the midclavicular line; these produce unsightly scars and are seldom justified.) One then dissects bluntly over the rib, to avoid the intercostal neurovascular bundle, and pops a blunt clamp through the parietal pleura. The pleural space is then explored digitally, and any adhesions that may exist are separated. Extensive adhesions require use of another chest wall site. One grasps a 34- or 36-Fr tube in the clamp, places the tube in the pleural space, and directs it either apically, for pneumothorax, or posteriorly, for hemothorax. The tube is then secured into place with 1–0 or 2–0 sutures and placed to water seal drainage, with an appropriate autotransfusion device interposed to collect blood.

Some practitioners tunnel one rib up from the incision to prevent leakage of air and fluid, but this is not recommended for thick-chested individuals. Some use trocars to place chest tubes, inserting them through a skin incision without digital exploration; this is extremely dangerous because there are patients who have adhesions of visceral to parietal pleura. Placement of a trocar in the lung parenchyma can cause near-instant death from an air embolus. Similarly, a great deal of force is required to push the trocar through the chest wall. Should too much force be expended, lung parenchymal puncture can easily occur.

Should the primary indication for tube thorocostomy be hemothorax, it must be recognized that adequate volume resuscitation must be initiated prior to drainage. The blood collection may offer some tamponade to the bleeding site, and drainage will not improve the situation. Similarly, one should take the time to prepare autotransfusion materials prior to emergent drainage of hemothorax. In cases of tension pneumothorax, of course, time is of the essence.

Anesthetic Aspects

Placement of a tube thoracostomy is very painful. There is no excuse for skimpy use of local anesthetic in an awake, stable individual. Local anesthetic use near the intercostal vascular system does produce relatively high serum levels; hence use of bupivacaine is contraindicated in this setting (see Chapter 9). The author recommends the infiltration of 3 mg/kg lidocaine (in a 70-kg person, this would be 21 ml of 1% lidocaine) along the area of incision, with thorough infiltration of the pareital pleura. One can avoid excessive edema in the area of dissection but retain anesthesia by injecting local anesthetic on either side of the area to be incised along the rib. If one insists on tunneling the tube to a higher rib, one should infiltrate the parietal pleura and intercostal areas at several rib levels.

Use of narcotic supplements as tolerated will also be appreciated by the awake, stable patient. Of course, if the patient's condition is unstable or if he is unconscious, anesthetic considerations become moot. The use of a local anesthetic such as lidocaine is quite safe, however, and it is the author's impression that its adequate use for tube thorocostomy is, unfortunately, rare.

CRICOTHYROIDOTOMY

Indications for this procedure have been discussed above. After a quick povidone-iodine preparation and hyperextension of the neck (if cervical spine work-up so allows), a lateral 2.5-cm incision is made below the thyroid cartilage prominence or Adam's apple and above the cricoid cartilage. The incision is carried down through the cricothyroid membrane. It is widened by a self-retaining retractor or by the handle of the scalpel. An appropriate airway (a small endotracheal tube will work perfectly adequately) is introduced, and the balloon is inflated. One must not neglect the usual maneuvers to ascertain proper placement of the airway (auscultation, observation of end-tidal CO_2 production, and so on). Bleeding vessels encountered during the dissection should be clamped initially if time permits and tied only after the airway is established. The procedure is relatively contraindicated in small children.

THOROCOTOMY

Indications

Patients with penetrating trauma who are moribund or in frank cardiac arrest require immediate thorocotomy. Patients with blunt trauma in cardiac arrest have a uniformly dismal prognosis, and thorocotomy for this indication is controversial. Patients with massive intra-abdominal bleeding who do not respond to resuscitative measures may benefit from cross-clamping of the thoracic aorta prior to definitive OR treatment. Patients with pericardial tamponade who do not respond to pericardiocentesis require thorocotomy.

Surgical Technique

After endotracheal intubation and positive pressure ventilation have been established, a left lateral incision is made below the nipple at the fourth or fifth intercostal space. It is carried over the rib into the chest cavity. A rib-spreading retractor is placed and the pleural cavity examined. Use of a headlight or an OR spotlight is essential. If massive hemothorax is present, the use of suction devices attached to an autotransfusion apparatus may be life saving. If cardiac rupture or tamponade exists or if open heart massage is required, the lung is retracted gently and the pericardium is incised longitudinally, care being taken to avoid the phrenic nerve and the great vessels. Cardiac laceration is repaired with mattress sutures placed with a large needle through Teflon pledgets. Sutures without pledgets may tear the cardiac wall. Care must be taken to avoid suturing coronary arteries.

Although the thoracic aorta may be compressed through the parietal pleura, if extreme hypotension demands clamping of the thoracic aorta, the pleura is incised and the aorta identified and clamped gently with a nontraumatic vascular clamp. Renal failure and paraplegia are common complications resulting from prolonged clamping of the suprarenal aorta.

Anesthetic Considerations

As mentioned above, endotracheal intubation and positive pressure ventilation are prerequisites for successful thorocotomy. Intravenous access and volume resuscitation are essential once the airway and hemorrhage are under control. The use of nondepolarizing muscle relaxants will become necessary as the patient regains blood pressure, as will the gradual institution of intravenous ketamine or narcotics. Intra-arterial monitoring should be established as soon as possible. Often a radial artery cutdown or femoral line are the sites of choice.

REFERENCES

1. Trunkey, D. D. Predicting the Community's Needs: Local Solutions to Local Problems. In J. G. West (ed.), *Trauma Care Systems.* New York Praeger, 1983. Pp. 5–10.
2. West, J. G., Trunkey, D. D., and Lim, R. C. Systems of trauma care: A study of two counties. *Arch. Surg.* 114:455, 1979.
3. West, J. G., Cales, R. H., and Gazzaniga, A. B. Impact of regionalization: The Orange County experience. *Arch. Surg.* 118:740–774, 1983.
4. Baxt, W. G., and Moody, P. The differential survival of trauma patients. *J. Trauma* 27:602–606, 1987.
5. Jacobs, L. M., Sinclair, A., Beiser, A., et al. Prehospital advanced life support: benefits in trauma. *J. Trauma* 24:8–13, 1984.
6. Ornato, J. P., Craren, E. J., Nelson, N. M., et al. The impact of improved emergency medical services and emergency trauma care on the reduction in mortality from trauma. *J. Trauma* 24:674, 1984.
7. Trunkey, D. D., and Lewis, F. R. *Current Therapy of Trauma—2.* Philadelphia: B. C. Decker, 1986. P. xi.
8. Boyd, C. R., Saleeby, R. G., Wood, K. W., et al. Payor mix of trauma patients at a rural-metropolitan regional trauma center: A three-year experience. *Ann. Emerg. Med.* 17:696–699, 1988.
9. Schwab, C. W., Young, G., and Camishon, R. C. Total DRG reimbursement: The demise of the trauma center (abstract). American Association of Trauma, Annual Meeting, Montreal, Canada, 1987.
10. Aprahamian, C., Thompson, B. M., Finger, W. A., et al. Experimental cervical spine injury model: Evaluation of airway management and splinting techniques. *Ann. Emerg. Med.* 13:584–587, 1984.
11. Majernick, T. G., Bieniek, R., Houston, J. B., et al. Cervical spine movement during orotracheal intubation. *Ann. Emerg. Med.* 15:417–420, 1986.
12. Podolsky, S., Baraff, L. J., Simon, R. R., et al. Efficacy of cervical spine immobilization. *J. Trauma* 23:461–465, 1983.
13. Magnaes, B. Clinical recording of pressure on the spinal cord and cauda equina.

Part 3: Pressure on the cervical spinal cord during endotracheal intubation in patients with cervical spondylosis. *J. Neurosurg.* 57:64–66, 1982.

14. Dunford, J. V. Spinal Cord Trauma. In W. G. Baxt (ed.), *Trauma.* Norwalk, Conn.: Appleton-Century-Crofts, 1985. P. 209.

15. Brieg, A. *Adverse Mechanical Tension in the CNS. An Analysis of Cause and Effect. Relief By Functional Neurosurgery.* Stockholm: Almqvist & Wiksell Int'l., 1978.

16. Bivins, H. G., Ford, S., Bezmalinovic, Z., et al. The effect of axial traction during orotracheal intubation of the trauma victim with an unstable cervical spine. *Ann. Emerg. Med.* 17:53–57, 1988.

17. Joyce, S. M. Cervical immobilization during orotracheal intubation in trauma victims. *Ann. Emerg. Med.* 17:145, 1988.

18. Dronen, S. C., and Syverud, S. A. Answering the airway management question. *Ann. Emerg. Med.* 17:1132–1133, 1988.

19. Wagner, R. C. Management of acute spinal cord injury. *Surg. Neurol.* 7:346–350, 1977.

20. Butler, A. B. Cervical Traction. In R. H. Wilkins and S. S. Rengachary (eds.), *Neurosurgery.* New York: McGraw-Hill, 1985. Pp. 1719–1722.

21. Holdsworth, F. Fractures, dislocations and fracture—dislocations of the spine. *J. Bone Joint Surg.* 52-A:1533–1551, 1970.

22. Grande, C. M., Barton, C. R., and Stene, J. K. Appropriate techniques for airway management of emergency patients with suspected spinal cord injury. *Anesth. Analg.* 67:710–718, 1988.

23. American College of Surgeons. *Advanced Trauma Life Support Course.* 1984.

24. Roven, A. N., and Clapham, C. C. Cricothyroidotomy. *Ear Nose Throat J.* 62:489, 1983.

25. Stewart, R. D. Airway Management. In D. D. Trunkey and F. R. Lewis (eds.), *Current Therapy of Trauma—2.* Philadelphia: B. C. Decker, 1986. Pp. 30–44.

26. Lewis, F. R. Prehospital Fluid Resuscitation. In D. D. Trunkey and F. R. Lewis (eds.), *Current Therapy of Trauma—2.* Philadelphia: B.C. Decker, 1986. Pp. 45–46.

27. Culling, R. D., Middaugh, R. E., and Mend, E. J. Rapid tracheal intubation with vecuronium. *Anesthesiology* 69(S):3A:A880, 1988.

28. Jarvis, A. P. Aids for easy cannulation. *Anesthesiology* 65:448–449, 1986.

29. McSwain, N. R., Garrison, W. B., and Artz, C. P. Evaluation of resuscitation from cardiopulmonary arrest by paramedics. *Ann. Emerg. Med.* 9:341–345, 1980.

30. Smith, J. P., Bodai, B. I., Hill, A. S., et al. Prehospital stabilization of critically ill patients: A failed concept. *J. Trauma* 25:65–70, 1985.

31. Pons, P. T., Honigman, D., Moore, E. E., et al. Prehospital advanced trauma life support for critical penetrating wounds to the thorax and abdomen. *J. Trauma* 25:828–832, 1985.

32. Aprahamian, C., Thompson, B. M., Towne, J. B., et al. The effect of a paramedic system on mortality of major open intra-abdominal vascular trauma. *J. Trauma* 23:687–690, 1983.

33. Copass, M. K., Oreskovich, M. R., Bladergroen, M. R., et al. Prehospital cardiopulmonary resuscitation of the critically injured patient. *Am. J. Surg.* 148:20–26, 1984.

34. Glaeser, P. W., Losek, J. D., Nelson, D. B., et al. Pediatric intraosseous infusions: Impact on vascular access time. *Am. J. Emerg. Med.* 6:330–332, 1988.

35. Katan, B. S., Olshaker, J. S., and Dickerson, S. E. Intraosseous infusion of muscle relaxants. *Am. J. Emerg. Med.* 6:353–354, 1988.

36. Lewis, F. R. Primary Assessment. In D. D. Trunkey and F. R. Lewis (eds.), *Current Therapy of Trauma—2*. Philadelphia: B.C. Decker, 1986. Pp. 60–69.

37. Karnauchow, P. N. Cardiac tamponade from central venous catheterization. *Can. Med. Assoc. J.* 135:1145–1147, 1986.

38. Suddleson, E. A. Cardiac tamponade: A complication of central venous hyperalimentation. *J. Par. Ent. Nutr.* 10:528–529, 1986.

39. Moore, F. D. *Metabolic Care of the Surgical Patient*. Philadelphia: W.B. Saunders, 1959.

40. Shires, T., Williams, J., and Brown, F. Acute change in extracellular fluids associated with major surgical procedures. *Ann. Surg.* 154:803–810, 1961.

41. Virgilio, R. W., Rice, C. L., et al. Crystalloid vs. colloid resuscitation: Is one better? *Surgery* 85:129–139, 1979.

42. Moss, G. S., Lowe, R. J., et al. Colloid or crystalloid in the resuscitation of hemorrhagic shock: A controlled clinical trial. *Surgery* 89:434–438, 1981.

43. Dawson, R. B. Colloid vs Crystalloid. In R. A. Crowley, A. Conn, and C. M. Dunham (eds.), *Trauma Care*. Vol. I. Philadelphia: J.B. Lippincott, 1987. Pp. 78–87.

44. Gammage, G. W. Crystalloid vs Colloid: Is Colloid Worth the Cost? In R. R. Kirby and D. L. Brown (eds.), *Anesthesia for Trauma*. Boston: Little, Brown, 1987. Pp. 37–60.

45. Carden, D. L., and Nowak, R. M. Disseminated intravascular coagulation in hypothermia. *J.A.M.A.* 247:2099, 1982.

46. Callaham, M. Heat Illness. In P. Rosen, F. J. Baker, R. M. Barkin, et al. (eds.), *Emergency Medicine*. St. Louis: C.V. Mosby, 1988. Pp. 693–717.

47. Merz, B. Malignant hyperthermia: Nightmare for anesthesiologists—and patients. *J.A.M.A.* 255:709–715, 1986.

48. Bivens, H. G., Knopp, R., Tiernan, C., et al. Blood volume displacement with inflation of anti-shock trousers. *Ann. Emerg. Med.* 11:409–412, 1982.

49. Gaffney, F. A., Thal, E. R., Taylor, W. F., et al. Hemodynamic effects of medical anti-shock trousers. *J. Trauma* 21:931–937, 1981.

50. Bellamy, R. F., DeGuzman, L. R., and Pedersen, D. C. Immediate hemodynamic consequences of MAST inflation in normo- and hypovolemic anesthetized swine. *J. Trauma* 24:889–895, 1984.

51. McSwain, N. E. Pneumatic anti-shock garment: State of the art 1988. *Ann. Emerg. Med.* 17:506–525, 1988.

52. Mateer, J. R., Thompson, B. M., Aprahamian, C., et al. Rapid fluid resuscitation with central venous catheters. *Ann. Emerg. Med.* 12:149–152, 1983.

53. Benumof, J. L., Trousdale, F. R., Alfery, D. D., et al. Large catheter sheath introducers and their side port functional usage. *Anesth. Analg.* 60:216–217, 1981.

54. Iserson, K. V., and Reeter, A. K. Rapid fluid replacement for severe hypovolemia—human subject trials. *West. J. Med.* 146:313–315, 1987.

55. Dawson, R. B. Transfusion: Volume Expansion, Oxygen Transport, Hemostasis, Transfusion Reactions, Autotransfusion. In R. A. Cowley, A. Conn, and C. M. Dunham (eds.), *Trauma Care*. Vol. II. Philadelphia: J.B. Lippincott, 1987. Pp. 131–141.

56. Sinclair, A., and Jacobs, L. M. Emergency department autotransfusion for trauma victims. *Med. Instrum.* 16:283–286, 1982.

57. Orr, M. D. Autotransfusion: Intraoperative scavenging. *Int. Anesth. Clin.* 20:97–119, 1982.

58. Committee on Trauma, American College of Surgeons. Blood and Fluid Replacement in Shock. In A. J. Walt (ed.), *Early Care of the Injured Patient*. Philadelphia: Saunders, 1982. Pp. 9–27.

59. Jacobs, L. M., and Hsieh, J. W. A clinical review of autotransfusion and its role in trauma. *J.A.M.A.* 251:3283–3287, 1984.
60. Timberlake, G. A., and McSwain, N. E. Autotransfusion of blood contaminated by enteric contents: A potentially life-saving measure in the massively hemorrhaging trauma patient? *J. Trauma* 28:855–857, 1988.
61. Jorden, R. C., and Barkin, R. M. Multiple Trauma. In P. Rosen (ed.), *Emergency Medicine.* St. Louis: C.V. Mosby, 1988. P. 169.
62. Miller, R. D., and Brizica, S. M. Blood, blood components, colloids and autotransfusion therapy. In R. D. Miller (ed.), *Anesthesia* (2nd ed.). New York: Churchill Livingstone, 1986. Pp. 1329–1367.
63. Telischi, M., Hoiberg, R., Rao, K. P. P., et al. The use of frozen, thawed erythrocytes in blood banking. *Am. J. Clin. Pathol.* 68:250, 1977.
64. National Institutes of Health. Fresh frozen plasma: Indications and risks. Consensus development conference statement. Vol. 5, No. 5, 1984.
65. Gravlee, G. P., and Hopkins, M. B. Blood Plasma Products. In N. Ellison and D. R. Jobes (eds.), *Effective Hemostasis in Cardiac Surgery.* Philadelphia: W. B. Saunders, 1988. Pp. 69–83.
66. Moseley, R. V., and Doty, D. B. Changes in the filtration characteristics of stored blood. *Ann. Surg.* 171:329, 1970.
67. Michel, R. P., LaForte, M., and Hogg, J. C. Physiology and morphology of pulmonary microvascular injury with shock and reinfusion. *J. Appl. Physiol.* 50:1227–1235, 1981.
68. Zauder, H. L. Massive transfusion. *Int. Anesth. Clin.* 20:154–170, 1982.
69. Durtschi, M. B., Haisch, C. E., Reynolds, L., et al. Effect of Micropore filtration in pulmonary function after massive transfusion. *Am. J. Surg.* 138:8, 1979.
70. Martin, B. A., Dahlby, R., Nicholls, I., et al. Platelet sequestration in lung with hemorrhagic shock and reinfusion in dogs. *J. Appl. Physiol.* 50:1306–1312, 1981.
71. Patterson, A. Massive transfusion. *Int. Anesth. Clin.* 25:61–74, 1987.
72. Barnes, A. Status of the use of universal donor blood transfusion. *Clin. Lab. Sci.* 4:147–160, 1973.
73. Crosby, W. H., and Akeroyd, J. H. Some immunohematologic results of large transfusions of group O blood recipients of other blood groups: A study of battle casualties in Korea. *J. Hematol.* 9:103–116, 1954.
74. Barnes, A. Transfusion of universal donor and uncrossmatched blood. *Bibl. Haemat.* 46:132–142, 1980.
75. Lefebre, J., McLellan, B. A., and Coovadia, A. S. Seven years experience with group O unmatched packed red blood cells in a regional trauma unit. *Ann. Emerg. Med.* 16:1344–1349, 1987.
76. Reitan, J. A., and Barash, P. G. Noninvasive Monitoring. In L. J. Saidman and N. T. Smith (eds.), *Monitoring in Anesthesia* (2nd ed.). Boston: Butterworth, 1984. Pp. 117–191.
77. Bedford, R. F., and Wollman, H. Complications of percutaneous radial artery cannulation: An objective prospective study in man. *Anesthesiology* 38:228, 1973.
78. Downs, J. B., Rackstein, A. D., Klein, E. F., et al. Hazards of radial artery catheterization. *Anesthesiology* 38:283, 1973.
79. Prys-Roberts, C. Invasive Monitoring of the Circulation. In L. J. Saidman and N. T. Smith (eds.), *Monitoring in Anesthesia* (2nd ed.). Boston: Butterworth, 1984. Pp. 79–115.
80. Baxt, W. G., Moody, P., Cleveland, H. C., et al. Hospital-based rotorcraft aeromedical emergency care services and trauma mortality: A multicenter study. *Ann. Emerg. Med.* 14:859–864, 1985.

81. Baxt, W. G., and Moody, P. The impact of a rotorcraft aeromedical emergency care service on trauma mortality. *J.A.M.A.* 249:3047–3051, 1983.
82. Urdaneat, L. F., Miller, B. K., Ringenberg, B. J., et al. Role of an emergency helicopter transport service in rural trauma. *Arch. Surg.* 122:992–996, 1987.
83. Bogetz, M. S., and Katz, J. A. Recall of surgery for major trauma. *Anesthesiology* 61:6–9, 1984.
84. Blacher, R. S. Awareness during surgery. *Anesthesiology* 61:1–2, 1984.
85. Simon, R. R., and Brenner, B. E. *Emergency Procedures and Techniques* (2nd ed.). Baltimore: Williams & Wilkins, 1987.

13. Head Injury

Kris Bjornson

Head injury is one of the more difficult problems facing trauma physicians in their practice. Frequently, these patients have serious multisystem diseases or are combative and uncooperative owing to the use of drugs or alcohol. However, most of them are young and healthy, and good patient care can be very rewarding for the physician.

In this chapter, we will first examine the incidence of head injury in the general population. A review of anatomy will follow to provide a more comprehensive picture of the areas of the brain that are involved in the formation of hematomas and the structures that are compressed during elevated intracranial pressure. Physiologic changes that occur in the event of trauma to the brain will also be noted. Last, we will review the pharmacologic agents used in the treatment of head injury and offer guidelines for the clinical definition of death.

Several studies have evaluated the incidence of head and spinal cord injury. These studies have looked at populations by age, sex, and external cause of injury and have analyzed the socioeconomic cost of these injuries. The National Head and Spinal Cord Injury survey [1] found an incidence of 204 per 100,000 population in 1974. The age group distribution showed the largest number of injuries in the 15- to 24-year-old group, with the 15 and under group the second most common. This occurrence rate was also borne out in Jennett's study, which looked at head injuries in Scotland, the Netherlands, and the United States [2]. The state of Rhode Island looked at all head injuries for the years 1979–1980 and found a rate of 152 per 100,000 population, with males having 206 and females 102 head injuries per 100,000 [3]. Head injuries were also examined in the county of San Diego, California, in 1978, which reported an incidence of 295 per 100,000 [4]. The external causes for these head injuries were broken down into three categories: motor vehicle, falls, and others. Motor vehicle accidents constituted the major cause of head injuries, with falls causing 60 percent as many head injuries as motor vehicle accidents.

Of interest was the finding in the San Diego study that motor vehicle accidents were associated with a higher percentage of concussive injuries and a lower percentage of intracranial hematomas than were found in injuries caused by falls or other events. It was concluded by Kalsbeek [1] that motor vehicle accidents cause severe primary brain damage because of the excessive force involved, whereas because the force of a fall is usually not as great, subsequent hematomas are more likely to form.

ANATOMY

The scalp provides a bony case for the brain and the other contents of the cranial cavity, which include the meninges, cerebral spinal fluid, and vascular supply, both venous and arterial. The cranial cavity has been divided into anterior, middle, and posterior cranial fossae. The anterior cranial fossa lodges the frontal lobes of the cerebral hemispheres. The middle cranial fossa contains the parietal, temporal, and occipital lobes of the cerebral hemispheres. The posterior fossa contains the cerebellum, the pons, and the medulla oblongata. The brain weighs between 1200 and 1400 gm. This constitutes 2 percent of body weight, but, with its high metabolism, the brain receives one-sixth of the cardiac output and one-fifth of the total oxygen consumption at rest.

The brain is bathed in cerebrospinal fluid (CSF), which is produced in the choroid plexus. Both secretion and transudation are involved in its production. The total volume of fluid is between 100 and 150 ml, and the normal pressure range is between 70 and 180 mm of saline in the lateral recumbent position (the usual position used for lumbar puncture). In the sitting position, the intracranial pressure is negative in the ventricles and equal to atmospheric pressure at the foramen magnum.

The CSF is secreted by the choroid plexus in the lateral ventricles and passes through the interventricular foramen to join fluid that is produced in the third ventricle. This fluid then passes through the aqueduct or foramen magnum to join fluid that is formed in the fourth ventricle. From here the fluid passes through the foramen of Luschka and the foramen of Magendie into the cerebellar medullary and pontine cisterns. Fluid passes caudally around the spinal cord at slow flow rates; however, there is faster flow through the subarachnoid space to the arachnoid granulations, where the fluid is then absorbed into the venous sinuses of the cranial dura.

The brain is surrounded by three membranes or meninges: the dura mater, the arachnoid, and the pia mater. The dura consists of an internal layer and an external layer. These are indistinguishable except where they are separated by venous sinuses. The internal layer has four processes that divide the brain into compartments; the falx cerebri, the tentorium cerebelli, the falx cerebelli, and the diaphragma sellae. The falx cerebri lies in the longitudinal fissure between the two cerebral hemispheres. It attaches to the crista galli in the front and fuses with the tentorium cerebelli in the rear. The superior portion of the falx cerebelli encloses the superior sagittal sinus, the lower portion of which contains the inferior sagittal sinus and the straight sinus. The tentorium cerebelli supports the occipital lobes of the cerebral hemispheres and divides the cranial cavity into the supratentorial cavity and the infratentorial cavity. The lateral edges form the lateral transverse sinuses and, with the falx cerebri, the straight sinus. The falx cerebelli divides the cerebellar hemispheres. The last process is the diaphragma sellae, which is the dural roof of the sella turcica and covers the hypophysis. The tentorial notch is the area between the edges of the tentorium cerebelli through which the brain passes; it is important because space-occupying lesions in either the supra- or infratentorial cavities can cause herniation through it.

The arachnoid and the pia mater, or leptomeninges, are united by trabeculae of connective tissue and form the subarachnoid space between their layers. It is in this space that the cerebrospinal fluid circulates. These three meninges form two spaces and one potential space, the epidural space, into which bleeding can occur from trauma. Progressing from an external point to an internal one, then, are the bony skull, the potential epidural space, the dura, the subdural space, the arachnoid, the subarachnoid space, the pia, and, finally, the cerebral cortex.

The arterial supply of the brain is provided by the two internal carotid and the two vertebral arteries. The internal carotid arteries divide into the middle cerebral and anterior cerebral arteries, and the two vertebral arteries join, forming the basal artery, which then divides to form the posterior cerebral arteries. These two systems are connected by the posterior cerebral artery and the internal carotid arteries. This blood supply completes the circle of Willis through the anterior communicating artery, which joins the two anterior cerebral arteries. This ingenious vascular supply provides protection for the brain when one or more of the major arteries becomes occluded.

PHYSIOLOGY

CEREBRAL BLOOD FLOW

There are two general types of arteries in the cerebral circulation: the conducting vessels and the penetrating vessels [5]. The conducting arteries bring blood to the resistance arteries and provide adequate perfusion pressure to these vessels. These arteries include the carotid system, including the middle, anterior, and posterior cerebral arteries, and the vertebral basilar arteries and their major tributaries. The penetrating vessels are arterioles that enter the brain parenchyma at right angles to the surface vessels. They are the vessels that are primarily responsible for autoregulation of the cerebral blood flow. Blood then traverses the parenchyma of the brain, draining through valveless cerebral veins into the dural sinuses. If the pressure of the cerebrospinal fluid exceeds the pressure in the small venous channels, blood will not flow. From the dural sinus the venous blood then enters the internal jugular vein and flows back to the central venous structures. From this description it can be seen that the cerebral perfusion pressure (CPP) is equal to the mean arterial pressure (MAP) minus the mean intracranial pressure (ICP):

$$CPP = MAP - ICP$$

Cerebral blood flow, cerebral perfusion pressure, and the cerebral vascular resistance are interrelated, of course, by a modification of Ohm's law, the cerebral blood flow being equal to the cerebral perfusion pressure divided by the cerebral vascular resistance. The cerebral blood flow is maintained at around 50 ml per 100 gm of brain tissue per minute [6].

AUTOREGULATION

Cerebral blood flow is amazingly constant. This has been attributed to four different mechanisms of blood flow control, which are autoregulatory, metabolic, chemical, and neurogenic in origin. Autoregulation of blood flow is constant over a wide range of cerebral perfusion pressures. Autoregulation is apparently accomplished by penetrating vessels that change their vessel diameter (Fig. 13-1). Perfusion pressure is relatively constant in normal brain tissue between approximately 60 and 150 mm Hg [7]. The arterioles appear to produce autoregulation by means of a myogenic response in the smooth muscle [8]. These arterial walls constrict when systemic arterial pressure is increased and dilate when pressure is decreased. Although there are sympathetic and parasympathetic nerve fibers that go to some of the arterioles of the brain, several studies have shown that the sympathetic system is not the main mechanism involved in autoregulation [9]. This observed arteriolar autoregulation also explains the consistent cerebral blood flow that is observed with mild elevations in ICP [10]. The response to changes in cerebral perfusion pressure has been shown to occur within 5 to 8 seconds [11].

Autoregulation does have a lower limit at which the cerebral blood flow becomes dependent on the cerebral perfusion pressure. This limit is nor-

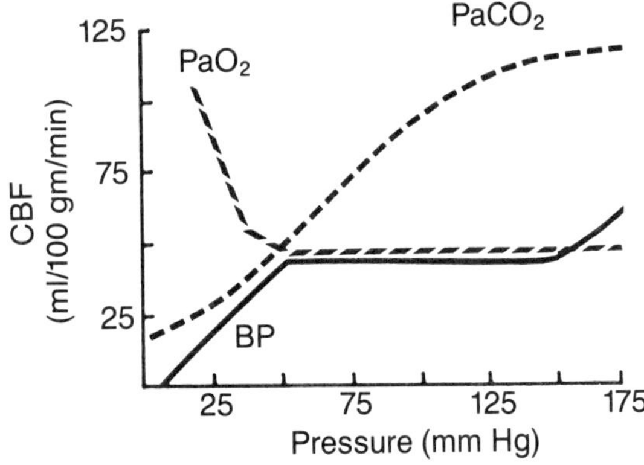

Fig. 13-1. Autoregulation of cerebral blood flow (CBF) with alterations of the PaCO2, PaO2, and mean blood pressure in the normal brain. (From R. D. Miller [ed.]. *Anesthesia* [2nd ed.]. New York: Churchill, Livingstone, 1986. With permission.)

mally approximately 60 mm Hg. It is at this pressure that the cerebral vasculature is maximally dilated. At approximately 40 mm Hg symptoms of cerebral ischemia begin to develop. The upper limit of autoregulation is around 150 mm Hg, at which pressure the cerebral vasculature is maximally constricted. Above this limit, forced dilatation of the arterioles occurs, and there is disruption of the blood-brain barrier.

Autoregulation occurs optimally in normal intact cerebral vessels and is decreased or abolished by trauma, ischemia, hypoxia, and hypercapnia. In patients with chronic hypertension the autoregulation curb is shifted to the right, and both the upper and lower limits of autoregulation are increased [12].

METABOLIC CONTROL OF CEREBRAL BLOOD FLOW

Cerebral blood flow (CBF) changes with the metabolic needs of the brain. There is a constant global metabolic demand for oxygen in resting wakefulness, but there are regional changes in oxygen uptake. It has been shown that there is a 30 percent increase in oxygen uptake in the area of the brain controlling the hand during hand movements [12]. It is also known that there are increases in cerebral blood flow during hypermetabolic disease states such as fever or seizures, and decreases with other states, e.g., coma. Several theories attempt to explain these metabolic changes. Most of them revolve around changes in concentrations of specific mediators that have vasoactive effects. The flow of hydrogen and potassium ions in the extracellular fluid surrounding the arterioles, for example, may have an effect on local cerebral blood flow. Adenosine, a potent vasodilator, is produced by the breakdown of adenosine triphosphate (ATP) and is another vasoactive mediator. Arachidonic acid, with the enzyme cyclooxygenase, has the metabolic products of thromboxane, which is a potent vasoconstrictor, and prostaglandins, which can be dilators as well as constrictors of cerebral resistance vessels.

CHEMICAL REGULATION

Chemical changes in cerebral blood flow are mediated primarily by the arterial carbon dioxide partial pressure ($PaCO_2$). The cerebral vessels dilate with increases in the $PaCO_2$ and constrict with decreases in $PaCO_2$. The change of cerebral blood flow is more dramatic with changes in the $PaCO_2$ than with changes in the neurogenic, metabolic, or autoregulatory mechanisms. The reactivity of the arterioles is not caused directly by carbon dioxide concentration but by variations in pH and consequently in hydrogen ion concentration within the cerebrospinal fluid and inside the wall of the arterioles [13,14]. It must be remembered that bicarbonate does not diffuse across the blood-brain barrier but that carbon dioxide gas is freely diffusible across this barrier. The change in cerebral blood flow is 2 ml/100 gm/min for each 1 mm Hg change in $PaCO_2$. This can bring about a fourfold change in cerebral blood flow between a $PaCO_2$ of 20 mm Hg and a $PaCO_2$ of 80 mm Hg. It can be appreciated, then, that changing the $PaCO_2$ is the easiest and most effective way of modifying cerebral blood flow. Lactic acidosis, local cerebral metabolism, and other pathologic states have the ability to change hydrogen ion concentration in the brain and thus change the cerebral blood flow. This produces an effective method of washing out metabolically produced carbon dioxide. In areas of increased cerebral function with high metabolism and high carbon dioxide production, the local vasculature dilates, eliminating these products of metabolism.

Chronic changes in $PaCO_2$ concentrations are buffered by bicarbonate concentrations in the CSF. These adaptive changes take 24 to 36 hours and will normalize the pH of the CSF [15–17]. The rapid response to carbon dioxide enables clinicians to control cerebral blood flow easily in the initial postinjury period by modifying ventilation. Acute alveolar hyperventilation, however, tends to become less and less effective with time as the bicarbonate level of the CSF adjusts to the lowered PCO_2 concentration in the blood. It is just as important to realize, on the other hand, that acute withdrawl of chronic hyperventilation will cause increased cerebral perfusion in a patient in whom the brain bicarbonate levels have been adjusted to a lowered $PaCO_2$ blood concentration. In acute situations there is a lower limit of $PaCO_2$, approximately 25 mm Hg, at which vasoconstriction can become severe enough to cause ischemia of the brain [18].

Oxygen has little influence on cerebral blood flow until the PaO_2 drops below 50 mm Hg. Below this level the brain starts to develop lactic acidosis, and, as mentioned earlier, the related increase in hydrogen ion causes cerebral vascular resistance to decrease and cerebral blood flow to increase.

NEUROGENIC CONTROL OF CEREBRAL BLOOD FLOW

There is slight neurogenic control of cerebral blood flow, but, when compared to the other means of regulation, neurogenic control plays only a small role in regulation. There is both sympathetic and parasympathetic innervation of the larger arterioles inside the brain tissue. The sympathetic fibers originate from the superior superficial ganglion, and the parasympathetic fibers originate from the facial nerve. Stimulation of both types of nerves either increases or reduces cerebral blood flow by 5 to 10 percent [20]. This amount of increased blood flow would correspond to a 2-mm Hg change in $PaCO_2$.

The major importance of sympathetic stimulation may lie in its effect of changing the lower portion of the autoregulation curve. It has been shown that cerebral blood flow is less during hemorrhagic hypotension than during pharmacologically produced hypotension. This effect may be due to an increase in sympathetic stimulation induced by hemorrhagic shock [21].

The obvious importance of cerebral blood flow is to bring oxygen and its major substrate, glucose, to the brain and to carry carbon dioxide away. The adult human brain consumes approximately 50 ml/min of oxygen. Glucose, the other essential substrate, is transported from the blood to the brain tissue by a carrier-mediated transport mechanism. Of these two substances, it is the deficiency of oxygen that causes unconsciousness if cerebral circulation is interrupted. With ischemia, the brain switches from aerobic to anaerobic metabolism, and lactic acid increases concomitantly. The effect of varying peri-ischemic glucose concentrations has been studied in cats and rats, in which cerebral ischemia was produced by cross-clamping the cerebral vessels. A significant increase in mortality was observed in animals with hyperglycemia. There were reduced values of ATP and phosphocreatine and increased lactate acid levels in those animals that received the glucose infusions [22–25]. Most probably, increased lactic acidosis caused by anaerobic metabolism in the presence of increased glucose substrate is the major offender. The important clinical inference from these studies is that glucose in the ischemic brain produces a negative outcome, and that glucose-containing solutions should not be used in the resuscitation of head-injured patients except in the presence of documented hypoglycemia and with frequent blood glucose determinations.

CARDIOVASCULAR RESPONSES

The cardiovascular system responds in many ways to head injury. This fact was first noted by Cushing when he described the triad of raised intracranial pressure, hypertension, and bradycardia in head-injured patients. This triad is seen late in patients with head injuries when the diastolic pressure is equal to the intracranial pressure in a patient who is usually brain dead. More often, tachycardia is the clinical presentation in conjunction with hypertension or normotension. Tachycardia with hypotension should be assumed to be secondary to hypovolemia and injury elsewhere in the patient and not a result of head injury until proved otherwise. It is now known that head-injured patients exist in a hyperenergic state, with catecholamine levels many times higher than normal. Clifton and coworkers [26] measured plasma norepinephrine and dopamine beta-hydroxylase levels in 48 patients for the first 7 days after head injury. They noted that in patients with multiple trauma the norepinephrine levels were usually elevated regardless of the Glascow coma score, and that in patients with isolated head injury the norepinephrine level was proportional to the Glascow coma score. The elevations of plasma norepinephrine and dopamine beta-hydroxylase were correlated in this study with elevations in blood pressure, pulse rate, and temperature. Levels of norepinephrine found in patients with Glascow coma scores of 10 or less (12 represents an alert, normal patient on neurologic examination) were in the range of norepinephrine levels found in patients who exercised on a treadmill to 80 percent of their maximal heart rate. Circulating catecholamine levels have been implicated in cardiac sequelae of head injury. McLoud and associates studied seven patients with diffuse isolated brain injury for cardiovascular effects [27]. They felt that these patients received optimal care and had no past history of cardiac disease. No anoxia was found in these patients, and yet 40 percent showed evidence of progressive myocardial ischemia. Two of these patients eventually died. One patient had an episode of ventricular tachycardia. Catecholamines were markedly elevated in all patients. At necropsy, physiologic evidence of myocardial damage was found in one of the patients who expired.

Hackenberry and associates studied 30 patients with severe head trauma and no spinal or chest injury [28]. Twenty-eight of the thirty patients showed elevated CK-MB activity. Of interest was the fact that the CK-MB remained elevated for at least 3 days after injury, suggesting that ongoing myocardial damage was occurring in these patients with severe head injuries. The authors felt that the underlying cause was elevated catecholamine levels.

Multiple abnormal electrocardiographic (ECG) findings have been noted in patients with head injuries. A review of this phenomenon by Frost showed that the QT interval was prolonged more than 440 msec in 60 percent of patients [29]. Tachycardia greater than 100 beats per minute (bpm) was noted in 45 percent, ST-segment depression in 20 percent, QRS prolongation in 15 percent, large U waves in 15 percent, ST-segment elevation in 15 percent, and ventricular extrasystolic beats in 10 percent of the patients studied.

Therapy must be aimed at adrenergic blockade. This can be accomplished with one of the beta-blockade drugs, propranolol, esmolol, or lobetalol. Narcotics are also useful in this situation, but it must be remembered that they do change the clinical physical examination picture and that they are contraindicated in spontaneously breathing head-injured patients.

RESPIRATORY RESPONSE TO HEAD INJURY

Respiratory disorders in the head-injured patient are quite common. At the time of injury and with loss of consciousness, respirations often cease. After a period of apnea, which can vary from patient to patient, respirations may return but with some significant changes from the patient's normal breathing pattern. Respiratory obstruction has been implicated as the primary cause of death in at least 15 percent of head-injured casualties [30]. Most patients, though, do not have increased $PaCO_2$ values by the time they arrive at the hospital, suggesting that obstruction causing hypoventilation is usually treated at the scene [31]. At the time of injury, gastric motility frequently ceases, making the possibility of regurgitation and salient aspiration very likely. All these patients must be considered to have full stomachs at the time of their injury. Although patients arriving were found not to have increased $PaCO_2$ values, they did have decreased PaO_2 values, 30 percent of them having PaO_2 values less than 65 while breathing room air on arrival at the hospital [32]. The underlying cause of this hypoxia was found to be shunt and $\dot{V}/\dot{Q}$ mismatch. Arterial-alveolar differences of more than 20 mm Hg were found in 80 percent of these patients. Neurogenic pulmonary edema has also been reported in head-injured patients, more commonly in patients with gunshot wounds to the head rather than blunt trauma. It is felt that the initial phase of this edema results from a centrally mediated massive sympathetic discharge [33]. This will cause vasoconstriction, hypertension, and a sudden shift of blood from the systemic circulation to the pulmonary circulation. With the large rise in the pulmonary capillary pressure, pulmonary edema ensues. This condition leaves the patient with abnormal pulmonary capillary permeability and edema that persists in spite of normal hemodynamic and cardiac function [32].

The most common derangement of respiration seen in the head-injured patient is hyperventilation. It has been proposed that this hyperventilation is primarily due to cerebral acidosis resulting from brain damage. These low PCO_2 values caused by hyperventilation may have detrimental effects on pulmonary gas exchange because low PCO_2 can contribute to bronchoconstriction and pulmonary vascular relaxation. This then tends to contribute to ventilation/perfusion inequality [32].

Several criteria have been suggested to define respiratory insufficiency. It is felt that if one or more of the following criteria are met, the patient should be intubated and assisted ventilation should be initiated:

1. Respiratory rate greater than 40 per minute or less than 10 per minute.
2. Irregular respiratory pattern.
3. Vital capacity less than 15 ml/kg.
4. Maximal inspiratory force less than -20 cm of H_2O.
5. Dead space–tidal volume (V_D/V_T) ratio of greater than 0.5.
6. Pulmonary shunt percentage greater than 15 percent.
7. $PaCO_2$ greater than 45 mm Hg or less than 25 mm Hg.

Hypoxia can be corrected by increasing the FiO_2. If the increased FiO_2 alone does not increase the PaO_2, positive end-expiratory pressure (PEEP) should then be added. Care must be taken in providing PEEP for these patients because it increases the central venous pressure, which will in turn increase the intracranial pressure.

INTRACRANIAL PRESSURE MONITORING

Three major techniques are presently used to monitor intracranial pressure. These are the epidural transducer, the subdural bolt, and the ventriculostomy tube. There are pros and cons in the use of each of these devices, but the important considerations are ease of placement, rate of infection, and accuracy of measurement of the true intracranial pressure.

The epidural transducer is placed between the dura and the inner surface of the cranial vault. Because the dura is not transgressed, this transducer has the lowest infection rate of the three major types. The major disadvantages of this tranducer are its exaggeration of the actual ICP and the difficulty of placing the monitor perfectly flat against the dura. Recalibration problems are also found with the epidural transducer.

Subdural bolts are placed by making an opening through the skull and the dura into the subdural space. A pressure sensor is then connected through fluid containing a tube to a transducer. The advantages of this method of measuring ICP are that it does not transgress brain tissue (as the interventricular catheter does) and that the bolt can easily be reset to zero to recalibrate it for continued measurement. There is still the possibility of infection with this catheter because the dura has been transgressed; however, infections secondary to this type of monitor are less severe than infections with an interventricular catheter [34]. When the bolt becomes occluded, there can be severe swelling of the brain, and an underestimation of high intracranial pressure results [35].

Interventricular pressure monitoring of ICP is the current gold standard. A small catheter is placed in the lateral ventricle after a burr hole has been drilled in the skull. The major problem associated with the interventricular catheter is infection, which has been shown to run between 8 and 10 percent [36]. Other problems with this catheter are bleeding and difficulty in placement, which is increased if the ICP is elevated and the ventricles have collapsed. This is the one method of ICP monitoring that also provides a therapeutic modality, i.e., cerebrospinal fluid may be removed if ICP is high. This method also offers the opportunity to check the compliance of the brain by injecting small quantities of normal saline through the catheter and observing changes in intracranial pressure.

The normal intracranial pressure is around 10 mm Hg. Pulsations may be noted on the pressure tracing that correspond to the heart rate and also to the respiratory pattern. Sustained values above 20 mm Hg should be considered moderate increases, and levels above 40 mm Hg severe increases in intracranial pressure.

Three distinctive wave patterns have been observed with this monitoring: A waves, or plateau waves (Fig. 13-2), B waves (Fig. 13-3), and C waves. A waves have been defined as intracranial pressure greater than 50 mm Hg that persists for 5 minutes. These increases are followed by decreases that bring the pressure back to the original level. The exact cause of these waves

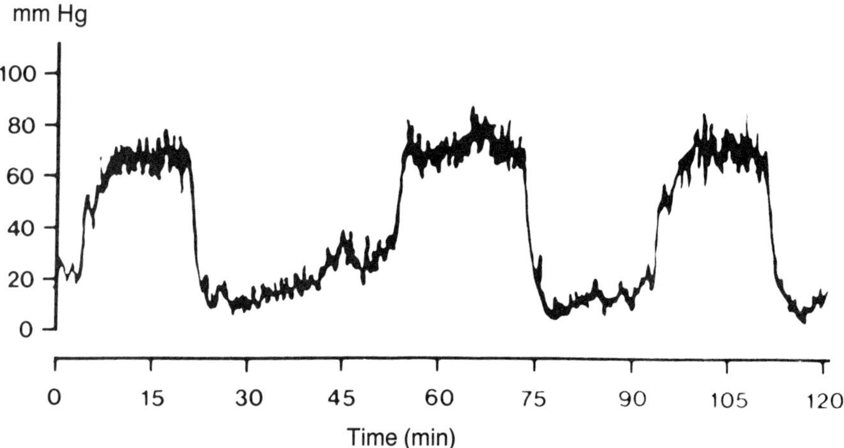

Fig. 13-2. Intracranial pressure A waves or plateau waves. (From W. Fitch and J. Barker [eds.]. *Head Injury and the Anaesthetist.* New York: Elsevier Science, 1985. With permission.)

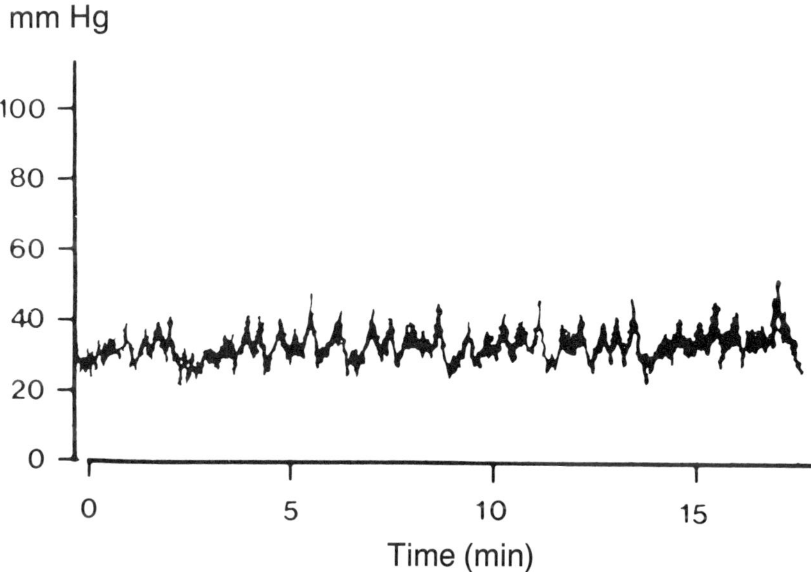

Fig. 13-3. Intracranial pressure B waves. (From W. Fitch and J. Barker [eds.]. *Head Injury and the Anaesthetist.* New York: Elsevier Science, 1985. With permission.)

is not completely understood, but it is known that they occur in association with a background of increased intracranial pressure. As compliance decreases, small volume changes produce large ICP increases. Because the cranial vault is nonexpansive, the brain can only compensate by producing less cerebrospinal fluid, absorbing more cerebrospinal fluid, decreasing blood flow, and reducing the volume of blood in the venous system. Increases in systemic arterial pressure seem to trigger these plateau waves [37]. The major clinical feature of a plateau wave is that the brain is at the point of decompensating completely when they occur, and if any therapeutic modalities are still held in at this point, they need to be initiated promptly.

B waves have much lower amplitude than A waves, and their time of duration is also much shorter. B waves last from 30 seconds to 2 minutes and usually have amplitudes of 10 to 15 mm Hg above the baseline ICP. They occur with a background of increased intracranial pressure in the 20- to 30 mm Hg range. The importance of B waves is the same as that of A or plateau waves because they also show decompensation in the ability of the brain to control intracranial pressure.

C waves occur at a rate of 5 per minute and are relatively small in amplitude; they are thought to correspond to variations in arterial pressure.

PATHOLOGY

The pathology of head injuries can be classified according to primary and secondary damage. Primary damage occurs at the time of impact, and there is little that therapy can do to change the outcome. However, each of the primary types of damage to the brain does have implications for secondary brain damage, which may be amenable to therapeutic intervention.

PRIMARY BRAIN DAMAGE

Primary brain damage can be subdivided into four groups: direct brain damage, polar damage, diffuse brain injury, and primary brain stem damage.

Direct brain damage occurs to the underlying brain from a depressed fracture or from a penetrating wound to the brain. Necrotic brain tissue in the area of the injury will swell owing to cytotoxic edema. The area around the necrotic portion usually will swell owing to vasogenic edema, and leakage of fluid into the brain will occur from damaged endothelium. There is also the possibility of hematoma formation secondary to this primary damage, as small cerebral blood vessels are torn or lacerated.

Polar damage occurs from brain contusion and laceration as the brain moves against the inner surface of the cranium. This most frequently happens in the frontal and anterior portions of the temporal lobes, but it may also occur in the occipital lobes. It is possible for this type of injury to cause a ruptured temporal lobe, in which there is acute subdural as well as inter-cerebral hemorrhage and contused brain. The difference between direct brain damage and polar damage is that no fracture or penetration of the cranium is needed to cause polar damage. These injuries tend to swell and to be accompanied by hemorrhage and edema, which act as space-occupying lesions.

Diffuse brain injury is a consequence of shearing forces at the time of injury that tear the nerve fibers. These injuries have been found as discrete lesions primarily in the corpus callosum and in the dorsal lateral quadrants of the rostral brain stem.

Primary brain stem damage is thought to be the cause of death in a significant portion of patients who succumb almost immediately to head injury. These patients have shearing of axonal nerve fibers and hemorrhage in the brain stem.

SECONDARY BRAIN DAMAGE

After primary damage has been done to the brain, there may be a cascade effect caused by secondary brain damage. Secondary damage has been classified as brain shift herniation, ischemic and hypoxic brain damage, and post-traumatic ventricular dilatation. It is in the group of patients with secondary brain damage that emergency intervention may prevent morbidity and mortality to the patient.

HERNIATION

Brain shift herniation results either from the formation of an intracranial hematoma or from swelling of contused brain. The type of herniation is dependent on which area of the brain is occupied by the lesion. Possible locations for hematomas or bleeding are the epidural space, the subdural space, the subarachnoid space, and in the cerebral parenchyma. If the lesion is unilateral and supratentorial, the cerebral hemisphere gradually enlarges and the sulci narrow, the gyri flatten, and the brain shifts across the midline. Because the falx cerebri is essentially nonmovable, swelling forces the cingulate gyrus against and then under the falx, causing herniation of the ipsilateral cingulate gyrus. Supratentorial herniation occurs primarily from a mass lesion shifting the medial portion of the ipsilateral temporal lobe through the incisura. The third cranial nerve stretches, causing its dysfunction, which is manifest by a dilated pupil on the ipsilateral side. If this condition continues, increased pressure on the midbrain causes characteristic bradycardia, increased mean arterial pressure, and Cheynes-Stokes respirations.

The classic description of an epidural hematoma is that of a patient who, rendered unconscious at the scene of the accident, regains consciousness briefly only to lose consciousness later. Usually a torn middle meningeal artery is the source of the hemorrhage. As this bleeding occurs, the dura is stripped from the inner surface of the skull, shifting the brain toward the opposite side of the head. Dilatation of the ipsilateral pupil occurs in approximately 80 percent of patients because the third nerve is compressed by the herniation of the temporal lobe through the tentorial notch [38]. There is usually progressive unconsciousness with weakness or decerebration of the contralateral extremity and Cheynes-Stokes respirations. This classic clinical picture may not be seen in patients with epidural hematomas. Jamieson and Yelland showed, in a series of 167 cases of extradural and epidural hematomas, that one-third of patients had the classic history, another third were unconscious from the time of injury and never regained consciousness, and the final third never became unconscious [39]. Epidural hematomas are usually arterial but may be venous in origin, from shearing of the diploic veins or emissary veins. The diploic veins flow from the scalp venous system through the cranium to communicate with the meningeal veins or venous sinuses of the dura mater. The incidence of epidural hematomas has been reported as between 5 and 15 percent of all intracranial hematomas in several large series [40]. Epidural hematomas, if diagnosed early, have been shown to have a very low mortality. Several institutions have reported less than 10 percent mortality when the initial diagnosis is made quickly [43].

Subdural hematomas are classified as either acute or chronic, acute hematomas being identified within 72 hours following trauma. Acute subdural hematomas are then classified as simple or complicated. A simple acute subdural hematoma is a collection of blood in the subdural space in which there is no underlying injury to the brain. A complicated subdural hematoma, on the other hand, has underlying cerebral contusion and laceration and carries a much graver prognosis. Simple hematomas are felt to be caused by tears in bridging veins. In complicated subdural hematomas, bleeding may be arterial from the surface of the brain and is associated with swelling from the contused or lacerated area. Patients with subdural hematomas account for about 26 to 63 percent of patients with mass lesions [40, 41].

The presentation of patients with acute subdural hematomas is quite varied. Much of this variation depends on whether the injury is acute or chronic. The clinical spectrum is broad. It extends from patients rendered unconscious at the time of injury and showing symptoms suggestive of mass lesions with hemiparesis, decerebration, and pupil enlargement to patients who never experience any loss of consciousness. Jamieson reported that 29 percent of patients with subdural hematomas that he treated had not had loss of consciousness [44].

Mortality after surgery for acute subdural hematomas ranges from 23 to 76 percent. This mortality increases dramatically to 100 percent if the subdural hematomas are bilateral or if there is a single subdural hematoma with multiple cerebral lacerations [44–48].

Seelig and others showed a reduced mortality if subdural hematomas were evacuated within 4 hours [49]. Given the high mortality noted in the previous references, and noting the lower mortality figures with early surgery, it is imperative for any head-injured patient with a possibility of a subdural hematoma to undergo CT scanning as soon as possible to determine the presence or absence of a surgical lesion.

There is some controversy regarding the best method of treating patients with subdural hematomas. Methodology or treatment is complicated primarily by the amount of contusion and edema present. Many neurosurgeons feel that small subdural hematomas with no associated midline shift or swelling do not warrant surgical intervention other than ICP monitoring. If there is a midline shift and the midline shift is not much greater than a small subdural hematoma, these patients again may not benefit from removal of the hematoma. When the patient has a midline shift caused by the hematoma, surgical intervention is required.

Chronic subdural hematomas may present weeks after a trivial head injury. Typically, the populations most commonly affected by this type of subdural hematoma are elderly patients who have cortical atrophy, patients on anticoagulant therapy, and patients with coagulation defects. The elderly patient with cortical atrophy is at increased risk of a shearing force that ruptures one of the bridging veins and subsequently causes a subdural hematoma. Because this is a low pressure bleed, the hematoma can accumulate over a prolonged period of time, giving the brain a chance to compensate and therefore not showing neurologic symptoms for weeks after the injury.

Freitag, Adams, et al., and Bruce et al., reported finding intracerebral hematomas in 13 to 22 percent of patients with mass lesions [41, 42, 45]. These lesions are usually located in the subfrontal and temporal regions of the brain. The CT scan is the most reliable method of identifying them. If these lesions are not fatal at the time of injury, there are two distinct periods of time when these patients are again at risk. The first is during the first 24 to 48 hours, when the patient's condition may slowly deteriorate. Then an event such as endotracheal suctioning or a seizure may produce renewed bleeding, with a sharp increase in intracranial pressure and possible herniation. The second period of risk is during delayed bleeding, which occurs after progressive recovery from a head injury at 10 to 14 days. This period coincides with physiologic lysis of a preexisting clot and renewed bleeding. Autopsies on this type of patient have shown that fresh hematomas are the cause of death [50]. Multiple intracerebral hematomas, if small, are usually not evacuated, but large hematomas, especially if they are solitary, should be evacuated surgically. The mortality for traumatic intracerebral hematoma was reported to be 42% in a study by Miller and associates [51].

Intracranial pressure, which may be supratentorial in nature, can also displace the cerebellar tonsils through the foramen magnum, causing herniation of the tonsils. Tonsillar herniation with subtentorial space-occupying lesions is also possible. These lesions tend to progress faster and produce fewer clinical signs before rapid deterioration of the patient results.

ISCHEMIC AND HYPOXIC BRAIN DAMAGE

Ischemic and hypoxic brain damage is usually induced by an increase in intracranial pressure from one of several causes. The brain receives inadequate amounts of blood and oxygen, which quickly leads to dysfunction of the intracellular metabolism of the brain and subsequent death of the brain cells. The primary cause of this dysfunction is brain swelling, which is found in the area adjacent to contusions and hematomas. Swelling may also occur diffusely over one or both of the cerebral hemispheres. This swelling appears to have one of two major causes. Congestive brain swelling may be due to an increase in the cerebral blood volume. Alternatively, edema may result from increased water content in the brain tissue itself.

A rapid increase in the cerebral blood volume may appear secondary to hypoxia, hypercapnia, or to a marked increase in the mean arterial blood pressure. Initially, the extra fluid is completely intravascular; this is not cerebral edema, only congestive brain swelling. Increased water content in cerebral tissue (cerebral edema) is usually caused by an increase in intravascular pressure, by a dysfunction of the blood-brain barrier that causes an increase in capillary permeability, or by a decrease in the osmotic pressure in the vascular space, leading to leakage of fluid into the extravascular tissue.

Post-traumatic epilepsy is a serious side effect of head trauma in which hypoxemia may develop. This in turn can lead to an increase in cerebral edema, which causes an increase in intracranial pressure and a concomitant decrease in blood flow to the brain.

POST-TRAUMATIC VENTRICULAR DILATATION

The third type of secondary brain damage is post-traumatic ventricular dilatation. This usually occurs several weeks to months after the head injury occurs. Kishore describes two types of ventricular dilatation [52]. The first of these is ventricular dilatation secondary to severe atrophy of the brain. This type of dilatation does not cause an increase in the severity of cerebral damage that has already occurred. It simply shows there has been widespread and diffuse cerebral injury secondary to the trauma. The second type of ventricular dilatation is of great importance because it is caused by the obstruction of the outflow of cerebrospinal fluid from the ventricles into the subarachnoid space. This obstruction may take place in the aqueduct between the lateral and third ventricles, or it may occur in the foramen of Luschka or the foramen of Magendie. Patients with this type of hydrocephalus usually show deterioration in mental status and need to have a ventricular peritoneal shunt placed to relieve the increased volume of fluid in the ventricles.

Understanding the relationship between the cerebral metabolic rate and the cerebral blood flow is of clinical importance. In the normal brain with normal ICP, the cerebral blood flow may increase or decrease in conjunction with increases and decreases in the cerebral metabolic rate. With an increase in cerebral metabolic rate, certain areas of the brain will receive increased amounts of lactic acid or carbon dioxide. This will cause dilatation of the cerebral arteries and increased cerebral blood flow to these areas. Normally, the increased rate of blood flow is easily accommodated by a compliant brain, but in pathologic states an increase in cerebral blood flow may cause an increase in intracranial pressure. A decrease in cerebral perfusion pressure will follow, and eventually a decreased flow of cerebral blood will result. The tissue metabolism changes from aerobic to anaerobic glycolysis, causing production of lactic acid, which is a mediator that stimulates a further increase in cerebral blood flow. It is of critical importance that in the pathologic state, the cycle of increased metabolism and increased blood flow is a downward spiral that leads to increased intracranial pressure and ultimately to brain death.

PHARMACOLOGY

In the following section, pharmacologic agents appropriate for the treatment of increased intracranial pressure in head-injured patients will be reviewed.

BARBITURATES

The barbiturates are known to cause a tandem decrease in both cerebral blood flow and cerebral metabolic rate. In a study by Steen and others, the cerebral metabolic rate (CMR) was reduced to approximately 50 percent of the awake state with barbiturates, but after this 50 percent reduction, continued administration of barbiturates did not further reduce the CMR [53]. In contrast, hypothermia reduces the cerebral metabolic rate in a direct fashion without such a threshold. Barbiturates appear to work by decreasing membrane excitability, thus causing a reduction in cerebral metabolism that is linked to brain function. They do not block metabolism related to cellular homeostasis. Because cerebral blood flow parallels the rate of cerebral metabolism, there is a concomitant decrease of up to 50 percent in cerebral blood flow. This mechanism gives the barbiturates a short-term capability to treat elevated intracranial pressure.

BENZODIAZAPENES

The benzodiazapenes, diazepam and medazolam, cause a decrease in both cerebral blood flow and cerebral metabolic rate. The mechanism of action of this group of drugs is multifaceted and includes serotonin antagonism, release of the gamma aminobutyric acid (GABA), facilitation of the neuronal activity of GABA, and decreased release and turnover of acetyl choline [54].

Cotev and Shalit slowly injected 15 mg of diazepam intravenously in eight patients suffering from head injuries [55]. Because of their injuries, the patients had cerebral blood flow rates that were at the lower end of the scale of normal for cerebral blood flow. However, it was noted that there was a 25 percent decrease in the mean cerebral blood flow rate after the injection. The cerebral metabolic rate was also evaluated in these patients, and it was found that the direct relationship between cerebral metabolic rate and cerebral blood flow as maintained both before and after the diazepam injection. Thus, diazepam decreases CMR.

When administered in a dose of 0.15 mg/kg, midazolam decreased CMR similarly and decreased cerebral blood flow by 33 percent in healthy volunteers [56]. Midazolam, 0.2 mg/kg, and diazepam, 0.3 mg/kg, were given to a group of dogs and no decrease in metabolic oxygen requirement was noted. Cerebral blood flow was reduced to approximately 55 percent of control at this dose. When the dose was increased to 10 mg/kg of midazolam and 7.5 mg/kg of diazepam, there was a dose-related decrease in cerebral metabolic oxygen consumption to a maximum of 55 percent. In this same study, a hypoxic mouse model was used to check for brain protection secondary to hypoxia. No decrease in the metabolic rate for oxygen was noted when midazolam was given to a group of mice. However, cerebral blood flow did decrease to approximately 55 percent of control values, and survival time increased 2.8 times that of control. Diazepam increased the survival time to 1.6 times that of control. By comparison, barbiturates increased the survival time to four times control [57]. It must be remembered that with both diazepam and barbiturates there is a decrease in respiratory drive, and the $PaCO_2$ is elevated. If these medications are used in the head-injured patient, ventilation must be controlled.

NARCOTICS

Narcotics tend to create minor changes in cerebral blood flow and in cerebral oxygen consumption. The ratio of cerebral blood flow to cerebral oxygen consumption appears not to change; rather, both decrease in a parallel fashion. Morphine given to normocapnic, normothermic dogs that had previously been anesthetized with less than 0.1 percent halothane and a 70:30 mixture of nitrous oxide and oxygen, showed a 15 percent decrease in cerebral metabolic oxygen consumption with a dose of 1.2 mg/kg of morphine. Cerebral blood flow was reduced to 50 percent of control at a dose of 0.6 mg/kg [54].

One of the newer synthetic narcotics, fentanyl, was administered to normocapnic, artificially ventilated rats that had been tracheotomized, paralyzed, and subsequently ventilated with 70 percent nitrous oxide and 30 percent oxygen. An IV bolus of fentanyl in doses of 25, 50, 100, and 200 μg/kg was followed by a slow IV infusion of the drug. There was a significant dose-related depression of approximately 40 percent in both cerebral blood flow and cerebral metabolic oxygen consumption compared to the nitrous oxide–ventilated controls [58].

KETAMINE

Ketamine is one of the few drugs that causes an abrupt increase in cerebral blood flow. There is also a simultaneous increase in the cerebral metabolic rate of oxygen consumption. There may be an increase in the mean arterial blood pressure, but this is not the only mechanism by which cerebral blood flow increases. Direct smooth muscular relaxation may cause the increase in cerebral blood flow, which then could cause an increase in ICP in patients with head injuries [59]. A 50 percent increase in cerebral blood flow and a less than 20 percent increase in the overall cerebral metabolic oxygen consumption has been reported. The dilatation resulting from ketamine administration has been studied and does not appear to be caused by adenosine, prostaglandins, cholinergic receptors, or beta-adrenergic receptors [60].

MUSCLE RELAXANTS

Muscle relaxants are used to facilitate intubation. These drugs fall into two major groups: the depolarizing muscle relaxants, of which succinylcholine is the most commonly used, and the nondepolarizing muscle relaxants, which include pancuronium, curare, vecuronium, and atracurium. Because of tachycardia, which is usually produced by pancuronium in intubating doses, and histamine release, which is seen with curare and in atracurium-intubating doses, many anesthesiologists are now using vecuronium for facilitating intubation.

Succinylcholine has the major advantage of producing superb muscle relaxation 60 seconds after injection. However, there are many disadvantages with the use of this drug. Bradycardia, asystole, and muscle fasciculations, which may transiently raise the central venous pressure and enhance the ICP, may occur. In addition, large increases in potassium ion in certain groups of patients have been noted. Succinylcholine has also been implicated in malignant hyperthermia. Messick et al. felt that the problems associated with use of succinylcholine in patients with increased intracranial pressure were secondary to inadequate anesthesia and lack of control of blood pressure and PCO_2 [54].

The pharmacologic, neuromuscular, and hemodynamic effects of atracurium and vecuronium have been studied. No changes were noted in cerebral metabolic rate, cerebral blood flow, or ICP with these drugs [61, 62].

ANTIHYPERTENSIVE DRUGS

Vasoactive drugs may have a significant effect on patients with intracranial hypertension. Systemic hypertension may be controlled by several different types of drugs. These include the smooth muscle relaxants, the beta blockers, and the calcium channel blockers. Nitroprusside and nitroglycerin are both smooth muscle relaxants. Nitroprusside produces equal effects on the arterial and venous vasculature, whereas nitroglycerin has a greater effect on the venous vasculature. Both compounds can increase the total cerebral blood flow until the blood concentration is increased enough to reduce the mean arterial pressure below the limits of autoregulation [63, 64]. The same effects have been noted with hydralazine. Approximately 15 mg of hydralazine was administered in one study to a group of patients, who were subsequently noted to have a 20 percent reduction in arterial pressure [65]. However, an increase in cerebral blood flow and an 11 percent increase in ICP also resulted. These effects correlated with a 20 to 30 percent decrease in cerebral perfusion pressure. With the use of any one of these three drugs, a decrease in systemic arterial pressure and an increase in cerebral blood flow occurs. This increased cerebral blood flow will continue until the systemic arterial pressure is reduced enough to cause a drop in cerebral blood flow. The level at which this happens is quite low and may be enough to compromise other body organs. This group of drugs does have a significant place in emergency medicine for treating hypertension but only in patients who have good cerebral compliance and are able to compensate for the increase in intracranial volume caused by the increase in blood flow.

Beta blockers such as propranolol or the new, short-acting drug esmolol, or combined alpha and beta blockers such as labetalol have not been shown to produce any significant alteration in either cerebral blood flow or cerebral metabolic oxygen consumption. Thus, such drugs should be considered first-line agents in the initial treatment of hypertension in the head-injured patient. This holds true unless there is a hemodynamic effect that results in a change in cerebral perfusion pressure that exceeds the limits of autoregulation [54].

GLASGOW COMA SCALE

A large number of different systems have been used to describe head-injured patients. An easy system was desired in order to follow patients'

Table 13-1. Glasgow coma scale

Sign	Response	Score
Eye opening	Spontaneous	4
	To speech	3
	To pain	2
	None	1
Best verbal response	Oriented	5
	Confused	4
	Inappropriate	3
	Incomprehensive	2
	None	1
Best motor response	Obey commands	6
	Localizes pain	5
	Withdrawal to pain	4
	Flexion to pain	3
	Extension to pain	2
	None	1

progress and, in addition, to facilitate comparisons of the different modes of therapy used in different institutions. The system that has gained the widest acceptance at the present time is the Glasgow Coma Scale (Table 13-1), which was proposed in 1974 by Teasdale and Jennett [66]. This scale enables observers to describe different levels of coma using the following three features: eye opening, motor response, and verbal response. It should be noted that no arbitrary levels of consciousness or anatomic correlations are used.

Eye opening is graded on a scale of 1 to 4, with 4 points given for spontaneous opening, 3 for opening in response to voice stimulus, 2 for opening in response to a painful stimulus, and 1 for no eye opening at all. (Spontaneous opening of the eyes is an indication that the brain stem is intact.) If a painful stimulation is used, it should be standardized. Application of pressure from a pen or pencil to the patient's nailbed has been advocated. After the patient has been maximally aroused, his verbal and motor responses are then assessed. Verbal responses are graded as oriented (5 points), confused (4 points), use of inappropriate words (3 points), incomprehensible sounds (2 points), and none (1 point). Normal, oriented conversation is considered present in the patient who is aware of concepts such as time and location and indicates a high level of brain function. Confused conversation encompasses a wide variety of responses, but the responses are somewhat appropriate. Inappropriate words are usually blurted out in an exclamatory manner, and incomprehensible sounds may occur in the form of moaning or groaning and represent a profound degree of brain dysfunction.

One of the major criticisms of the Glasgow Coma Scale involves the evaluation of the verbal response. Patients who are intubated are unable to speak, and some young children may refuse to speak because of fear or other emotional reasons.

Motor response is based on response of the arms to varying stimuli. There are six levels by which motor response is graded. These are obeying a command (6 points), localizing pain (5 points), withdrawing from pain (4 points), decorticate flexing (3 points), decerebrate extension (2 points), and no movement at all (1 point). In patients who do not obey commands, the motor response is first tested by the standard stimulus to the nailbed and then by pressure applied to the supraorbital notch. To distinguish between an attempt to localize pain and abnormal flexion that occurs with supraorbital stimulus, the hand must move above the chin if the patient is truly localizing pain and not manifesting the decorticate flexion response. Withdrawing from pain may be evaluated by applying standard pressure on the nailbed. Abnormal extension and flexion may be elicited with supraorbital notch pressure. The total score ranges from 3 for the least responsive to 15 for the most responsive. There is a close correlation between the outcome of head injury and the Glasgow Coma score [67].

The Glasgow Coma Scale has been used and accepted worldwide. In 1978, Langfitt, in an editorial in the *Journal of Neurosurgery,* urged that the Glasgow Coma Scale be adopted by neurosurgical units throughout the world to evaluate patients with head injuries. Bearing this in mind, all patients need an initial baseline for their progress to be followed through their hospital course. This baseline measurement should be performed by the emergency physician at the time of the patient's admittance to the emergency department.

CEREBRAL PROTECTION

Several agents that provide brain protection after a hypoxic or ischemic event have been evaluated. The primary insult is a decrease in available oxygen to the cerebral parenchyma. This in turn switches the brain from aerobic to anaerobic metabolism and provides much less ATP for metabolism. There have been multiple reports on different modalities for treatment of cerebral hypoxia. Care must be taken in interpreting these because many studies utilize preinsult therapy, whereas in clinical practice, treatment is always given after the insult. An exception to this statement would be treatment given in the operating room, when ischemia or the possibility of microemboli can at times be foreseen. The major modalities presently in use are hypothermia, barbiturates, and calcium channel blockers.

HYPOTHERMIA

It has long been known that hypothermia will protect the brain during periods of ischemia or hypoxia. Hypothermia is routinely used in cardiac surgery and has proved to be of great value in this setting. Metabolic oxygen consumption at 37°C was reported by Michenfelder in 1958 to be two and one-half times that found at 27°C [68]. The only practical way to provide rapid and controllable hypothermia is by means of cardiopulmonary bypass, which provides total corporeal hypothermia. However, this creates numerous problems for multiple organ systems, including a lowered fibrillation threshold, reduced kidney function, and metabolic acidosis.

The second major problem with providing hypothermia is the systemic heparinization needed for cardiopulmonary bypass. It would be risky, to say the least, to heparinize a patient who has just suffered multiple trauma or has an isolated head injury.

Although inducing hypothermia in a head-injured patient is impractical, prevention of hyperthermia is essential. Hyperthermia may result from injury to the brain stem or the hypothalamic region or from blood in the ventricular system. The other source of hyperthermia is exposure to a high ambient temperature. Pyrexia unrelated to infection has been reported in as many as 15 percent of head-injured patients. Patients with pyrexia should be treated with acetaminophen and cooling blankets. If shivering develops, it may be treated with narcotics, chloropromazine, or promethazine.

BARBITURATES

The use of barbiturates in brain preservation has been studied extensively during the past 15 years. There are many appealing aspects of barbiturates as agents for brain preservation. Barbiturates cause decreases in cerebral metabolic rate, cerebral blood flow, and intracranial pressure. They also lead to diminished vasogenic cerebral edema, lowered intracellular lactate, depressed glucose utilization by cells, inhibition of glycolysis, inhibition of mitochondrial respiration, and uncoupling of oxidative phosphorylation. However, there is a price paid for all these beneficial effects. There are decreases in cardiac output and cardiac contractility, and there may be associated hypotension that is refractory to vasopressors.

Much of the confusion surrounding the use of barbiturate coma came from early reports of barbiturates used in monkeys subjected to global ischemia. In 1975, Bleyaert et al. demonstrated that monkeys subjected to global ischemia for 16 minutes had less neurologic deficit if they were pretreated with sodium thiopental, 90 mg/kg. This infusion was begun 5 minutes postischemia and was completed by 65 minutes postischemia [69]. This same experiment was tried by other investigators. Grisvold and colleagues used pigtailed monkeys but were unable to reproduce the results [70]. Marshall et al., in a study of head-injured patients in 1979, showed that some improvement occurred in those who were treated with barbiturate coma [71]. The methodology used in these studies has been criticized, and, in an effort to increase the validity of the results, randomized clinical studies were performed on both patients after cardiac arrest and patients after severe head injury. Patients with severe head injuries were placed in a randomized control trial of prophylactic pentobarbital therapy by Ward and associates [72]. The pentobarbital was started as soon as possible after the head injury, regardless of the intracranial pressure, and continued for a prescribed period of time. Fifty-three consecutive head-injured patients were placed in this study. Twenty-six were placed in the control group and 27 received pentobarbital. Except for the pentobarbital therapy, all patients were treated with the same protocol and received aggressive resuscitation, prompt diagnosis and treatment of mass lesions, and related intensive care. The researchers found no difference between the groups in the incidence of elevated ICP, the duration of ICP elevation, or the response of ICP elevations to treatment. There were significant differences, however, in complications found in the group receiving pentobarbital. Fifty-four percent of the pentobarbital-treated group had arterial hypotension compared with only 7 percent in the untreated group. The authors concluded that they could not recommend the prophylactic use of pentobarbital coma in the treatment of patients with severe head injuries.

In the status post cardiac arrest study there were 262 initially "comatose" survivors [73]. These were split into two groups. The control group received standardized brain-oriented intensive care, and the second group received sodium thiopental, 30 mg/kg. The results revealed no statistically significant differences between treated groups in mortality, survival with good cerebral recovery, or survival with permanent severe neurologic damage. The results of this study do not support the use of sodium thiopental for brain resuscitation after cardiac arrest.

To further complicate the issue, Nussmeier and colleagues were successful in demonstrating that barbiturates provide some cerebral protection when the barbiturate is given prior to cardiopulmonary bypass [74]. In this study, the authors were able to show that sodium thiopental significantly decreased neuropsychiatric complications from open ventricle cardiac surgery requiring cardiopulmonary bypass. Eighty-nine patients randomly received sodium thiopental in a dose sufficient to maintain electroencephalographic silence throughout the period from before atrial cannulation to termination of bypass. Ninety-three control patients received only fentanyl in anesthesia. By the tenth postoperative day, all neuropsychiatric dysfunction had resolved in the thiopental group but persisted in 7.5 percent of the control group. This was felt to be the first demonstration of cerebral protection by a barbiturate in humans. Because hypothermia was not used during bypass, the study has been criticized, and acceptance of this treatment has been correspondingly slow. As in previous studies, hypotension in barbiturate-treated patients required significantly more treatment with cardiac inotropes and vasopressors. A key factor in this study, however, is that the barbiturate was given prior to the insult. At this time, there is still no good support from the literature for placing head-injured or cardiopulmonary arrest patients in barbiturate coma for cerebral protection.

STEROID THERAPY

Use of steroids was advocated in the 1970s for severely head injured patients. It had been known for some time that steroids reduced intracranial pressure in patients with brain tumors and associated peritumor cerebral edema. It was felt that steroids stabilized the cell membranes and reduced the amount of edema and therefore the intracranial pressure. Several studies examined the use of steroids in head injured patients in the late 1970s. Both high and low doses of steroids were evaluated. Gudeman et al. examined the hypothesis that an abrupt increase in cortical steroid dose in patients with severe head injury would cause a detectable reduction in intracranial pressure within 48 hours [75]. They studied 20 consecutive patients with severe head injury, 12 of whom had had surgical decompression of a mass lesion. All of the patients were artificially ventilated and had continuous monitoring of intracranial pressure and intermittent testing of cerebral compliance by measurement of the volume pressure response. The patients received 40 mg of methylprednisolone every 6 hours for the first 12 hours after admission and then received a single dose of 2 gm and then 500 mg every 6 hours for the next 24 hours. The drug was then tapered rapidly. No significant change in intracranial pressure or volume pressure response could be detected during 24 to 48 hours of this high-dose steroid therapy. The course of intracranial pressure fluctuation and the final outcome in these patients were not significantly different from those observed in a previous group of 262 patients managed without the high doses of steroids. There was, however, a 50 percent incidence of gastric hemorrhage and an 85 percent incidence of hyperglycemia with glucosuria in the 20 steroid-treated patients.

Cooper and colleagues investigated both low-dose dexamethasone therapy at 16 mg/day and high-dose therapy at 96 mg/day in head-injured patients, and showed that there was no significant difference between the groups in intracranial pressure or outcome [76]. In light of these findings, steroid therapy cannot be recommended in patients with severe head injuries because there are no data to show significant differences in either outcome or control of intracranial pressure.

CALCIUM CHANNEL BLOCKERS

Calcium channel blockers have recently been advocated for the treatment of complete global cerebral ischemia [77]. After a period of cerebral ischemia, there is a marked increase in cerebral blood flow hyperperfusion that lasts 10 to 15 minutes after restoration of blood flow. Following this there is a prolonged period of hypoperfusion, and it is for this hypoperfusion phase that the calcium channel blockers have been advocated. Flunarizine was initially touted as a drug that could ameliorate this postischemic hypoperfusion state [78]. In subsequent studies, however, this action could not be confirmed [79]. Nimodipine has been shown to improve outcome when given to primates after complete cerebral ischemia by Steen and others [80]. Twenty-seven monkeys were subjected to 17 minutes of complete cerebral ischemia followed by 96 hours of intensive care treatment. Fourteen of these monkeys received nimodepine, 10 μg/kg 5 minutes post ischemia, followed by a nimodepine infusion, 1 μg/kg/min for 10 hours. At the end of 96 hours, only 2 of the 10 control subjects had apparently normal levels of consciousness, and all had major neurologic deficits. Of the treated animals, 11 had a normal level of consciousness, and four of these had no detectable neurologic deficits; a fifth had only a slight motor deficit. Calcium channel blockers have also been shown to be beneficial in treating cerebral vasospasm in humans after subarachnoid hemorrhage and in increasing cerebral blood flow in humans with cerebral vascular disease [81]. There have been no good human studies, however, on the use of calcium channel blockers after complete cerebral ischemia. Thus, presently such therapy can be regarded only as an interesting experimental modality that will require more study until it can be added to clinical practice. Initially positive animal studies were also seen with the barbiturates, but later such therapy was shown to have no therapeutic value in clinical medicine.

TREATMENT OF HEAD INJURY

AIRWAY

With the foregoing information in mind, how are severe head injuries best treated? As in cardiopulmonary resuscitation, the basics need to be followed. First and foremost is treatment of the airway. Rose and colleagues reviewed 116 case studies looking for avoidable factors that contributed to death after head injury [82]. They found, in decreasing order of occurrence, delayed treatment of hematoma, airway obstruction, hypotension, poorly controlled epileptiform activity, and meningitis as preventable factors contributing to death. Early intubation should follow the criteria given for respiratory insufficiency earlier in the chapter. Gildenberg and Malkela examined the effect of early intubation and ventilation on outcome in patients with head trauma and found that the mortality in the group intubated within 1 hour of injury was 22.5 percent, whereas mortality in patients intubated 1 hour or longer after injury was 38.4 percent [83]. Early intubation not only prevents hypoxia and provides prophylaxis against vomiting and aspiration, it also allows the treating physician to initiate hyperventilation.

Rapid sequence induction is the safest modality that allows endotracheal tube placement without causing trauma or an increase in intracranial pressure. Oral intubation is the quickest and easiest route for placement of an endotracheal tube; it also provides the least trauma and the smallest probability of an increase in intracranial pressure. Nasotracheal intubation carries the risk of traumatic epistaxis as well as vomiting and aspiration when the endotracheal tube reaches the nasopharynx. If the nasopharynx is not properly anesthetized, there will be a large increase in intracranial pressure as the tube passes through this area. First, the patient should be mask ventilated with 100% oxygen as cricoid pressure is applied to prevent vomiting and aspiration. Administration of IV sodium thiopental can blunt the ICP-raising stimulus of intubation. The dose varies from 1 to 5 mg/kg depending on the cardiovascular stability of the patient at the time of intubation. Lidocaine, 1 mg/kg IV, also is helpful in preventing increases in intracranial pressure before placement of the endotracheal tube [84]. There is controversy about which of the neuromuscular blocking drugs should be used to facilitate intubation. Succinylcholine is considered by many to be the muscle relaxant of choice. The dose of succinylcholine is 1 to 1.5 mg/kg. The drug can provide ideal muscle relaxation for intubation in 60 seconds and has a duration of paralysis of 5 to 10 minutes, with full recovery in 12 to 15 minutes. The brief duration of action of succinylcholine is due to its rapid hydrolysis by pseudocholinesterase, which is an enzyme found in the plasma and liver. The advantage of using succinylcholine for rapid sequence induction lies not only in its rapid onset but also in its rapid hydrolysis. This provides a margin of safety in the event that the trachea cannot be intubated. If the patient is preoxygenated, 1 to 2 minutes will be available for safe placement of the tube in the trachea after the onset of paralysis in most patients. If the trachea cannot be intubated, the patient can be ventilated with a bag and mask with continued cricoid pressure until there is spontaneous reversal of the effects of succinylcholine.

An oral airway or other adjunct device may be needed to assist in ventilating the patient with a mask during this period of paralysis. There may be episodes of prolonged neuromuscular blockade from succinylcholine in patients who have atypical forms of pseudocholinesterase. This genetic variant is relatively uncommon and is often found in family members. Low levels of pseudocholinesterase are found in some patients with liver disease, pregnancy, or cancer and in patients who have ingested cholinesterase inhibitors such as organophosphates. As a rule, such patients still recover quickly from succinylcholine administration, whereas those with atypical forms often require several hours of mechanical ventilation while the drug is metabolized in the liver.

The most common cardiovascular side effect of succinylcholine is sinus bradycardia. This is more prominent in children than in adults. The likelihood of sinus bradycardia increases if a second dose of succinylcholine is given. Children, especially infants, should receive atropine sulfate in a dose of 0.01 mg/kg before receiving succinylcholine. Adults should receive atropine in the same dose if a second dose of succinylcholine is required.

Hyperkalemia has also been reported in patients receiving succinylcholine who have burns, trauma, spinal cord damage, or neuromuscular disease [85]. The period of risk for the burn patient is between 10 and 60 days after the burn. The blunt trauma patient with muscle damage appears to have stable serum potassium levels until about 1 week after injury, at which time the level may increase dramatically, or even fatally, with an infusion of succinylcholine. Patients with neuromuscular disease may also have an increased serum potassium level after administration of succinylcholine. This appears to be more prominent in patients with progressive diseases such as muscular dystrophy. Hyperkalemia after succinylcholine may also be noted in patients with hemiplegia or paraplegia secondary to upper motor neuron lesions. The period of vulnerability appears to be within the first 6 months after motor neuron damage.

Succinylcholine is a depolarizing muscle relaxant. It causes muscle fasciculations if patients are not pretreated with a small dose of nondepolarizing muscle relaxant. It has been noted that up to 89 percent of patients who receive succinylcholine without this pretreatment complain of muscle pains at the conclusion of anesthesia [86]. Myoglobinuria after succinylcholine has been noted, indicating muscle damage [87]. Pretreatment of the patient with pancuronium, 0.5 to 1 mg IV, or curare, 2 to 3 mg IV, prior to administration of succinylcholine can help to prevent some of these side effects. Fasciculations, elevation of intraocular pressure, and elevated intragastric pressure may also be ameliorated with this regimen [88].

Because of the side effects of succinylcholine, other neuromuscular blockers have been advocated for rapid sequence induction. Vecuronium is this author's personal choice for a muscle relaxant in this situation. The priming principle was advocated by Schwartz et al. to shorten the time of satisfactory conditions for tracheal intubation. The initial dose of vecuronium used was 0.015 mg/kg, followed 6 minutes later by 0.05 mg/kg. This technique shortened the time to intubation from 61 seconds to 21 seconds [89]. This result has not been born out in other studies, however [90]. It has been noted that the time to intubation has been shortened by using larger intubating doses, i.e., 0.25 mg/kg. This increase is possible because of the lack of adverse side effects from vecuronium. Cricoid pressure needs to be applied during this period of time, and careful ventilation with 100% oxygen should also be carried out. The major problem with using vecuronium by this or other regimens mentioned earlier in this volume in this setting is failed intubation. If, however, the physician is comfortable with managing airways, the side effects of succinylcholine are eliminated by the use of the nondepolarizing drug. No change in heart rate or blood pressure is associated with the use of vecuronium, and there is also no histamine release with this drug.

Once the endotracheal tube has been placed, hyperventilation should be instituted and the $PaCO_2$ lowered to 30 mm Hg. If the patient is showing signs of increased intracranial pressure, mannitol should be started at 0.25 mg/kg. This dose has been shown by Marshall et al. to cause the same reduction in ICP as higher doses, i.e., 0.5 to 1 mg/kg [91]. Lasix, 1 mg/kg IV, has been shown to cause a greater volume and rate of water loss than mannitol alone [92].

TREATMENT OF HYPERTENSION

If the patient has shown signs of catecholamine hyperactivity with tachycardia, T-wave changes, or hypertension, beta blockade is recommended with incremental doses of propranolol or labetalol. Propranolol may be given in 1-mg IV boluses every 3 to 5 minutes until the desired response is achieved. Labetalol is recommended in a dose of 20 mg IV, or 0.30 mg/kg in a 70-kg patient, by slow intravenous injection over a 2-minute period. The maximum effect usually occurs within 5 minutes, and additional injections of 40 mg or 80 mg may be given at 10-minute intervals until the desired supine blood pressure is achieved, or a total of 300 mg of labetalol has been injected.

Labetalol has some alpha-blocking effects that could increase cerebral blood flow. Further study is needed in this area, but at present there is little clinical evidence that this objection is more than theoretical.

Esmolol, a new beta blocker, may also be used for hypertensive therapy in the head-injured patient. The drug is distributed as 2.5 gm in 10 ml of diluent, which is injected into 250 ml of IV solution. This results in a solution with a drug concentration of 10 mg/ml. To initiate treatment, a loading dose of 500 μg/kg over 1 minute is administered followed by a 4-minute maintenance infusion of 50 μg/kg/min. If an adequate therapeutic effect is not observed within 5 minutes, the same loading dose is repeated and is followed with a maintenance infusion of 100 μg/kg/min. Because esmolol is rapidly metabolized by hydrolysis of its ester linkage, the effect of this drug is usually gone or substantially reduced within 10 minutes. This drug offers the advantages of a beta blocker that is readily reversible, which is not possible with propranolol or labetalol. Because head-injured patients may have other painful injuries, narcotic therapy should also often be instituted in conjunction with ventilation as needed.

TREATMENT OF SEIZURES

Control of seizures is of utmost importance because seizure activity greatly increases metabolic oxygen consumption. Tonic-clonic status epilepticus should be stopped as soon as possible. Mortality rates as great as 50 percent have been reported after tonic-clonic status epilepticus when the seizures have lasted longer than 60 minutes [93]. It has been shown that there is permanent damage to cells in the hippocampus, amygdala, cerebellum, thalamus, and middle cerebral cortical layers after 60 minutes of convulsive activity. This cell damage has been noted even if animals have been ventilated and metabolic side effects have been corrected.

The prescribed sequence of drugs for treatment of status epilepticus has been detailed by Delgado-Escuator and others in an excellent review article [93]. Diazepam is the first drug of choice and should be given no faster than 2 mg/min IV until seizures stop or until a total of 20 mg has been given. Infusion of IV phenytoin at a rate no greater than 50 mg/min to a total of 18 mg/kg should then be started. The main side effects of phenytoin are hypotension and QT interval prolongation in the ECG. If either develops, the infusion should be slowed to 25 mg/min. If the seizures persist after both diazepam and phenytoin have been given, intravenous phenobarbital is recommended, with a continuous infusion at a rate of 100 mg/min until the seizure stops or until a loading dose of 20 mg/kg has been given. If the seizure continues, a general anesthetic with halothane or isoflurane in conjunction with neuromuscular blockade is then recommended [84]. If the patient is already paralyzed, some type of continuous EEG monitoring is indicated because tonic-clonic movements would, of course, not be visible. Again, it has been shown that even with neuromuscular blockade, if there is seizure activity in the brain there most probably is cell damage.

CONTROL OF ELEVATED INTRACRANIAL PRESSURE

Treatment of refractory, elevated ICP can be very frustrating for the physician and, of course, ultimately fatal for the patient. It not only leads to decreased cerebral perfusion pressure but also causes structural brain damage from gross herniation or subtle contusion.

Various modalities that lower elevated ICP have been discussed throughout this chapter. These include hyperventilation, positioning (i.e., elevating the head of the bed to 30 degrees), and pharmacologic therapy with barbiturates or diuretics. A remaining treatment that may lead to lowered ICP is the prevention of ongoing secondary damage from hyperglycemia, hypoxia, uncontrolled hypertension or hypotension, or unrecognized epileptiform activity (see above). If all fails and the ICP remains at 25 to 30 or more mm Hg, consideration should be given to surgical intervention. Because of the shape of the cerebral compliance curve (see Fig. 13-4), there is a point at which very small changes in cerebral volume lead to very large changes in ICP. This may benefit therapy as well as exacerbate errors. Thus, if patient's brain is physiologically lying on this "knee" of the compliance curve, a small amount of CSF may be released from a ventriculostomy catheter with good results.

Finally, a previously unrecognized hematoma may be evacuated. As stated earlier, of the preventable causes identified by Rose and colleagues [82] as contributing to death after head injury, the primary one was delayed treatment of hematoma. Therefore, early CT scan should be performed promptly after initial ED stabilization, and repeat CT scans should be considered as needed.

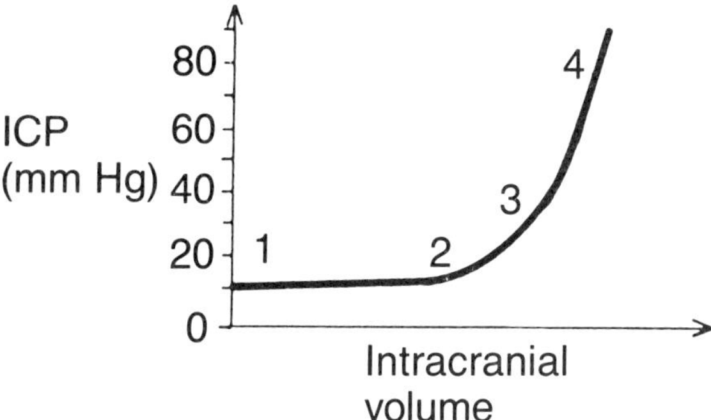

Fig. 13-4. Intracranial compliance. The brain is compliant between 1 and 2, but from 2 to 4 compliance is lost, and small changes in volume cause large changes in intracranial pressure (ICP). (From R. D. Miller [ed.]. *Anesthesia* [2nd ed.]. New York: Churchill Livingstone, 1986. With permission.)

Avoidance of iatrogenic elevation of ICP is also a consideration. Circumferential endotracheal tube taping or lateral rotation of the head may obstruct cerebral venous drainage. Use of PEEP may also restrict venous outflow. Vasodilators such as nitroprusside should be avoided if possible. Finally, reiterative, compulsive observation of the treatment modalities mentioned above must be made. Hyperventilation, elevation of the head, mannitol or furosemide diuresis, and barbiturate therapy must be monitored carefully. Serum glucose levels, arterial blood gas tensions, and serial electroencephalograms and CT scans should be followed.

DETERMINATION OF DEATH

With the advent of modern medical technology, there has been considerable debate about the definition of death. Guidelines for determination of death were published in 1982 in *Critical Care Medicine* [85]. Medical consultants to the President's Commission for the Study of Ethical Problems in Medicine and Biomedical and Behavioral Research devised a uniform definition of death. "An individual who has sustained either: (1) irreversible cessation of circulatory and respiratory functions, or (2) irreversible cessation of all functions of the entire brain including the brainstem, is dead. A determination of death must be made in accordance with accepted medical standards [94].

CRITERIA FOR DETERMINATION OF DEATH

An individual presenting with the findings in either section A below (cardiopulmonary) or section B (neurologic) is dead. In either case, a diagnosis of death requires that demonstration of both cessation of functions, as set forth in subsection 1, and irreversibility, as set forth in subsection 2.

A. An individual with irreversible cessation of circulatory and respiratory functions is dead.
   1. Cessation is recognized by an appropriate clinical examination.
   2. Irreversibility is recognized by persistent cessation of functions during an appropriate period of observation and/or trial of therapy.
B. An individual with irreversible cessation of all functions of the entire brain, including the brainstem, is dead.
   1. Cessation is recognized when evaluation discloses findings of a and b:
      a. Cerebral functions are absent, and
      b. Brainstem functions are absent.
   2. Irreversibility is recognized when evaluation discloses findings of a, b, and c:
      a. The cause of coma is established and is sufficient to account for the loss of brain functions, and
      b. The possibility of recovery of any brain functions is excluded, and
      c. The cessation of all brain functions persists for an appropriate period of observation and/or trial of therapy.

Determination of brain death takes on special importance in the setting of isolated, severe neurologic insult when organ donation is considered. It is imperative in this setting that potentially reversible metabolic or pharmacologic causes of brain death be ruled out. In addition to having two physicians sign statements attesting to irreversible neurologic function, some jurisdictions require cerebral perfusion scans documenting cessation of cerebral blood flow, or hypercapnic apnea tests in which apnea is demonstrated at PCO_2 of 60 mm Hg.

REFERENCES

1. Kalsbeek, W. D., McLaurin, R. L., Harris, B. S. H., III et al. National head and spinal cord injury survey: Major findings. *J. Neurosurg.* 53:S19, 1980.
2. Jennett, B., and Teasdale, G., et al. Spearhead injuries in three countries. *J. Neurol. Neurosurg. Psychiat.* 40:291, 1977.
3. Fife, D., Faich, G., Hollinshead, W., et al. Incidence and outcome of hospital-treated head injury in Rhode Island. *Am. J. Publ. Health* 76:773, 1986.
4. Klauber, M. R., Barrett-Connor, E., Marshall, L. F., et al. The epidemiology of head injury. *Am. J. Epidemiol.* 113:500, 1981.
5. Sundt, T. M., Siekert, R. G., Piepgras, D. G., et al. Bypass surgery for vascular disease with carotid system. *Mayo Clin. Proc.* 48:719, 1976.

6. Kety, S. S., and Schmidt, C. F. The nitrous oxide method for the quantitative determination of cerebral bloods flow in man: Theory, procedure and normal values. *J. Clin. Invest.* 27:476, 1948.

7. Messick, J. M., Newberg, L. A., Nugent, M., et al. Principles of neuroanesthesia for the non-neurosurgical patient with CNS pathophysiology. *Anesth. Analg.* 64:143, 1985.

8. Eklof, B., Ingvar, D. H., Kagstrom, E., et al. Persistence of cerebral blood flow through autoregulation following chronic bilateral cervical sympathectomy in the monkey. *Acta Physiol. Scand.* 82:172, 1971.

9. Waltz, A. G., Yamaguchi, T., and Regli, F. Regulatory responses of cerebral vasculature after sympathetic denervation. *Am. J. Physiol.* 221:298, 1971.

10. Haggendal, E., Lofgren, J., Nilsson, N. J., et al. Effects of varied cerebral spinal fluid pressure on cerebral blood flow in dogs. *Acta Physiol. Scand.* 79:262, 1970.

11. Greenfield, J. C., Rembert, J. C., and Tindall, G. T. Transient changes in cerebral vascular resistance during the Valsalva maneuver in man. *Stroke* 15:76, 1984.

12. Lassen, N. A., and Christensen, M. S. Physiology of cerebral blood flow. *Br. J. Anesth.* 48:719, 1976.

13. Olesen, J. Contralateral focal increase of cerebral blood flow in man during arm work. *Brain* 94:635, 1971.

14. Elliott, K. A. C., and Jasper, H. H. Physiological salt solutions for brain surgery; studies of the local pH and PO vessel reactions to buffered and unbuffered isotonic solutions. *J. Neurosurg.* 6:140, 1949.

15. Lassen, N. A. Brain extracellular pH: The main factor controlling cerebral blood flow. *Scand. J. Clin. Lab. Invest.* 22:247, 1968.

16. Plum, F., and Siesjo, B. K. Recent advances in CSF physiology. *Anesthesiology* 42:708, 1975.

17. Fencl, V., Vale, J. R., and Broch, J. A. Respiration and cerebral blood flow in metabolic acidosis and alkalosis in humans. *J. Appl. Physiol.* 27:67, 1969.

18. Severinghaus, J. W., Chiodi, H., and Eger, E. I. Cerebral blood flow in man at high altitudes: The role of cerebral spinal fluid pH and normalization of flow in chronic hypocapnia. *Circ. Res.* 19:274, 1966.

19. Harp, J. R., and Wollman, H. Cerebral metabolic effects of hyperventilation and deliberate hypotension. *Br. J. Anesth.* 45:256, 1973.

20. Alm, A., and Bill, A. The effect of stimulation of the cervical sympathetic chain on retinal oxygen tension and on uveal, retinal, and cerebral blood flow in cats. *Acta Physiol. Scand.* 88:84, 1973.

21. Fitch, W., Mackenzie, E. T., and Harper, A. M. The effects of decreasing arterial blood pressure on cerebral blood flow in the baboon; influence of the sympathetic nervous system. *Circ. Res.* 37:550, 1975.

22. Todd, M. M., Chadwick, H. S., and Shapiro, H. M. Outcome after cardiac arrest; the role of plasma glucose. *Anesthesiology* 55:A265, 1981.

23. Rehncrona, S., Rosen, I., and Siesjo, B. K. Brain lactidosis and ischemic cell damage; biochemistry and neurophysiology. *J. Cerebral Blood Flow Metab.* 1:297, 1981.

24. Ginsberg, M. D., Welch, F. A., and Budd, W. W. Deleterious effect of glucose pretreatment on recovery from diffuse cerebral ischemia in the cat. *Stroke* 2:347, 1980.

25. Siemkowicz, E., and Jgedde, A. Postischemic coma in the rat; effects of different pre-ischemic blood glucose levels on the cerebral metabolic recovery after ischemia. *Acta Physiol. Scand.* 110:225, 1980.

26. Clifton, G. L., Ziegler, M. G., and Grossman, R. G. Circulating catecholamines and sympathetic activity after head injury. *Neurosurgery* 8:10, 1981.
27. McLoud, A. A., Neil-Dwier, G., Mayer, C. H., et al. Cardiac quality of acute head injury. *Br. Heart J.* 47:221, 1982.
28. Hackenberry, L. E., Minner, M. E., Rea, G. L., et al. Biochemical evidence of myocardial injury after severe head trauma. *Crit. Care Med.* 10:641, 1982.
29. Frost, E. A. M. Cardiorespiratory effects of central nervous system derangements. *Anesthesiol. Clin. North Am.* 5(3):507, 1987.
30. Frost, E. A. M. The intensive care of the neurosurgical patient. *Semin. Anesth.* 1:340, 1982.
31. Miller, J. D., Sweet, R. C., Narayan, M. D., et al. Early insults to the injured brain. *J.A.M.A.* 240:439, 1978.
32. Miller, J. D., Butterworth, J. F., and Gudema, S. W. K. Further experiences in the management of severe head injury. *J. Neurosurg.* 54:289, 1981.
33. Theodore, J., and Robin, E. D. Pathogenesis of neurogenic pulmonary edema. *Lancet* 2:749, 1975.
34. Rosner, M. J., and Becker, D. P. Intracranial pressure monitoring: Complications and associated factors. *Clin. Neurosurg.* 23:494, 1976.
35. Mendelow, A. D., Rowan, J. O., Murray, L., et al. A clinical comparison of subdural screw pressure measurements with ventricular pressure. *J. Neurosurg.* 58:45, 1983.
36. Mayhall, C. G., Archer, N. H., Lamb, V. A., et al. Ventriculostomy related infections: A perspective epidemiologic study. *N. Engl. J. Med.* 310:553, 1984.
37. Rosner, M. J., and Becker, D. P. Origin and evolution of plateau waves. Experimental observations and a theoretical model. *J. Neurosurg.* 60:312, 1984.
38. Galbraith, S. C. Age distribution of extradural hemorrhage without skull fracture. *Lancet* 1:1217, 1973.
39. Jamieson, K. G., and Yelland, J. D. N. Extradural hematoma; report of 167 cases. *J. Neurosurg.* 29:13, 1968.
40. Maloney, A. F. J., and Whatmore, W. J. Clinical and pathological observations in fatal head injuries; a five year survey of 173 cases. *Br. J. Surg.* 56:23, 1969.
41. Frietag, E. Autopsy findings in head injuries from blunt forces. *Arch. Pathol.* 75:402, 1963.
42. Adams, J. H., Graham, D. I., Scott, G., et al. Brain damage in fatal non-missile head injury. *J. Clin. Pathol.* 33:1132, 1980.
43. Bruce, D. A., Schut, L., Bruno, L. A., et al. Outcome following severe head injury in children. *J. Neurosurg.* 48:679, 1978.
44. Jamieson, K. G., and Yelland, J. D. N. Surgically treated traumatic subdural hematomas. *J. Neurosurg.* 37:137, 1972.
45. Bruce, D. A., Gannarelli, T. A., and Langfitt, T. W. Resuscitation from coma due to head injury. *Crit. Care Med.* 6:254, 1978.
46. Fell, D. A., Fitzgerald, S., Moiel, R. H., et al. Acute subdural hematomas; Review of 144 cases. *J. Neurosurg.* 42:37, 1975.
47. Moiel, R. H., and Caram, B. C. Acute subdural hematoma; a review of 84 cases, six year evaluation. *J. Trauma* 7:660, 1967.
48. Talalla, A., and Morin, M. A. Acute trauma subdural hematoma; A review of 100 consecutive cases. *J. Trauma* 11:771, 1971.
49. Seelig, J. M., Becker, D. P., Miller, J. D., et al. Traumatic acute subdural hematoma. Major mortality reduction in comatose patients treated within four hours. *N. Engl. J. Med.* 304:1511, 1981.
50. Baratham, G., and Dennyson, W. G. Delayed traumatic intercerebral hemorrhage. *J. Neurol. Neurosurg. Psychiat.* 35:698, 1972.

51. Miller, J. D., Becker, D. P., Ward, J. D., et al. Significance of intercranial hypertension in severe head injury. *J. Neurosurg.* 47:503, 1977.
52. Kishore, P. R. S., Lipper, M. H., Miller, J. D., et al. Post-traumatic development of hydrocephalus in patients with severe head injury. *J. Neuroradiol.* 16:261, 1978.
53. Steen, P. A., Newberg, L., Milde, J. H., et al. Hyperthermia and barbiturates: individual and combined affects on canine cerebral oxygen consumption. *Anesthesiology* 58:527, 1983.
54. Messick, J. M., Newberg, L. A., Nugent, M., et al. Principles of neuroanesthesia for the non-neurosurgical patient with CNS path physiology. *Anesth. Analg.* 64:143, 1985.
55. Cotev, S., and Shalit, N. N. Affects of diazepam on cerebral blood flow and oxygen uptake after head injury. *Anesthesiology* 43:117, 1975.
56. Forester, A., Juge, O., and Morel, D. The effects of medazolam on cerebral hemodynamics and cerebral vasomotor responsiveness to carbon dioxide. *J. Cerebral Blood Flow Metab.* 3:246, 1983.
57. Nugent, M., Artu, A. A., and Michenfelder, J. D. Cerebral metabolic vascular and protective affects of medazolam, a maleate. *Anesthesiology* 56:172, 1982.
58. Carlsson, C., Keykhah, M., Smith, D. S., et al. Influence of high dose fentanyl on cerebral blood flow and metabolism. *Acta Physiol. Scand.* 113:271, 1981.
59. Shapiro, H. M., Wyte, S. R., and Harris, A. B. Ketamine anesthesia in patients with intracranial pathology. *Br. J. Anesth.* 44:1200, 1972.
60. Fukuda, S., Murakawak, T., Takeshita, H., et al. Drug effects of ketamine on isolated canine cerebral and mesenteric arteries. *Anesth. Analg.* 62:553, 1983.
61. Unni, V. K. N., Gray, W. J., and Young, H. S. A. Effects of atracurium on intracranial pressure in man. *Anaesthesia* 41:1047, 1986.
62. Minton, M. D., Stirt, J. A., Bedford, R. F., et al. Intracranial pressure after atracurium in neurosurgical patients. *Anesth. Analg.* 64:1113, 1985.
63. Marsh, N. L., Shapiro, H. M., Smith, R. W., et al. Changes in neurologic status and intracranial pressure associated with sodium nitroprusside administration. *Anesthesiology* 51:336, 1979.
64. Ghani, G. A., Sung, Y. F., Weinstein, M. S., et al. Effects of intravenous nitroglycerin on the intracranial pressure and volume response. *J. Neurosurg.* 58:562, 1983.
65. Overgaard, J., and Skinhoj, E. Paradoxical cerebral hemodynamic effect of hydralazine. *Stroke* 6:402, 1975.
66. Teasdale, G., and Jeannette, B. Assessment of coma and impaired consciousness. A practical scale. *Lancet* 2:81, 1974.
67. Teasdale, G., Parker, L., Murray, G., et al. Comparing a series of head injured patients. *Acta Neurosurg.* 28:205, 1979.
68. Michenfelder, J. D., and Theye, R. A. Hyperthermia: Effect on canine brain and whole body metabolism. *Anesthesiology* 29:1107, 1968.
69. Bleyaert, A. L., Nemoto, E. M., Stezoski, S. W., et al. Amelioration of postischemic encephalopathy by sodium thiopental after 16 minutes of global brain ischemia in monkeys. *Physiologist* 18:145, 1975.
70. Grisvold, S. E., Safer, P., Hendricks, H. L., et al. Thiopental treatment after global brain ischemia in pigtailed monkeys. *Anesthesiology* 60:88, 1984.
71. Marshall, L. F., Smith, R. W., Shapiro, H. M. The outcome of aggressive treatment in severe head injuries. Part II: Acute and chronic barbiturate administration in the management of head injury. *J. Neurosurg.* 50:26, 1979.

72. Ward, J. D., Becker, D. P., Miller, J. D., et al. Failure of prophylactic barbiturate coma in the treatment of severe head injury. *J. Neurosurg.* 62:382, 1985.

73. Abramson, N. S., Safar, P., Detre, K. M., et al. (Brain Resuscitation Clinical Trial I Study Group). Brain resuscitation; A clinical trial one study group, Randomized clinical study of thiopental loading in comatose survivors of cardiac arrest. *N. Engl. J. Med.* 314:397, 1986.

74. Nussmeier, N. A., Arlund, C., and Slogoff, S. Neuropsychiatric complications after cardiopulmonary bypass: Cerebral protection by a barbiturate. *Anesthesiology* 64:165, 1986.

75. Gudeman, S. K., Miller, J. D., and Becker, D. P. Failure of high dose steroid therapy to influence intracranial pressure in adults with severe head injuries. *J. Neurosurg.* 51:301, 1979.

76. Cooper, P. R., Moody, S., Clark, W. K., et al. Dextramethasone and severe head injury. *J. Neurosurg.* 51:307, 1979.

77. White, B. C., Winegar, C. D., Wilson, R. F., et al. Possible role of calcium blockers in cerebral resuscitation: a review of the literature and synthesis for future studies. *Crit. Care Med.* 11:202, 1983.

78. White, B. C., Gadzinski, D. S., Hoehner, P. J., et al. Effect of flunarzineon canine cerebral cortical blood flow and the vascular resistance post-cardiac arrest. *Ann. Emerg. Med.* 11:119, 1982.

79. Newberg, L. A., Steen, P. A., Milde, J. H., et al. Failure of flunarizine to improve cerebral blood flow on neurologic recovery in a canine model of complete cerebral ischemia. *Stroke* 15:666, 1984.

80. Steen, P. A., Gisvold, S. E., Milde, J. H., et al. Nimodipine improves outcome when given after complete cerebral ischemia in primates. *Anesthesiology* 62:406, 1985.

81. Allen, C. S., Ahn, H. S., Perziosi, T. L. J., et al. Cerebral arterial spasm—a controlled trial of nimodipine in patients with subarachnoid hemorrhage. *N. Engl. J. Med.* 308:619, 1983.

82. Rose, J., Valtonen, S., and Jennett, B. Avoidable factors contributing to death after head injury. *Br. Med. J.* 2:615, 1977.

83. Gildenberg, P. L., and Malkela, M. E. The Effect of Early Intubation and Ventilation on Outcome Following Head Trauma. In *Symposium of Neuro Trauma, Charlottesville, Virginia.* New York: Raven, 1982.

84. Stoelting, R. K. Circulating changes during direct laryngoscopy and tracheal intubation. Influence of duration of laryngoscope with or without prior lidocaine. *Anesthesiology* 47:381, 1977.

85. Miller, R. D., and Savarese, J. J. Pharmacology of Muscle Relaxants and Their Antagonists. In R. D. Miller (ed.), *Anesthesia* (2nd ed). New York: Churchill Livingstone, 1986. Pp. 889–943.

86. Brodsky, J. B., Brock-Unte, J. C., and Samuels, S. I. Pancuronium pretreatment and post-succinylcholine myalgias. *Anesthesiology* 51:259, 1979.

87. Ryan, J. F., Kagen, L. J., and Hyman, A. I. Myoglobinemia after a single dose of succinylcholine. *N. Engl. J. Med.* 285:824, 1971.

88. Miller, R. D. The advantages of giving D-tubocurarine before succinylcholine. *Anesthesiology* 37:568, 1972.

89. Schwartz, S., Llias, W., Lachner, F., et al. Rapid tracheal intubation with vecuronium: The priming principle. *Anesthesiology* 62:388, 1985.

90. Silverman, D. C., Swift, C. A., Hartmann, K. A., et al. Onset of blockade with vecuronium alone or combined: A reassessment under uniform controlled conditions. *Anesthesiology* 69:3A, A881, 1988.

91. Marshall, L. F., Smith, R. W., Rauscher, L. A., et al. Mannitol dose requirements in brain injured patients. *J. Neurosurg.* 48:169, 1978.

92. Schettini, A., Stahurski, B., and Young, H. F. Osomotic and osmotic-loop diuresis in brain surgery: Effects on plasma and CSF electrolytes and ion excretion. *J. Neurosurg.* 56:679, 1982.
93. Delgado-Escueta, A. V., Wasterlain, C., Treiman, D. M., et al. Management of status epilepticus. *N. Engl. J. Med.* 306:1337, 1982.
94. President's Commission for the Study of Ethical Problems in Medicine. Guidelines for the determination of death. *Crit. Care Med.* 10:62, 1982.

14. Legal Issues

Benjamin Shwachman

The area of law as applied to medicine, specifically anesthesiology and emergency medicine, could literally encompass volumes. I shall attempt in this chapter to cover certain basic issues that seem to come up often. The reader should keep in mind that under our federal system of law, the law can vary from state to state, and individual state law and/or applicable federal law should be checked. In addition, although the law of a sister state is binding only in that one state, it is "secondary authority" in other states and often becomes the law or the basis of law in other states.

DEFINITIONS—TORT

A tort is defined as a civil wrong [1]. There are obviously many types of torts. The tort of "medical malpractice" is actually the tort of negligence. The economic impact of tort on our lives in recent years has been considerable and is the subject of much heated debate and acrimony, particularly in medicine. Consider just the following few items from newspapers:

1. *The Wall Street Journal,* Jan. 11, 1988: A U.S. General Accounting Office report found that Florida's average paid claim on behalf of physicians in 1984 was $140,594, dwarfing New York's $104,810, California's $61,774, and the national average of $56,739.
2. *The Arizona Republic,* March 20, 1988: The [Medical Malpractice Insurance rate increase] would mark the fourth double-digit insurance rate increase for Arizona doctors in 4 years.
3. *The Sacramento Bee Final,* April 6, 1988: In Dade County, FL in 1987 the average malpractice premium . . . was $165,000, up from $30,000 in 4 years.

   Twenty-five percent of Florida physicians are sued annually.

   The average amount paid in lawsuits increased eight times between 1975 and 1985, from $13,000 to $103,000. The average Florida jury award was $250,000.

   [It cost] $40,000 to defend even a frivolous lawsuit in Florida.

ELEMENTS OF THE TORT OF NEGLIGENCE

To prove the tort of negligence the plaintiff must show the following elements:

1. That *duty* existed between the plaintiff and the physician,
2. That there was a *breach* of this duty,
3. And that the breach was the *cause in fact.*
4. And that it was the *proximate cause*
5. Of the *harm* that resulted.

The punishment for commission of this tort is monetary damages to make the plaintiff "whole." We will now look at some individual problems in this area.

ISSUES IN THE TORT OF NEGLIGENCE

RES IPSA LOQUITOR

Res ipsa loquitor means "the thing speaks for itself." To get the court to issue an instruction of res ipsa loquitor the following must be shown:

1. The event must be of a kind that ordinarily does not occur in the absence of someone's negligence.
2. It must be caused by an agency or instrumentality within the *exclusive* control of the defendant.
3. It must not have been due to any voluntary action or contribution on the part of the plaintiff [2].

Res ipsa loquitor, although recognized in most jurisdictions, has caused considerable confusion about the meaning of the term and what benefits the plaintiff derives when it is applied [3]. It is thus not too surprising that doctors are also confused. In California Evidence Code 646 was passed to help clarify the matter.

In trials there are two burdens. One is the burden of producing evidence, and the other is the burden of proof. Thus, for example the plaintiff in a tort case has the burden of presenting evidence and the burden of producing proof. Res ipsa loquitor is a presumption affecting the burden of producing evidence. It does not prove guilt.

Therefore, when the plaintiff has established the three conditions above, the jury is required to find that the accident resulted from the defendant's negligence *unless* the defendant comes forward with evidence that would support a contrary finding. If the defendant produces evidence that he is not negligent or that if he was negligent, such negligence was not the proximate cause of the accident, then the presumptive effect of the doctrine vanishes. But remember, although the presumptive effect of the doctrine disappears, because it does not apply to guilt the jury could still, from the facts presented, find that there was a lack of due care and find for the plaintiff in a negligence action [2].

Now look at the three criteria. Note that the first criterion would rule out application of the doctrine to issues involving correct diagnosis and treatment. Whether or not a diagnosis or treatment was correct is not something that "ordinarily does not occur in the absence of someone's negligence." These questions require an expert, and thus generally res ipsa loquitor is inapplicable. When a sponge or instrument is left in the abdomen or injury to a body part not involved in the treatment or surgery occurs, then the doctrine may apply. Obviously, the applicability of the doctrine is very narrow.

The rarity of an injury will not in itself result in a res ipsa loquitor instruction by the court because of the first criterion. For example, in *Silverson v. Weber* [4] involving a vesicovaginal fistula that occurred following a hysterectomy, the court refused to apply res ipsa loquitor saying:

> The fact that a particular injury suffered by a patient as the result of an operation is something that rarely occurs does not in itself prove that the injury was probably caused by the negligence of those in charge of the operation.

The second criterion of this doctrine makes matters rather difficult for the case of a plaintiff filing suit against multiple defendants. The question concerns the issue of who had "exclusive control of the instrumentality or agency" causing the accident.

In *Ybarra v. Spangard* [5] a patient was put to sleep for an appendectomy and awoke with a shoulder injury. Res ipsa loquitor was applied against the multiple defendants in this case. The defendants argued that the plaintiff could not show who was responsible or who had exclusive control of the instrumentality causing the injury. The Supreme Court of California in essence imposed the burden of explanation on the defendants [6].

Thus, in *O'Connor v. Bloomer* [7] the assistant surgeons were granted a summary judgment in a malpractice action involving a heart valve case. The patient had agreed to the implantation of a particular valve. Someone failed to order the valve, and another valve was implanted. The court stated that, in regard to res ipsa loquitor, the defendants had shown that they had no responsibility for, or control of, the availability of the heart valve, and so the court refused to apply res ipsa loquitor.

CONSENT

Although the issue of consent itself may not seem difficult, certain aspects of it present problems. It has been recognized in numerous cases that the performance of an operation or other treatment without first obtaining any consent may fall within the concept of assault and battery as an intentional tort [8]. Remember that intentional torts are not covered by malpractice insurance, and punitive damages can be assessed in the case of an intentional tort.

There is a so-called model law on consent, and individual state law should be consulted, since states may or may not adopt all or parts of this law. Other states may have their own laws on consent. Similarly, forms for consent have been prepared by the American Medical Association (AMA) and are also to be found in legal references. Individual state laws cover issues of capacity and should be reviewed by the emergency physician.

Consent to medical treatment may be express or implied from the circumstances [9]. In *Grannum v. Beard* [10] the court said:

> The rule is well established that in surgical cases consent to such procedure must be obtained from either the patient, or, if the patient is under some disability, from a near relative capable of giving consent.
>
> Such consent may be manifested in a number of ways: as an express consent the patient may sign a formal written permission or agree orally; he may give implied authority by his conduct, as in voluntarily submitting to an operation or by failing to object.
>
> The mental capacity necessary to consent is a question of fact to be determined from the circumstances of each individual case.
>
> The law will presume sanity . . . and competency.

Generally, one who has reached the age of majority can give an effective consent unless the physician knows of some temporary or permanent abnormality or disability [11]. This of course can be a difficult question of fact.

Generally, except in an emergency, a surgeon will be liable for an assault if he operates on a child without the consent of the latter's parents [12].

Baker v. Welsh [13] is an interesting case. Here a 17-year-old boy from a Michigan farm went to Grand Rapids, Michigan to have a tumor removed from his ear. He was accompanied to the doctor's office and to the hospital by adult relatives. He died under anesthesia. The father sued, saying that the boy was not of age to consent and he, the father, had not consented. The court held that consent for an operation on a minor child will sometimes be implied from the fact that adult relatives of a child are present. This case was decided in 1906, and the decision might be different today.

More recently, in *Tabor v. Scobee* [14] the court said:

> Where an operation on a child without prolonged delay appears to a physician to be necessary only a reasonable and diligent effort on the part of the physician to find parents of a patient and advise them of the situation is required.

It is also a general rule that one cannot consent for medical care for his or her spouse. The relationship of husband and wife does not in itself make one spouse the agent of the other [15].

Emergency Consent

Prosser's textbook on *Tort* [16], a veritable bible on tort law, sums up the area of emergency consent very succinctly. The following excerpt is taken from this text.

> ... It has been asserted that a physician ... has implied consent to
> deliver medical services, including surgical procedures, to a patient in
> an emergency where the following apply:
>
> (a) The patient must be unconscious or without capacity to make a
> decision, while no one legally authorized to act as agent for the patient
> is available;
>
> (b) Time must be of the essence, in the sense that it must reasonably
> appear that delay until such time as an effective consent could be ob-
> tained would subject the patient to a risk of a serious bodily injury or
> death which prompt action would avoid; and
>
> (c) Under the circumstances, a reasonable person would consent,
> and the probabilities are that the patient would consent.

Although in older cases "dire" emergencies had to exist, today courts
probably would not insist on that unless the treatment itself carried a risk
of loss of bodily function [15]. For example, in *Gravis v. Physicians and
Surgeons Hospital* [15] the court said:

> We recognize the rule that consent will be implied where the patient
> is unconscious or otherwise unable to give express consent and an im-
> mediate operation is necessary to preserve life or health. In the absence
> of exceptional circumstances, however, a surgeon is subject to liability
> for assault and battery where he operates without the consent of the
> patient or the person legally authorized to give such consent.

Informed Consent

Even given the capacity to consent, such consent must be an informed consent. Originally, when an informed consent was found to be lacking the
matter was treated as an intentional tort. Since about 1960 these cases have
been treated as a negligent breach of the standard of care (duty) [17]. This
change is critical because intentional torts are usually not covered by insurance and can carry punitive damages.

Although some have held that the duty to disclose is that which a good
doctor in good standing in the medical community would disclose, a landmark California case disagreed. In *Cobbs v. Grant* [18], the court stated that
the physician owes the patient a duty of "reasonable disclosure of the available choices with respect to the proposed therapy and of the dangers in-
herently and potentially involved in each."

The court stated that a mini course in medicine is not necessary, nor is it
necessary to disclose very low incident risks. The scope of the communication to the patient, then, must be measured by the patient's need, and that
need is whatever information is material to the decision.

It must be proved by the plaintiff that had such revelation been made,
consent would not have been given. Importantly, the court said that this
issue is *not* whether or not the patient in the instant case would have con-

sented but what a "prudent person" would have done after being fully informed.

The court also laid down the following rules and exceptions:

1. There must be a causal connection between the failure to inform and the injury to the plaintiff.
2. The physician need not inform the patient when the patient requests that he not be informed.
3. No information of remote dangers need be given when such dangers are commonly appreciated to be remote in a simple procedure.
4. When a reasonable person would be so upset by the disclosure that such person would not be able to weigh the risks dispassionately, information can be withheld.

Please note that the standards expected of the physician and the method of analyzing the patient's comprehension will vary considerably from state to state and should be reviewed.

Refusal To Consent

So far we have discussed an injury to a patient that occurs after consent to a test or treatment. What about a physician's liability when a patient refuses a test or treatment and then suffers the result of *not* being treated or tested?

In *Truman v. Thomas* [19] a woman refused a Papanicolaou test and died of cervical cancer at age 30. The court stated, in ruling for the plaintiff, that a doctor must warn the patient not only of the inherent risks of a procedure but also of the risks of a decision not to undergo the treatment or test.

THE DUTY TO WARN

In light of the physician's knowledge of a patient's problem or problems, what is the physician's duty to others? Reports of certain communicable diseases are required, and the physician should check individual state and local law for a listing of reportable diseases. But what about situations not covered by state or local laws? In *Derrick v. Ontario Community Hospital* [20] the court held that the physician and not the hospital had a duty to warn others immediately exposed to a patient with a contagious disease.

In another case involving the shooting death of a third person by a mentally disturbed patient Tarasoff I [21], the court said

> ... we conclude that a doctor treating a mentally ill person, just as a
> doctor treating a physical illness, bears a duty to use reasonable care to

give threatened persons such warnings as are essential to avert foreseeable danger arising from his patient's condition or treatment.

In Tarasoff II [22], a rehearing of the original case, the court seemed to restrict itself to psychotherapists [23]. The court, retreating from an absolute duty to warn, said:

> In our view, however, once a therapist does in fact determine, or under applicable professional standards reasonably should have determined, that a patient poses a serious danger of violence to others, he bears a duty to exercise reasonable care to protect the foreseeable victim of that danger. While the discharge of this duty of due care will necessarily vary with the facts of each case, in each instance the adequacy of the therapist's conduct must be measured against the traditional negligence standard of the rendition of reasonable care under circumstances.

We should keep in mind that it is possible, given the right set of circumstances, that the courts might impose this duty on the emergency physician.

The emergency physician should thus be aware that, if a physician using reasonable care would have foreseen that a patient presented a serious danger of violence to another, the physician may be found to have a duty to protect an unsuspecting potential victim by warning such a person of the danger.

Many jurisdictions also have statutes allowing the immediate temporary detention of unstable individuals, and these should be reviewed. See for example, the Lanterman Petris Short Act, California Welfare and Institution Code Sec. 5000-5404.1.

IMMUNITY FROM TORT SUIT—GOOD SAMARITAN LAWS

Writing in the *California Law Review,* Stiepel [24] made the following points:

1. Under traditional common law there is no duty to aid another in peril. Once such aid is rendered, then a duty arises to use reasonable care.
2. Beginning in California in 1959, and then subsequently in all the states and the District of Columbia, Good Samaritan laws have been enacted.
3. These laws protect physicians from civil liability when they offer their professional services under emergency conditions. These

statutes basically are designed to encourage physicians to respond to medical emergencies when they have no legal obligation to do so.

Although some statutes have strayed, the basic concept is whether or not a duty exists between the patient and physician. The issues here are well demonstrated by two California cases: *Colby v. Schwartz* [25] and *McKenna v. Cedars of Lebanon Hospital* [26]. The Colby case held that no protection existed under California's statutes for emergency physicians or the "back up" panel treating emergency patients as part of their normal course of practice. In short, these physicians had a preexisting duty to all persons who came to their emergency rooms.

Contrast this with the case of Dr. McKenna, who was in the hospital visiting one of his patients when he came to the aid of a convulsing patient. He gave the patient IV diazepam and the patient suffered a cardiac arrest. McKenna was protected by California's Good Samaritan statute because he was a true volunteer "who by chance and on an irregular basis" came upon or was called to render emergency care.

The next issue is location. In the *McKenna* case the court held that the immunity provided by the statute held, regardless of the location of the emergency. However, one must be aware that in a number of states location is important, and, in fact, emergency departments are excluded in some of these states.

These Good Samaritan statutes have been expanded, interestingly, in some states to include more than the volunteer. Thus in California, defying the original rationale to provide immunity to the true volunteer, California Health and Safety Code Section 1317 provides civil liability immunity to all members of the cardiopulmonary resuscitation team. This team obviously has a preexisting duty to the patient and at least partially contradicts the reasoning cited in the above cases.

It is thus critical for the emergency physician and anesthesiologist to review local state law, not merely for the physician's own status but also for the status of others who may be sought in consultation.

TORT REFORM—THE ANSWER

In 1969, as malpractice litigation in California rose by 25 percent, Howard Hassard and James Ludlum, attorneys for the California Medical Association (CMA) and the California Hospital Association (CHA), respectively, conceived the idea of applying arbitration to the malpractice litigation process rather than standard litigation. A study of arbitration done by Duane Heinz [27] was set up in July 1969 by CMA and CHA. The experiment covered eight southern California hospitals in the Los Angeles area. Some 498,190 admissions from 1970 through June 1975 were covered and analyzed. The results showed a smaller number of claims, quicker resolution (lower legal fees), and almost 15 percent lower costs per closed claim. For reasons that continue to baffle this author, it is only in California, to my knowledge, that the Cooperative of American Physicians has an active arbitration program, and frankly, this is of recent vintage.

In 1975, following explosive events in California—a doctor's strike, no insurance available or available only at enormous costs—the state passed the Medical Injury Compensation Reform Act (MICRA). MICRA, while not a complete answer, has been regarded as model legislation. It has certainly stabilized malpractice insurance premiums in California, as documented by the *Wall Street Journal* report quoted at the beginning of this chapter.

The law provides for 90 days' notice prior to the commencement of a suit, permits the introduction of evidence of collateral source recovery, a $250,000 cap on damages for noneconomic (pain and suffering) damages, an effective statute of limitations, a limitation on contingency fees, and provisions for arbitration. In addition, the law sharply tightens physician disciplinary procedures, including reporting of hospital actions restricting or suspending privileges, to a newly constituted Board of Medical Quality Assurance, which replaced the old Board of Medical Examiners.

Further legislation and study should be done. For example, plaintiff bar charges on a per hour basis can be estimated by dividing the settlement or judgment by the number of hours worked by the defense bar. This assumes that the defense bar expends a volume of time similar to that of the plaintiff bar. No reasonable calculations have been done in this area, the problem being that the insurance companies refuse to release the number of hours expended by the defense bar, or even to do the work and release final data.

Medical malpractice is still a very active area in California despite the stabilization of premiums by MICRA. A recently negotiated truce between the plaintiff bar, physicians, manufacturers, and insurers has cooled what would have been an election battle on a $40 million ballot initiative.

TRANSFUSION ISSUES

The problems faced by the emergency physician and anesthesiologist in treating Jehovah's Witnesses are well known. Recently, because the AIDS crisis and the attendant hysteria, others besides Jehovah's Witnesses are refusing blood. In *Randolph v. City of New York* [28], Mrs. Randolph, a Jehovah's Witness, was admitted for elective cesarean section. The record was quite clear that she was appropriately informed about the possible need for blood, and she competently requested that no blood be given under any circumstances. At surgery she was found to have a placenta previa and placenta accreta, and a hysterectomy was attempted. In the process massive bleeding ensued. The patient went into shock due to irreversible blood loss and expired. Prior to her death the anesthesiologist had asked the City Corporation Council for permission to give blood and on obtaining such permission proceeded to give blood.

There were two basic questions here: (1) First, the plaintiff contended that blood should have been started earlier despite Mrs. Randolph's refusal. (2) Assuming that she was not in irreversible shock when the transfusion was started, was the transfusion performed negligently and was this negligence the proximate cause of her death? If she was in irreversible shock at the start of the transfusion, then the manner of transfusion would, of course, have been irrelevant. Most interesting was the fact that the plaintiff and both the majority and minority court views coincided in deciding that, if blood had not been administered and if her instructions had been obeyed, no liability would have ensued.

In any event, the majority opinion held that Mrs. Randolph's death was not proximately caused by any negligence in administration of blood but that by her refusal to allow blood she had gone into irreversible shock, and thus, irreversible shock resulting from her refusal to accept blood was the proximate cause of her death. The attitude of the court as evident in the following paragraph is interesting:

> To this writer, to require a physician to stand by helplessly while a patient is dying, and when it is too late to save the patient, the doctor is instructed to proceed to use his skills to save her, and to then attempt to apply liability for his actions, is just unacceptable.

The minority opinion of the court held, however, that the anesthesiologist could have been found negligent in the blood administration process and that evidence was given at trial that could have allowed the jury to find that the woman was not in irreversible shock at the time of the start of the transfusion. The minority noted that, with respect to the transfusion itself, it took 45 minutes to give one transfusion when, with a larger bore catheter and a pressure bag, a unit of blood could have been given in 10 to 15 minutes. The attitude of the court was very important in this case, in the author's opinion. But what would the court's attitude have been if AIDS and not religion had been involved? The answers may be forthcoming in the next few years.

A final interesting case occurred in Washington D.C. [29]. Here a judge approved permission for the physicians to give blood to a woman with a bleeding ulcer. The court felt that she was not competent at the time to decide, and, although her husband refused to permit the transfusion, the court stated "If . . . a parent has no power to forbid the saving of his child's life, a fortiori the husband of the patient . . . had no right to order the doctors to treat his wife in a way so that she would die."

In addition, the court noted that the woman had a 7-month-old child, and although "the state as parens patriae will not allow a parent to abandon a child, [and] so it should not allow this most ultimate of voluntary abandonments."

This case should be viewed with some caution because there were significant arguments subsequently about procedural aspects [30]. Again, the author believes that attitudes entered the picture. The issue of refusal to receive blood transfusions continues to result in law suits.

RIGHT TO DIE—PULLING THE PLUG

Classically, deciding whether a person was dead or not was rather simple. When breathing ceased, the heart stopped, the brain died, and the patient was declared dead. With modern technology, things became more difficult. In the August 5, 1968 [31] issue of the *Journal of the American Medical Association,* an attempt was made to delineate when death occurred in the light of advanced technology. This was the Report of the Ad Hoc Committee of the Harvard Medical School To Examine the Definition of Brain Death. The characteristics of a permanently nonfunctioning brain were listed as:

1. Unreceptivity and unresponsivity—even the most intensely painful stimuli evoke no vocal or other response, not even a groan, withdrawal of a limb, or quickening of respiration.
2. No movements or breathing. Criteria for establishing apnea were spelled out for the patient on a ventilator.
3. No reflexes.
4. The flat electroencephalogram (EEG) was listed as confirmatory, and its use for this purpose was described.

The famous case of Karen Quinlan [32] simply did not fit the Harvard criteria. She had, for example, some movement, she reacted to light and sound and noxious stimuli, she blinked her eyes, she would grimace, make stereotyped sounds and cries, and she had chewing motions. But she was decerebrate. Was she dead?

Karen Quinlan had suffered two severe (about 15-minute) periods of apnea under unexplained circumstances and was given ineffectual mouth-to-mouth resuscitation by friends. There was no question that she was in a persistent vegetative state and exhibited the usual pattern of a decerebrate individual. The issues presented by the case were: (1) Could her father be appointed as her legal guardian, and (2) Could he turn off her respirator and allow her to die?

The state's concern was the preservation and sanctity of human life and the defense of the right of the physician to administer medical treatment according to his best judgment. When courts, expressing the state's interest, had acted to permit physicians to treat patients (e.g., in the blood transfusion cases) there was hope of a salvageable life. But here the court noted that the "State's interest ... weakens and the individual's right to privacy grows as the degree of bodily invasion increases and the prognosis dims. Ultimately there comes a point at which the individual's rights overcome the State interest." Simply put, the court felt that Karen had a constitutionally guaranteed right to privacy, and such right included a right to refuse medical treatment.

Because Karen was not competent to assert her right to privacy, how could this right be asserted? The court felt that the guardian, family, and attending physicians could conclude that there would be no recovery from the vegetative state, and after consultation and agreement by a hospital Ethics Committee, life support could be withdrawn. The use of an Ethics Committee to consult and confirm was favored by the court to ease the potential civil and criminal liabilities of the physician in these cases. Physicians are not immunized for their actions as are judges. "Judges," said Lord Coke, a famous judge of several centuries ago, "are only to make an account to God and the King."

These matters are still evolving as states seek to reach a resolution. The law continues to develop, albeit sometimes painfully. Consider the following hypothetical situation. A patient enters the emergency or operating room, is sedated or given a general anesthetic, and a procedure is performed. During the procedure or in the recovery period, the patient has a cardiac arrest and is resuscitated. It is then discovered that the patient is in a persistent vegetative state. The plaintiff's attorney alleges negligence and after a few years a judgment is paid. A short time later the patient dies, and the physician is sued again for wrongful death and pays yet another judgment.

Suppose, on the other hand, that the physician faced with this tragedy withholds fluids and other life-sustaining measures, and the patient dies in a week or two. Now only one cause of action—wrongful death—remains and only one judgment. Thus the physician has mitigated his damages.

The author has reason to believe that this was the thought process of the district attorney in the Barber case, in which he charged the physicians with murder. It must be emphasized that no such charges of negligence, murder, or any other criminal action or intent were ever proved against any of the individuals involved in the Barber case.

In *Barber v. Superior Court* [33] two physicians were charged with murder for withholding and removing life-sustaining devices and fluids in a patient in a persistent vegetative state. The patient had entered the hospital for closure of a colostomy and anastomosis. Several months earlier he had had the colostomy done for acute diverticulitis with perforation.

The appellate court in this case stated that

> ... a physician is authorized under the standard of medical practice
> to discontinue a form of therapy which in his medical judgment is use-
> less. ... If the treating physicians have determined that continued use
> of a respirator is useless, then they may decide to discontinue it without
> fear of civil or criminal liabilities. By useless is meant that the continued
> use of the therapy cannot and does not improve the prognosis for re-
> covery.

The issues delineated by this court, then, are who determines at what point
further treatment is of no reasonable benefit to the patient and who can
direct termination of the treatment. The court dismissed the murder
charges and held that although no formal conservatorship existed, the wife
was the proper surrogate to act for the patient, and judicial approval to
withdraw treatment was not legally required.

An important lesson to be learned from the *Barber* case is that when a
tragedy such as this occurs district attorneys may look at the case in the
context of the criminal law. It thus behooves a physician, faced with this
unfortunate situation, to contact and work with legal counsel immediately.
Had this been done quickly in the *Barber* case, the physicians might never
have had to go through this travail.

Other cases in this area are still being argued and appealed. See for example, In Re Conservatorship of Drabick Hoo2349 as reported in the *Los
Angeles Daily Journal* Thursday, April 14, 1988.

CARDIAC RESUSCITATION—TO QUIT OR NOT TO QUIT

The patient in the emergency department who has a cardiac arrest with
attempts made to resuscitate him will be involved in one of the following
three situations:

1. The patient is successfully resuscitated.
2. The patient is successfully resuscitated but has residual brain damage. If the damage is severe the case resembles the Karen Quinlan
   case discussed above.
3. The resuscitation efforts fail to establish an electrical pattern consistent with cardiac ejection.

In this last situation there are then two questions: (1) When does the
physician quit? (2) Who makes the decision to quit?

In regard to the first question of when to quit, it is clear from various
cases that termination of extraordinary medical means of sustaining the life
of a comatose patient who has no chance of recovery, which termination

will in all medical probability accelerate the patient's death, will result in no criminal liability because the ensuing death will then be considered expiration from existing natural causes [34]. Patients in acute cardiac arrest are comatose, and if cardiac resuscitation fails if one stops, death, however defined, would obviously be of "existing natural causes."

One should realize, however, that the resuscitative measures and decisions, as with all of medicine, can be reviewed by the courts from the standpoint of the tort of negligence. Here the court will apply the elements of negligence as cited earlier in this chapter to determine if indeed there was negligence.

The standard used in negligence cases is the "reasonable man" standard. Perfection is not required. In *Baldor v. Rogers* [35] the court noted, "The doctor is obligated only to use reasonable skill and he fulfills his obligation if he uses methods approved by others of the profession who are reasonably skilled." Of interest, one should note that the court in Baldor also said, "If the treatment used is approved by a 'respectable minority' of the medical profession" that would relieve the defendant of the charge of malpractice."

As for the second question, this author knows of no definite answer from a court case. However, given the immediacy and nature of the problem, he firmly believes that the decision of the physician to stop will be respected.

CONTRACTS, PRIVILEGES, AND ANTITRUST ISSUES

HOSPITAL STAFF PRIVILEGES

The traditional view of private organizations limited them to contract and tort legal theories only. In short, these were private entities and as such were not subject to the standards of governmental agencies under the constitution or under the common law. In the 1960s it became clear that this concept simply could not be allowed to stand with respect to certain types of private enterprise that had developed in our modern technologic world [36, 37]. Thus, the courts began to look at the common law concept of the "status" of the organization and the individual.

In feudal times the law looked to the status of individuals and ascribed duties to them. Some of these linger today, such as parent-child and landlord-tenant. The law then moved away from this interpretation, allowing individuals to set their own duties freely through the concept of contracts. Recently, courts have said that individuals on medical staffs or in labor unions are not really freely setting the terms of their contracts (bylaws), and thus regardless of the bylaws, the law must ascribe duties to the parties in the interest of fairness.

Thus it has been held that certain organizations, including hospital and professional societies, affect the "public interest" to such an extent that their relationships with individuals would be subject to judicial review as a matter of public policy [38, 39]. Further, it has been held that these organizations must afford to their applicants and members "fair procedure." Fair procedure, although not due process, is very similar, yet it allows flexibility without the formal constraints of due process [38]. It is this author's opinion that the courts are moving to a full due process standard.

A classic demonstrative example in this area is the Pinsker I [39] and Pinsker II [40] cases. In Pinsker I the California court held that the orthodontist society to which Dr. Pinsker had applied and which had rejected him was an organization affecting the public interest, and therefore the application process was subject to judicial review. In Pinsker II the court determined that the society had to use fair procedure.

Again ". . . Membership decisions of hospital staff associations whether in public or private hospitals must be rendered pursuant to minimal requisites of fair procedure required by established common law principles."

The Pinsker cases, by the way, represent one reason why physicians become frustrated with the law. To reach the Supreme Court, the Pinsker I case took 5 years and the Pinsker II case took another 7 years. After 12 years the court did not order acceptance of his application but laid out certain legal criteria and directed the society to "reconsider his application." Obviously, Dr. Pinsker must have really wanted to join the Society.

It thus now appears that memberships on medical staffs and in certain professional organizations are subject to review under procedures covered by concepts of fundamental fairness. It is also probable that medical staff bylaw provisions can provide contracts that permit physicians to waive many of their rights.

Emergency physicians are often under contract, and these contracts may provide for the arbitrary removal of their staff privileges concomitant with their loss of the contract. The Joint Commission on Accreditation of Hospitals (JCAH) Manual of 1985 provided, for example:

> In the case of physicians or other individuals actively serving in administrative responsible capacities in the hospital pursuant to a contract, the continuation of clinical privileges may or may not be made contingent on continuance of the contractual arrangement.

Unfortunately, some attorneys have suggested that the contract clause surrendering fairness in the privilege review process be used as a bargaining chip in contract negotiations [41].

Although loss of the contract effectively means a loss of privileges, many emergency physicians and anesthesiologists would prefer that economics and privileges be kept separate. Privileges they feel, relate to competency. Bylaws should thus be checked to be sure that privileges are independent of the contract.

ANTITRUST LAWS AND POLICY

Scarcely any text touching on medicine and law today can be written without discussing antitrust. Antitrust is not so much a matter of law as it is the legal expression of a fundamental economic policy of the United States. The basic concern of this policy as expressed by law is competition. The courts have turned more and more in recent decades to analyzing economic theory as they review antitrust law and develop antitrust policy.

In medicine we are dealing, usually, with two basic antitrust laws, the Sherman Act administered by the Department of Justice, and the Federal Trade Commission Act administered by the Federal Trade Commission. Although the Acts overlap and both agencies can usually file suits, each agency respects the others' jurisdiction and does not enter when one agency is acting or has acted.

The Sherman Act basically provides that (1) Every contract, combination in the form of trust or otherwise, or conspiracy in restraint of trade or commerce among the several States, . . . is hereby declared to be illegal. Any person involved in these contracts, trusts etc. is guilty of a felony and subject to fines and imprisonment. (2) Every person who shall monopolize, or attempt to monopolize, or combine or conspire with any other person or persons, to monopolize any part of the trade or commerce among the several States, . . . shall be deemed guilty of a felony and subject to fines and imprisonment.

The Federal Trade Commission Act under Sec. 5 (a)(1) says simply that "Unfair methods of competition in or affecting commerce, and unfair or deceptive acts or practices in or affecting commerce, are hereby declared unlawful." Here the Commission issues a cease and desist order, the violation of which is punishable by up to $10,000 per day for each day of violation and for each violation.

The above are simplistic statements of the acts and penalties. It is obvious that the penalties for violation can be severe.

Private actions constitute a major part of the antitrust caseload of the federal courts [42]. The Clayton Act (passed in 1914 to supplement the Sherman Act) Sec. 4 states "That any person who shall be injured in his business or property by reason of anything forbidden in the antitrust laws may sue therefore . . . and shall recover" [triple damages, costs of suit and attorney fees].

Finally, it is important to understand that the states are immune from antitrust law, and in some cases activities authorized and/or regulated by the states can be immune from the antitrust laws.

Antitrust law was at one time thought not to be applicable to the "learned professions." Such is certainly not the case today. The courts have determined that the practice of medicine is subject to and will be reviewed under the antitrust laws. Preferred provider organizations (PPOs), health maintenance organizations (HMOs), independent physicians associations

(IPAs), and fee-reviewing activities by medical organizations have all been the subject of review by antitrust authority.

Recently, for example, peer review activities came under antitrust review in *Patrick v. Burget* [43]. The U.S. District Court in Oregon held that the state action exemption did not apply to peer review activities. The reviewing physicians were held liable for ostensibly using peer review to choke off competition and hence violate the antitrust laws. They were hit with a judgment in excess of $2 million. This judgment was reversed by the appellate courts. Congress then moved to protect the peer review process by passing the Health Care Quality Improvement Act of 1986. By conforming to the act reviewing physicians could gain considerable protection.

The act requires that, in return for the antitrust protection, the hospital must provide notice to the physician of the proposed action, the reasons for the action, notification of the physician's right to request a hearing, 30 days advance notice of a hearing, a list of witnesses, a hearing before an arbitrator, hearing officer, or panel of individuals not in direct economic competition with the physician, and fair procedure during the course of the hearing including the right to be represented by an attorney, the right to call, examine, and cross examine witnesses, and the right to a written determination [44].

Although all that may seem complicated, this author believes these requirements are basic standards of fair play under our Anglo-American system of fairness. Nevertheless, many hospitals are in opposition.

The law also requires reporting of disciplinary actions to the Secretary of the Department of Health and Human Services. A number of states, such as California, have similar reporting requirements.

Currently in California, the California Medical Association is attempting to opt out of the law and is trying to pass a law with an even greater level of fairness. For example, by simplifying certain procedures legal fees for defense and time would be reduced under the California proposal. Again, hospitals are opposed.

Finally, the United States Supreme Court, on May 16, 1988, reversed the appellate court's decision in *Patrick* and held that the physicians on the peer review panel were not immune to antitrust. The author believes that the appellate court felt that the physicians did not give Patrick a fair hearing. Congress subsequently suggested what the basis of a fair hearing is when it spoke by passing the Health Care Quality Improvement Act. Before one condemns the court's actions you are urged to read the *Patrick* case and then form your own opinion of the need for a remedy.

CONCLUSION

Anesthesiology and emergency medicine are practices of medicine. It is obvious that much of what the law says about one applies to the other as it does to medicine in general. We have tried in this chapter to cover some basic issues, knowing that we could not possibly cover the entire subject or even come close in one chapter. It is hoped that we have supplied some answers and piqued the reader's interest enough so that he or she will search for more information.

The sciences never change, remaining as God made them. It is our understanding of the sciences that changes. Law, on the other hand, changes substantively in response to people, a changing environment, and circumstances. Despite what some may say, the hallmark of American-Anglo Saxon law is an attempt to achieve fairness. It is our hope that we have shown this attempt in some small degree in this chapter. As for the lack of perfection in our system of law we offer the following:

> Abraham to the Holy One: If Thou desirest the world to endure, there can be no absolute justice, while if Thou desirest absolute justice the world cannot endure, yet Thou wouldest hold the cord by both ends, desiring both the world and absolute justice. Unless Thou foregoest a little, the world cannot endure. Genesis, Midrash Rabbah 39.6 (Levi).

REFERENCES

1. *Black's Law Dictionary* (4th ed.). St. Paul, Minn.: West Publishing, 1957.
2. West Annotated Evidence Code Sec. 646 Law Revision Commission Comment 1970 Ed. St. Paul: West Publishing.
3. McCold, A. H. Negligence Actions Against Multiple Defendants, 7 *Stan L. Rev.* 480 at 482 (July 1955).
4. *Silverson v. Weber,* 57 Cal. 2d 834 at 839 (1962).
5. *Ybarra v. Spangard,* 93 Cal. App. 2d 43, 208 P.2d 445, (1949).
6. McCold, A. H. Negligence Actions against Multiple Defendants, 7 *Stan. L. Rev.* 480 at 484 (July 1955).
7. *O'Connor v. Bloomer,* 116 Cal. App. 3d 385, 172 Cal Rptr. 128 (1981).
8. 61 AM JUR 2d Physicians and Surgeons Sec. 178, page 308.
9. *Bradford v. Winter,* 215 Cal. App. 2d 448; 30 Cal Rpt. 243 (1963).
10. *Granum v. Berard,* 70 Wash. 2d 304; 422 P. 2d 812 (1967).
11. Prosser, W. L., and Keaton, W. P. *Prosser And Keaton On Torts* (5th ed.). St. Paul: West Publishing, 1984. P. 114.
12. 61 AM JUR 2d Physicians and Surgeons Sec. 178, page 308.
13. *Bakker v. Welsh,* 108 NW 94 (1906).
14. *Tabor v. Scobee,* 254 SW 2d 474 (1951).
15. *Gravis v. Physicians and Surgeons Hospital of Alice,* 427 S.W. 2d 310 (1968).
16. Prosser, W. L., and Keaton, W. P. *Prosser and Keaton On Torts* (5th ed.). St. Paul: West Publishing, 1984. P. 117.
17. Prosser, W. L., and Keaton, W. P. *Prosser and Keaton On Torts* (5th ed.). St. Paul: West Publishing, 1984. P. 190.
18. *Cobbs v. Grant,* 8 Cal 3d 229, 104 Cal. Rptr. 505, (1972).
19. *Truman v. Thomas,* 27 Cal. 3d 285, 165 Cal. Rptr. 308 (1980).
20. *Derrick v. Ontario Community Hospital,* 120 Cal. Rptr. 566, 47 Cal. App. 3d 145 (1975).

21. *Tarasoff v. Regents of the University of California* 118 Cal Rptr 129, 529 P 2d 553 (1974).
22. *Tarasoff v. Regents of the University of California* 17 Cal. 3d 425, 131 Cal. Rptr. 14 (1976).
23. Seligman, B. Untangling Tarasoff—*Tarasoff v. Regents of the University of California. 29 Hastings L.J.* 179 (1977) at page 183.
24. Stiepel, H. R. Good Samaritan And Hospital Emergencies 55 S. *Cal. L. Rev.* Jan. 1981, 417 at page 417.
25. *Colby v. Schwartz* 78 Cal. App. 3d 885, 155 Cal Rptr 631 (1979).
26. *McKenna v. Cedars of Lebanon Hospital* 93 Cal. App. 3d 282, 155 Cal. Rptr. 631 (1979).
27. Heintz, D. H. An Analysis of the Southern California Arbitration Project January 1966 Through June 1975, DHEW Publication No. (HRA)77-3159, Washington, D.C.: U.S. Government Printing Office, 1977.
28. *Randolph v. City of New York,* 501 N.Y.S. 2d 837, A.D. 1 Dept. (1986).
29. *Application of President and Director of Georgetown College,* 118 App. D.C. 80, 331 F 2d 1000. See also 9 A. L. R. 3d 1367 case and discussion.
30. 9 A. L. R. 3d Supplement 1391—1398 Sec 3.
31. Report of the Ad Hoc Committee of the Harvard Medical School to Examine the Definition of Brain Death. A Definition of Irreversible Coma *J.A.M.A.* 205:85-88, 1968.
32. *In the Matter of Karen Quinlan, An Alleged Incompetent,* 355 A. 2d 647 (1976).
33. *Barber v. Superior Court,* 147 Cal. App. 3d 1006 (1983).
34. 55 Am. Jur. 2d Right to Die Right to Life Sec 31 page 28 New Topic Service.
35. *Baldor v. Rogers,* 81 S. 2d 658 (1954).
36. Tobriner, M. O., and Grodin, J. R. The Individual And The Public Service Enterprise In The New Industrialized State, 55 *Calif. L. Rev.* 1247 (1967).
37. Sloss, P. F., and Becker, R. G. The Organization Affected With A Public Interest And Its Members—Justice Tobriner's Contribution To Evolving Common Law Doctrine, 29 *Hastings L. J.* 99 (1977-1988).
38. *Anton v. San Antonio Community Hospital,* 19 Cal 3d 802, 140 Cal. Rptr. 442 (1977).
39. *Pinsker v. Pacific Coast Society of Orthodontists,* 1 Cal. App. 3d 160, 81 Cal. Rptr. 623, 460 P. 2d 495 (1969).
40. *Pinsker v. Pacific Coast Society of Orthodontists,* 12 Cal. 3d 541, 116 Cal. Rptr. 245 (1974).
41. Allen Polsby and Reed, *The Health Lawyer* Fall, 1985, Vol 2 No. 4 at page 6. Medical Staff Privileges And Radiology Contracts: Do Practice Rights Survive Hospital Contracting Decisions?
42. Sullivan, L. A., *Antitrust.* St. Paul: West Publishing, 1977.
43. *Patrick v. Burget,* 800 F. 2d 1498 (9th Cir 1986).
44. *The Health Lawyer 3 (1):18.* The Chairman's Corner, Anderson H.H. See also the Health Care Quality Improvement Act of 1986, 42 USCS Sec. 11101-11152 (1986).

15. Disaster Medicine

Glenn S. Vanstrum

It has become a standard yearly routine in hospitals in the United States to have a mock disaster drill. Usually organized by the emergency medicine department, a scenario is developed, e.g., "victims" of a large earthquake are brought to the hospital, and triage and organizational protocols are reviewed and practiced. Such drills are certainly important and deserve increased attention from other specialties. Unfortunately, they are usually performed in a perfunctory manner, the Joint Commission of the Accreditation of Hospitals regulation is satisfied, and everyone returns to their routines with great relief. Why does a lack of preparation and commitment to such foresighted activities often exist?

To get at this question, one might first define a disaster as an unexpected calamity that overwhelms existing resources. It is thus an extremely relative term. Even a single patient, for example, a cardiac transplant patient in whom a donor heart has failed, an artificial heart is placed, and a 15 blood volume coagulopathy results, can easily qualify as a disaster for an operating room and blood bank. There are few hospital emergency departments that would not be extremely stressed by the simultaneous admission of six critically injured victims of a bus accident. In a sense, the daily work load of an emergency department or operating room is nothing but a continuous string of individual disasters. Thus, the mere thought of multiple victims from a plane crash or natural disaster such as an earthquake invokes a sort of mental numbing on the part of health care professionals. Most are tired enough as it is with the reality of the daily work load and simply tune out any thoughts of some hypothetical problem.

As one contemplates ever increasing magnitudes of disaster, one might start with a vehicle accident, for example, a bus or train crash. In such a situation, major problems will be extrication, scene triage, and appropriate distribution of patients to receiving hospitals. Most communities can absorb such calamities, in the sense that, with the exception of some isolated rural areas, there should be adequate resources to provide medical care close to the standard of care which any individual patient might normally expect to receive. Airplane crashes are similar because, although they might involve more victims, the reality of such occurrences is that most patients are unsalvageable. An exception to this rule was the 1982 Air Florida crash in the Potomac.

A major natural disaster, such as an earthquake or tsunami, can provide a much greater stress to a community and create near total disruption of a given societal fabric for a considerable period of time. The 1985 Mexico City earthquake is a good example of this; the quake, 8.1 on the Richter scale, produced destruction of three of the city's largest hospitals and 10,000 deaths, with some 30,000 casualties [1]. Although international rescue and medical aid brigades composed of some 50,000 individuals responded to the calamity, reconstruction of the city will take many years.

Manmade disasters such as the Chernobyl nuclear explosion, or the Bhopal explosion, can also create major health problems over a wide area involving, depending on the scattered effluents, many countries. The true extent of the legacy of such disasters will never be known because environmental carcinogens create long-term genetic loads that are impossible to quantitate.

As one continues to consider a widening spectrum of disasters, one reaches disasters of such a scope that, in a sense, everyone on the planet is involved, and there is really no noninvolved, "outside" area from which victims may expect, however, late, some relief or medical assistance. Historically, one thinks of the two world wars and of the bubonic plague. One might argue that in spite of the devastation created by such events, there were still many areas relatively unaffected; for example, the plague was isolated to Europe primarily, and fighting during World Wars I and II was concentrated in certain areas. The United States proper, for example, with the exception of Pearl Harbor, was spared the ravages of both wars. Realistically, when one thinks of such all-encompassing disasters today, one thinks of a war between two "super" powers with "super" weapons, such as nuclear bombs and missiles, biologic warfare, chemical warfare, and the like. Such a war would inevitably involve noncombatant nations and their people, through such phenomena as nuclear winter, disseminated radiation, carcinogens, and disease, not to mention disruption of the normal flow of trade, commerce, and the general fabric of human interaction we call civilization.

One might even continue beyond such frightening speculations to consider, for the sake of completeness, that our star, the sun, also has a finite lifespan, be it in billions of years, and the earth itself could be swallowed up in a supernova or impact with a comet or some other heavenly body. Perspective, of course, is the key here, and to worry or prepare for such phenomena is, of course, ridiculous. However, we do have control over our own activities, and we do have control, collectively, over such manmade disasters as nuclear war. We can expect terrific natural disasters such as earthquakes to continue to occur, and we can expect our daily workload to be punctuated with rare but periodic, gut-wrenching perturbations of large numbers of patients.

There are ample areas in which emergency medicine and anesthesiology intersect with this background. Severely injured multiple disaster victims generally require either operation, analgesia, decontamination, or airway management. Before such treatment can be rendered, the process of triage, or assignment of victims according to severity of injury, must occur. Before triage can take place, communication and dispatch of medical personnel must occur. To ensure that these things happen in a timely manner during a chaotic situation, prior planning, practice drills, and adequate stocking of materials must be ensured. Because there is a wide spectrum of disasters and because we live in a world with finite resources, all of the above must be preceded with careful analysis and philosophic decision making (e.g., providing the greatest good for the greatest number versus preserving certain key people even if heroic measures are required). At each step, both specialties need to become involved and to interject their particular perspective. Although it might seem logical to discuss disaster management by beginning with the philosophic underpinnings, this area contains the most controversy and, especially, disagreement about the preparations for nuclear disaster. Hence, we will begin our discussion with organization, communication, and triage and treatment modalities, and consider preparation and philosophy last.

DISASTER TREATMENT CONSIDERATIONS

DISASTER ORGANIZATION

Any consideration of international disaster organizations must include the International Red Cross, the charitable relief organization that plays a major role in many worldwide disasters. The World Association for Emergency and Disaster Medicine (WAEDM), formerly the Club of Mainz, is a think tank that produces a journal (*JWAEDM*) and encourages scientific and scholarly investigation of disaster management. It has recently joined the National Association of Emergency Medical Service Physicians (NAEMSP) to produce the journal *Pre-hospital and Disaster Medicine.*

At a national level, the armed forces medical services play a reserve role in a major disaster. Because economic limitations have inhibited the military's own need for surge capacity, the Department of Defense (DoD) initiated the Civilian-Military Contingency Hospital System (CMCHS) in 1980, in which civilian hospitals agree to accept military patients exceeding the capacity of DoD and Veterans' Administration (VA) hospitals. CMCHS is of limited utility for civilian disaster, however [2]. A new agency, the Federal Emergency Management Agency (FEMA), was established in 1979 to consolidate the various federal bureaucracies involved in disaster management. It achieved considerable notoriety for its controversial Crisis Relocation Planning, in which urban areas would be emptied over several days, in anticipation of nuclear attack (critics have noted that several days is considerably longer than the minutes it takes a missile to be launched and reach its target [3, 4]. The National Disaster Medical Service (NDMS) was designed in 1981 to be a coordinating body built from a partnership of federal agencies such as FEMA, the VA, the Public Health Service, the DoD, and state and local governments and the private medical sector. Charged with addressing interstate medical care for catastrophic disasters [1, 2, 5], the NDMS is developing a response for "a maximum plausible incident," which they have defined as a very large California earthquake (100,000 casualties) but specifically not victims of nuclear war [2]. This important system, which is still under development, will attempt to provide rapid mobilization of

150 disaster medical teams, each with three 29-person teams of physicians, nurses, medical technicians, and support personnel. These teams will be transported by a combination of military and civilian aircraft to some 100,000 precommitted civilian hospital beds. NDMS is still in the preliminary planning stages, but in spite of the many problems such as a program faces, not the least of which is the problem of lack of vacancies of the committed hospital beds, one must acknowledge the importance of support from the emergency and anesthesiology medical community for such a system.

At a state level, declaration of a state of emergency from the governor can assist in qualifying relief areas for federal funding from the Federal Disaster Relief Act, but actual state-organized disaster relief is variable. It is at the county and urban levels that the bulk of present day disaster organization and preparation exists in the United States, which should give insight into the sorts of limited disasters for which we are prepared. Coordination between fire, police, hospital, transport, communication, and utility personnel is crucial, and communication is a central and vulnerable prerequisite to such coordination. Traditional lines of communication, such as telephones, are traditionally overloaded or destroyed and are next to useless in many disasters. Hence, the importance of radio communication is apparent.

The fire and police departments are necessary first responders to a disaster site. Only when they have designated safe areas can medical personnel enter a site. Many disasters require highly skilled technical assistance to determine the safety of an area, e.g., a chemical bioengineer in the case of a toxic spill, or a health physicist in the case of a nuclear accident. The role of medical commander is assumed by the first competent medical person arriving at a scene, and an order of succession should be established, e.g., EMT-1, paramedic, R.N., M.D. A medical commander should establish a medical command post and identify the scene commander (usually a fire department public safety officer), a triage officer, and a transport officer. Locations that must be identified include the medical command center, casualty collection points, casualty loading areas, transport staging areas, and base hospitals. All medical personnel on scene are organized through the medical command post into triage teams initially and treatment teams later.

On September 9, 1988, the first San Diego exercise of the NDMS, which integrates many of these disaster components, was held in San Diego County. Participants included 19 local civilian hospitals, the San Diego Naval Regional Medical Center, and the Miramar Naval Air Station. The scenario was a large earthquake in the San Francisco Bay Area, with an airlift of 225 victims to San Diego.

This ambitious exercise was a learning experience for all concerned. Triage, transportation, and communication systems were tested, and problems were identified. Although this was the first drill of the San Diego NDMS, a final conclusion was still made that the number of casualties (225) was excessive for the level of preparedness existing (NDMS After Action Report, San Diego, Sept. 9, 1988). This conclusion underscores the tremendous effort needed to coordinate multiple organizations in the handling of multiple casualties and the importance of such drills in expanding awareness of disaster medicine.

TRIAGE

Implying a division into three groups by its French root, triage today usually involves assigning a patient to one of four groups: dead or expectant (black tag), critical or requiring immediate intervention (red tag), urgent but without immediate life-threatening injury (yellow tag), and walking wounded (green or white tag). Fundamental to all triage is the concept of allocation of limited resources [6]. This requires some knowledge of existing supplies and the extent of the disaster and medical response on the part of the triage teams. For example, it does little good to classify a patient with labored and ineffective respiration as critical and to intubate that patient if there is neither a ventilator nor an individual with a bag and mask available. Generally, patients who are apneic should be considered dead and labeled as such [7]. It is also dangerous to underclassify patients who may well deteriorate. For example, a patient with a fresh femoral fracture may initially appear quite stable and present as an urgent patient but may then deteriorate or even die in time owing to bleeding without resuscitation. As a rule, triage takes precedence over nearly all forms of treatment, especially as the scope of the disaster widens.

TREATMENT

As discussed in Chapter 12, the relative merits of "scoop and run" versus on scene treatment are still being debated without a clear consensus on either one. It is doubtful whether meaningful field studies comparing these two modalities will ever be accomplished in the field of disaster medicine, given the unexpected nature of the events and the need for prior preparation. The military leans toward the scoop and run approach, due primarily to considerations of "enemy fire" [8]. Civilian disasters often present risk from delayed explosion, radiation contamination, or earthquake aftershock, which may support such reasoning. Whether initial treatment takes place on the scene or at some removed medical staging area, the usual trauma management sequences are followed, with consideration being given to limited resources in both equipment and personnel.

The limiting factor in the provision of definitive care for multiple severely injured casualties is often the number of operating rooms that can be run [9]. Problems identified with past disaster responses revolve around timeliness and appropriateness of medical aid [1]. Care that is supplied within the first 24 hours is most important, and aid arriving later often can do little

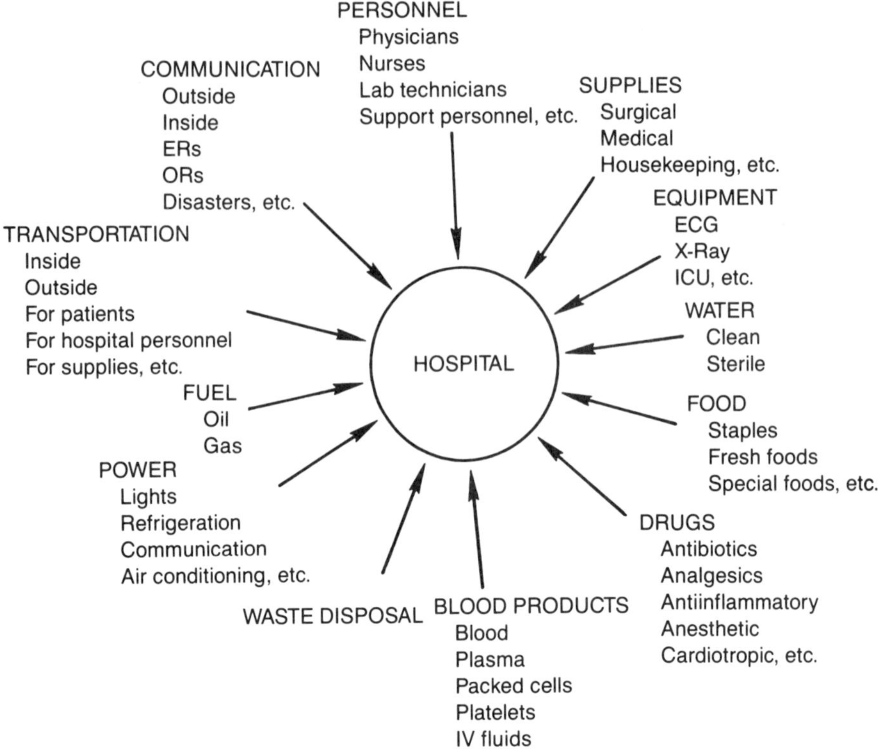

Fig. 15-1. Factors on which the proper functioning of a hospital depend. (From F. Solomon and R. Q. Marston [eds.]. *Medical Implications of a Nuclear War.* Washington, D.C.: National Academy Press, 1986. With permission.)

to save life or limit disability. Especially in the case of earthquakes, in which trapped victims must be freed and treated rapidly to avoid morbidity and death, the emergency phase for disaster medical care is limited to the 3 or 4 days after impact [10]. In past disasters there has often been an embarrassment of unnecessary materials and superfluous volunteers. Such inappropriate aid responses has prompted the call for the formation of completely self-sufficient and rapidly mobilized medical teams that can converge on a disaster from the outside and provide care without clogging and confusing existing medical systems that are overloaded [1] (Fig. 15-1).

Should field or MASH-type packaged disaster hospitals be available, prime considerations include sterilization equipment, adequate lighting, power, water, and safety from further involvement in the disaster [11]. Placement of adjacent OR tables can allow a single anesthesiologist to handle several patients simultaneously should personnel requirements dictate this. This would usually require the use of some type of ventilator, most feasibly a lightweight pressure type ventilator. Use of regional anesthetic techniques has obvious attraction in the disaster setting [12] because once an effective block is rendered with a nontoxic dose of local anesthetic, less attention may be required than with general anesthesia using unfamiliar equipment. As an airway and local anesthetic expert, and as a physician with some surgical training, an emergency physician might be expected to function as either surgeon or anesthesiologist, should triage and resuscitation be well underhand and help needed in the OR.

ANESTHESIA CONSIDERATIONS IN DISASTER MEDICINE

It is difficult to discuss disaster in general terms because the scope and range of potential disasters is so large. Boulton has produced an excellent summary of the topic and reiterates three goals of anesthesia in such conditions: (1) Preserve the life of the patient, (2) keep the patient free from pain, and (3) in so far as the first two goals are met, provide the best possible conditions for surgery [13]. If a disaster does not overwhelm existing hospital resources, the usual choices and considerations in normal hospital-based trauma anesthesiology hold true. Airway management, fluid resuscitation, and, if the patient's condition allows, provision of analgesia, amnesia, and hypnosis by the use of inhalational or intravenous drugs would proceed as usual.

Should an overwhelming disaster such as an earthquake or war exceed standard hospital resources, certain priorities in supplies and management take precedence (Table 15-1). Oxygen and simple oxygen delivery systems take precedence over complex anesthetic machines and volatile agents. Fluid therapy and intravenous lines must be allocated carefully. Intravenous drugs such as ketamine, which generally supports blood pressure except in the event of catechol and volume depletion and which provides excellent analgesia and amnesia for such procedures as burn wound care, tube thoracostomy, and so on, have proved themselves in such major disasters as the Iran earthquake of 1978 [14]. In an IV dose of 0.5 to 2 mg/kg, ketamine has a half-life of about 2 to 3 hours.

Table 15-1. Disaster anesthesiology supplies

Airway equipment
    Endotracheal tubes, stylets, laryngoscopes, batteries and bulbs, oral and nasal airways, bag-valve-masks, oxygen cylinders, regulators, tubing, stethoscopes.
Intravenous therapy
    Tourniquets, alcohol swabs, intravenous catheters, intravenous tubing, crystalloid solution, syringes, needles.
Drugs
    Ketamine, atropine, morphine, pancuronium, lidocaine, epinephrine
Monitoring equipment
    Manual blood pressure cuffs, precordial stethoscopes

Although ketamine has been said to spare respiratory effort, recent studies have shed some new light on this statement. Shulman et al. demonstrated that the maintenance of oxygenation observed in children anesthetized with ketamine but breathing spontaneously was caused by a delay in expiratory flow that seemed to maintain functional residual capacity and thus oxygenation [15]. However, this delay in expiratory flow may be gained at the expense of decreased carbon dioxide expiration. Bourke and colleagues have shown that ketamine does depress respiration and leads to carbon dioxide retention but in a much less potent manner than morphine [16]. Thus, when one also considers the increased salivary gland secretion and increased intracranial blood flow induced by ketamine, it is clear that a physician must be very careful indeed in using the drug in anesthetic doses without endotracheal intubation and positive pressure ventilation. Head-injured patients should not receive ketamine (see Chapter 5).

The increased sympathetic tone seen with ketamine is produced by secondary release of endogenous catecholamines, as in the function of ephedrine and metaraminol. It is important to emphasize that hypotension has been reported in hypovolemic, volume-depleted patients and that the drug should be carefully titrated.

Use of morphine is important in disaster management, but care must be taken to avoid unskilled use of the drug. Subcutaneous injection in cold patients can lead to overdose with later rewarming, and, as with ketamine but more so, use in shock patients can induce hypotension or cardiovascular collapse. Local anesthetics can also play a role, as previously mentioned, if adequate injection equipment exists [12]. Muscle relaxants are near-essential to abdominal surgery, and they imply, of course, the use of endotracheal intubation and positive pressure ventilation by some means.

Thus, it is clear that anesthesia in disaster medicine is fundamentally different from the normal practice of anesthesia, especially for disasters in developing countries. Nevertheless, treatment modalities used in routine practice should be preserved even if in simplified form if at all possible. Airway management with manually powered devices and simple oxygen delivery systems, fluid resuscitation, and inexpensive, well-known drugs such as ketamine, lidocaine (for regional anesthesia), pancuronium, and morphine, are the mainstays of resuscitology and pain control for large numbers of casualties. Some have recommended the stockpiling of atropine as well because many deadly toxic warfare compounds utilize acetylcholine esterase inhibitors [11]. The use of all of these items should be familiar to emergency physicians as well as anesthesiologists.

Some general considerations regarding trauma patients require emphasis. The possibility of a full stomach and cervical spine injury still hold. Hypothermia is a major enemy as always, and blankets must be stockpiled. If feasible, blood transfusion requires some sort of warming system, even if tubing is simply coiled in a jug of warm water. As discussed in Chapter 12,

in a mass casualty situation it is probably preferable to use type O blood
rather than take chances on clerical errors with type-specific blood.

The use of explosive anesthetic agents such as ether or cyclopropane has
been banned in the United States but still occurs in some countries, as do
explosions and patient deaths from their ignition [17]. A recent poll of anesthetists in Great Britain revealed that 4 of 144 (3 percent) physicians used
ether in their practice regularly, and cyclopropane was used regularly by 62
of 144 (43 percent) [18]. The author has worked in a hospital in Cuzco,
Peru where some extra ventilation was provided to the OR by a large hole
in the roof secondary to an ether explosion. Obviously, if the surgical team
uses electrocautery, the use of such agents is foolhardy and extremely dangerous. In the uncertain environment of a disaster, great opportunity for
ignition exists. Hence, even though these agents are inexpensive and can
be used with a minimum of equipment, their use is to be deplored, especially by those inexperienced in explosion prevention and because the
above-mentioned intravenous drugs can be used much more safely.

PREPARATION—PRACTICE, PSYCHOLOGY, AND PHILOSOPHY

PRACTICAL CONSIDERATIONS

In the above section, a list of needed supplies for disaster anesthesiology
and emergency medicine was outlined (Table 15-1). This list was not complete by any means because it included only the "bare bones" requirements
for the practice of anesthesiology in an emergency catastrophic setting. Left
out were important items for surgical care, such as dressings (especially
burn dressings), surgical instruments, sterilization equipment (if only boil-
ing fresh water), stretchers, chest tubes, suture, tape and other sundry items
that are taken for granted in the normal course of hospital affairs. The essential nature of auxiliary power supplies for lighting and sterilization
equipment, as well as storage of ample fresh water supplies should be re-
emphasized. San Diego County, for example, has provided for the storage of
many of these items through three modalities. First, a collection of 13 package disaster hospitals, complete with electrical generators, medical supplies,
woolen blankets, and so on are dispersed throughout the county. Second,
approximately 50 U.S. Navy Phase I medical bandage kits have been dispersed, each with about 21 square feet of storage of wound, burn, and fracture supplies. Finally, some 45 first-aid stations have been deployed, each
with 720 cubic feet of storage of litters, blankets, medical supplies, and
dressings.

Central to such preparation is frequent periodic inspection and replacement of expired sterile solutions, drugs, oxygen cylinders, and so on. To say

this is costly, both financially and in terms of labor, is to understate the issue. County officials certainly do their best to keep these supplies current, yet one must suspect that even in the best of hands, these supplies look better on paper than they do in actuality. San Diego, like most U.S. cities, is hardly London during the World War II blitz. It takes constant use and a sense of urgency to optimize disaster storage and supplies, not to mention personnel organization and training.

PHILOSOPHIC AND PSYCHOLOGICAL CONSIDERATIONS

Humans learn from experience, in accordance with behavioral laws, as do most successful intelligent species. We seek positive reinforcement and avoid negative reinforcement. To allow these laws of behavior to work requires experience or feedback from disaster events to accrue with some frequency. Thus, most preparations are made for events that, for any given county or nation, have been experienced before. Counties and cities prepare for bus, train, and plane crashes. In California, earthquakes are actively prepared for and are not considered merely a hypothetical possibility because everyone living there has experienced tremors and knows that a major quake could occur. On a national level, countries that were victims of unprovoked surprise attacks in World War II, such as both the United States and the U.S.S.R., are extremely sensitive to defense issues and have amassed huge arsenals in hopes of deterring further such events.

The underlying philosophy for disaster preparation varies. Although most medical triage references seem to be based on the principle of "the greatest good for the greatest number," such programs as the protection of the President and Cabinet in times of national emergency (i.e., nuclear attack) and the provision of defensive caverns for the armed forces command, control, communications and intelligence (C_3I) centers in places such as the NORAD Cheyenne Mountain Fortress indicate that national planners have made some judgments about the importance of protection of certain individuals. In no other area of disaster medicine do these issues of philosophy and psychology seem to spark as much emotion and controversy as they do in regard to the preparation for nuclear war. Because physicians have become increasingly involved in these debates, this subject is discussed in detail below.

DISASTER PREPARATION AND NUCLEAR WAR

BACKGROUND

Scientists, of course, were involved in the invention of the fission and fusion bombs, the former being developed amid the relatively straightforward moral climate of World War II. It was clear that an all-out effort from all countries was required to stop the aggressive Axis, and it was a question of either developing the bomb first or succumbing to its use by Hitler. By the time the bomb was ready for use, however, Hitler had been defeated and Japan was close to defeat. Although Leo Szilard, the Hungarian physicist who was the initiating force behind the whole World War II nuclear program, joined with other scientists to entreat Truman to use the bomb only after negotiation and a demonstration, the forces behind using it on people (civilians for the most part) were too strong for the new president. Although most people in the United States believe that the prevention of multiple American casualties from an invasion of Japan was the moral rationale for the use of the bomb, other pressing reasons for its use, such as the intimidation of the U.S.S.R., may have been even more cogent at the time. These events have recently been documented objectively and thoroughly by Kurzman [19]. Physicians, as a sort of subsection of scientists, first became involved in nuclear war at Hiroshima and Nagasaki in 1945, the only places to date where wartime fission bombs have been exploded. John Hersey's *Hiroshima* contains graphic descriptions of the valiant but mostly futile attempts of surviving Japanese physicians to treat victims of the instant devastation and later, the radiation sickness, that these weapons produced [20].

Following World War II, the Cold War saw the development of thermonuclear or fusion weaponry, which made the fission bombs of 1945 seem puny by comparison. Atmospheric testing produced such pollution that a consortium of physicians in the United States called Physicians for Social Responsibility (PSR) formed in the early 1960s and lobbied successfully on many fronts, contributing, ultimately, to the Nuclear Test Ban treaty, which limits testing to underground regions.

Throughout the 1960s, 1970s, and 1980s many political perturbations have occurred, East-West relations have frozen and thawed, then frozen again, many new nations have joined the dubiously illustrious club of countries-with-the-bomb, and many "small" wars have been and are being fought. Yet, strangely enough, given our race's warlike tendencies, there has yet to be a war between two countries with the nuclear bomb. This may be due simply to physics. The destructive energy unleashed by fission and especially fusion reactions is several orders of magnitude greater than the energy released by conventional means. After all, the sun warms the solar system by means of fusion. There is no history and no experience with nuclear war—hence, it is a large unknown. The awesome power of any individual weapon, however, is well known, as is its radioactive residue. Thus, fear of retaliation and the knowledge that a nation would destroy whatever real estate it was attacking (and most wars are fought for territorial reasons) have prevented such a war. Unfortunately, it has not prevented the tremendous stockpiling of the weapons nor kept the technology at bay. Currently, there are some 50,000 nuclear weapons in the world's arsenals, about 20,000 of which are the huge strategic variety. Development of multiple independent reentry vehicles (MIRV) and other advanced technologic devices now allow the possibility of attacking an enemy's missile silos themselves. Because this would be advantageous only if the missiles were still there, these are considered "first use" weapons and have led to "launch on warning" decision times based on minutes and seconds, with increasing reliance placed on computerized attack systems. The dubious morality of first-strike weaponry and fears of computer malfunction and accidental nuclear war have increasingly concerned many [21, 22].

In answer to this situation, a number of physician groups have formed and reformed. PSR has become very active, and its membership has skyrocketed in the past 10 years. It has also spread to form an international organization, the International Physicians for the Prevention of Nuclear War (IPPNW), which serves to bring together physicians from at least 50 countries, including the United States and the U.S.S.R. These groups have not existed without a great deal of controversy and opposition. Starting from careful research into the medical effects resulting from a single 1-megaton blast [23] and extending that to analyses of the synergistic effects of a large-scale nuclear war, it has been their conclusion that effective medical treatment of nuclear war victims is impossible. Hence, it is a "party platform" of these organizations to downplay the ability of physicians to treat or to prepare to treat victims of such an event and instead to concentrate efforts on prevention. Although the Nobel Peace Prize was awarded to IPPNW in 1985, much criticism of the organization followed this award.

The insistence on focusing on prevention efforts has angered some, who feel that this decision plays into the hands of a Soviet regime with superior conventional forces in Europe. The idea that prevention should overshadow disaster preparation [24, 25] for any type of nuclear explosion has angered others [26], who feel that this is morally irresponsible and that physicians must be realists and pragmatists and should be ready for anything. In California an organization, Doctors for Disaster Preparedness, was formed in response to these concerns. These critics also point out the possibility of an isolated explosion by, say, a terrorist group. To examine this problem objectively, current knowledge about the medical situations following a nonmilitary nuclear power accident, an isolated 1-megaton nuclear blast, and a nuclear war will be briefly reviewed below, followed by a discussion of the involved psychological, ethical, and practical issues of preparation for such disasters.

MEDICAL RESPONSE TO NONMILITARY NUCLEAR DISASTER

On April 26, 1986 the worst accident in the history of nuclear power occurred at the Chernobyl nuclear power station in the U.S.S.R. Because of improved communication between Soviet and American medical communities, a number of lessons of use to all disaster physicians were learned from this disaster. As the radioactivity was contained and the populace evacuated, the first priority of treatment was the provision of care to persons with non-nuclear–related thermal injuries and blast injuries, which led to two immediate deaths. Radiation injuries, which eventually led to 29 deaths, were not immediately life threatening [27].

The second priority was assessment of the radiation dose received by the victims, which was based on biologic dosimetry, i.e., onset of nausea and vomiting and serial measurement of granulocyte and lymphocyte counts [28]. Thus, if a patient became nauseated within one half-hour of exposure, 600 to 1600 rads was the predicted dose; within 1 hour, 400 to 600 rads; 2 hours, 200 to 400 rads. Although a 50 percent mortality is expected with a 500-rad acute dose, at Chernobyl, with the benefit of such supportive measures as isolation, gastrointestinal tract decontamination, antimicrobial therapy and transfusion, at least 21 of the 50 patients (42 percent) estimated to have received considerably more than 500 rads survived. Bone marrow transplants, which required operation with general anesthesia, played a minor role in this disaster [27, 28].

Reduction of exposure to patients at risk was a final major priority. This included both internal and external decontamination attempts and use of potassium iodide as treatment for exposure to iodine-131 [27]. The danger of on-site triage and treatment was emphasized by the death of a young physician from acute radiation absorbed solely from victims with high burdens of internal contamination and contaminated skin. Dispersion of victims from the scene to hospitals as far away as Moscow for decontamination was felt to provide optimal management in this case. In summary, an incredible amount of personpower was mobilized to treat a relatively small number of casualties at Chernobyl, but the results were judged exemplary, for the most part. The ultimate health effects of the disaster, however, were not limited to the local area but were global in consequence [27].

MEDICAL EFFECTS OF A 1-MEGATON URBAN BLAST

The focus will now shift from peacetime accidents to war. In the transition from conventional explosives to first, fission, and finally fusion explosives, the increments of energy released have increased by many orders of magnitude. Many thousands of these weapons exist, and the destructive energy released by multiple explosions would have no historical equivalent. To make the effects of nuclear war more comprehensible, military planners and civil defense specialists have usually examined the effects of a single weapon on a single target. The standard unit of measurement is tons of trinitro-toluene (TNT), and thus, 1 megaton equals the force released by 1 million tons of TNT. In predicting the anticipated medical casualties from a single "medium"-sized warhead of 1 megaton, one must first know if the explosion is an air burst, in which explosive effects predominate, or a ground burst, in which radiation effects predominate. An international symposium was held by the Institute of Medicine of the National Academy of Sciences (NAS), in September, 1985, to present and discuss new studies on the potential health effects of nuclear war. The results of these studies have been published [29] and reviewed by Leaf and Relman [30, 31]. They should be familiar to any disaster planning physician. One of the findings of this august body was that the estimates initially used by civil defense planners concentrated on blast effects from air bursts and failed to consider mortality from resultant firestorms and fire winds. Thus, it is known that blast overpressure of 5 psi is uniformly fatal, and, using "cookie-cutter" radius models based on the area of this overpressure, it had been assumed that everyone within a 7-km radius (150 square kilometers) of a 1-megaton air burst would be killed (Fig. 15-2).

Firestorms were created in Hiroshima, Dresden, Hamburg, and Tokyo during World War II. In each of these cities, the rising superheated air created gale force winds. It is not surprising that the temperature generated by a fusion thermonuclear explosion, tens of millions of degrees centigrade, hotter than the sun's surface (6000°C) [32], would create a tremendous firestorm over such a large mass of incendiary material as a large urban area. Although weather conditions would modify the size of such firestorms, it is now predicted that the actual area for 100 percent fatalities would be from an 8-km radius (heavy precipitation) to a 15-km radius (clear weather) [33]. Thus the lethal area during average conditions would be some 380 km squared. In a 2-km penumbra surrounding this area there would be 50 percent fatalities and 33 percent severe injuries.

H. J. Geiger, a public health physician at New York University, has considered these hypothesized conditions for a city such as Detroit, with 3.86 million people in its metropolitan area [32]. He states that conservative estimates of initial fatalities are 939,000 people killed (24 percent) after such an explosion, with another 1,145,000 (30 percent) seriously injured. Obviously, the latter group would be the target group for disaster relief. Unfortunately, it is estimated that only some 5000 of Detroit's available 18,000 hospital beds would be intact, and more than 80 percent of the physicians would be killed or wounded [32]. Similar percentages were reported from Hiroshima and Nagasaki (Figs. 15-3, 15-4). Communications would be totally disrupted, by both the disruptive effect of the electromagnetic pulse on solid-state equipment (see below) and by blast and fire effects. Water and power supplies would also be destroyed. The majority of medical supplies, such as the ones described earlier that are cached in San Diego, would be destroyed or unobtainable.

The usual functions of triage and evacuation would be complicated by the ever-present danger of radiation. As discussed above, vomiting within 1 hour indicates that about 500 rads have been absorbed [34], and one may presume that the patient has received a near-lethal dose. But with the many confounding variables that would affect the immune system after a nuclear explosion, from increased disease vectors, contaminated water, and even

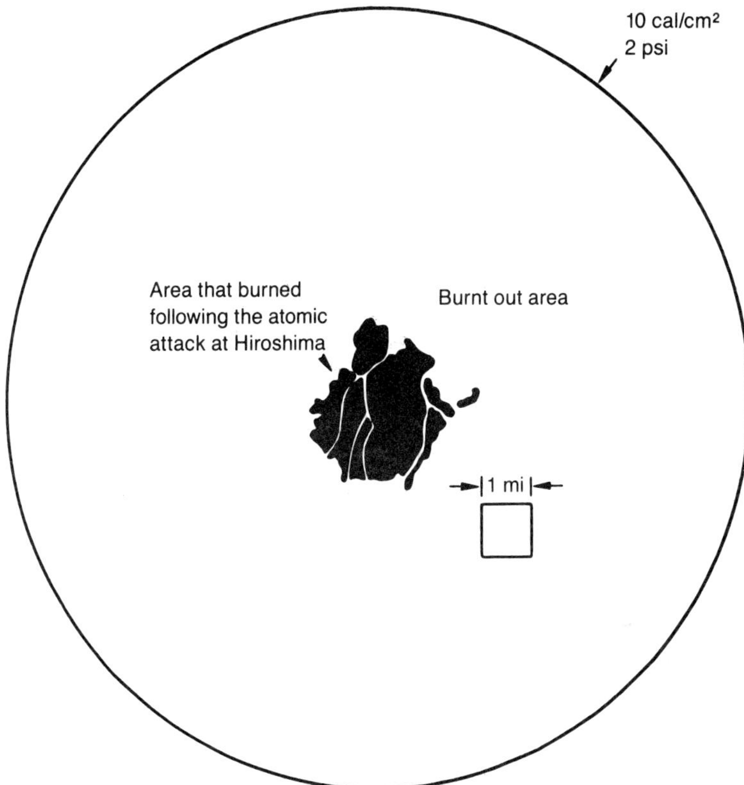

Fig. 15-2. The area over which a mass fire could be initiated from the combined blast and thermal effects of a 1000 kiloton detonation at a height of burst of 8000 feet (about 2440 m). The outer circle is highly speculative, as heat from the fireball (10 calories/cm² at the outer circumference) might only initiate scattered and isolated fires in highly combustible, exposed materials. However, the 2-psi blast effects at the outer circumference would result in considerable interior and exterior damage to wooden residential homes. The disruption from blast effects could then initiate many secondary fires that would also contribute to the growth of a mass fire of unprecedented scale. By comparison, the silhouette shown in the center of the diagram is the area that burned following the atomic bombing of Hiroshima. (From F. Solomon and R. Q. Marston [eds.]. *Medical Implications of a Nuclear War.* Washington, D.C.: National Academy Press, 1986. With permission.)

the inevitable psychological depression, it has been predicted that considerably less radiation in the event of a large blast would be fatal [29]. The proper treatment of radiation victims, which includes washing, protection of medical personnel, and careful disposal of contaminated wash water, clothing, and the like [34], would be difficult, to say the least, in such a circumstance.

Should such a blast be isolated, caused by, for example, a terrorist attack or a nuclear accident, we might assume that the medical resources of the

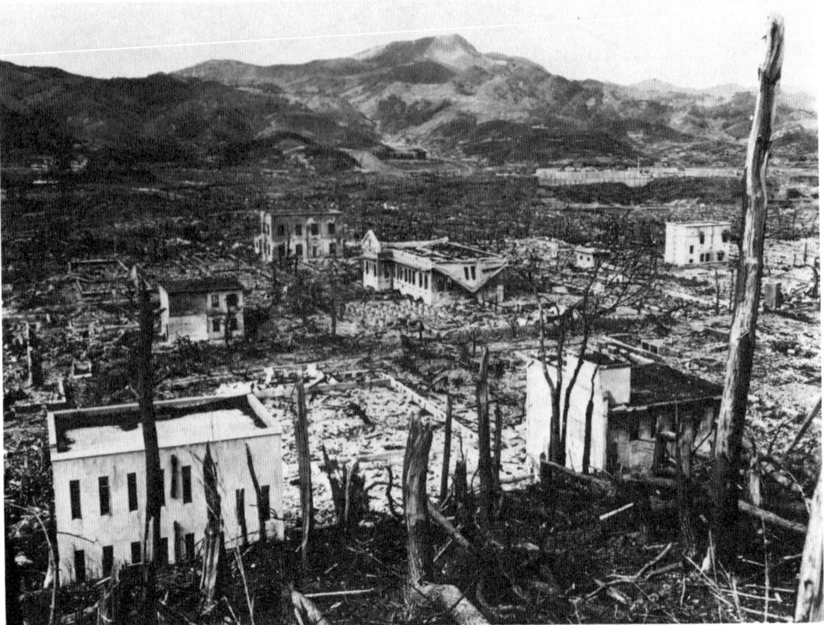

Fig. 15-3. Nagasaki Medical College was located on this hill, 1900 feet from the hypocenter. The wooden structure was demolished instantly and burned out. In the ruins of the five auditoriums the bodies of professors and students were found where they had been at the moment of the blast, on platforms and at desks. The total death toll, including the hospital, was 535 students, 42 of the teaching staff, 315 employees and nurses—892 in all. (From Hiroshima-Nagasaki Publishing Committee, U.S. Army returned materials. Shiba, Japan. The photograph was taken in November, 1945.)

nation could be brought to bear to assist in caring for this unprecedented number of casualties. Unfortunately, many of the injuries would include burn injuries, which require greater investment of hospital resources and hospital time than any other traumatic injury. Burn injuries in the United States result in the hospitalization of more than 100,000 patients annually and require 2 million bed-days [35]. San Diego, as an example, has no more than ten dedicated beds for burn patients in its burn unit, most of which are currently occupied. To mobilize burn care for the half-million simultaneously burned patients from such an explosion in Detroit would require an international health effort the likes of which has never before been known.

MEDICAL EFFECTS OF MULTIPLE NUCLEAR EXPLOSIONS

Much discussion in recent years among certain defense analysts has revolved around such concepts as "nuclear war fighting," in which nuclear

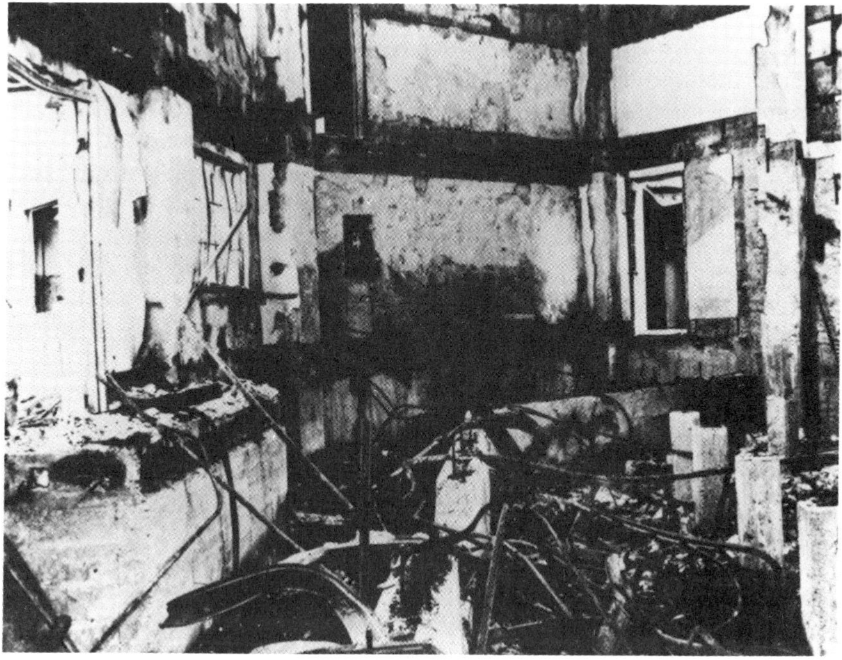

Fig. 15-4. The interior of the operating room at Nagasaki University Hospital, 2200 feet from ground zero. Fire has consumed the floor, the balcony, and all seats and has distorted the metal railings and pipe. (Office of the U.S. Strategic Bombing Survey.)

war is somehow contained to either tactical battlefields or used solely against an enemy's nuclear missile silos (counterforce doctrine) [3]. It is difficult to project just what would happen in a nuclear war, but certain facts make a rapid escalation to all-out use of vast amounts of current arsenals very likely. First, there is the problem of communications, command, control and intelligence (C_3I, in military jargon). A single large nuclear detonation in the atmosphere causes an electromagnetic pulse, with peak fields of 50,000 volts per meter [36], which would render most solid-state equipment for thousands of miles inoperable. Although attempts are being made to shield equipment from this pulse effect, the phenomenon is difficult to control and even more difficult to test. In addition, the nuclear submarine force, if submerged and undetectable, is extremely difficult to communicate with. Submarines trail a long radar antenna for the use of low-frequency radio communication [37], but such communication would be very vulnerable. Thus, in the chaos surrounding a nuclear war, the decision of whether or not to fire a submarine's missiles could well rest with each individual commander. Second, there is the launch-on-warning philosophy intrinsic to the MIRVed technology we now possess. Thus, if one country does not fire first and empty its silos, it is vulnerable to the other country's counterforce attack. Third, one can only guess at the psychological impact the destruction of an entire city would have on any country's leadership.

Thus, there is, unfortunately, good reason to think that under present circumstances, a limited nuclear war would escalate rapidly. What would be the synergistic effect of many nuclear explosions? Beyond the obvious combined destruction of multiple warheads and the inability to produce the above discussed international rescue effort required for a single nuclear explosion, there are new and disturbing considerations. Climactic disturbances, first suggested by Ehrlich and others [38] and Turco et al. [39], have now been accepted as probable in the scientific community [29]. The soot raised into the atmosphere by firestorms (which would most probably result even if nonurban areas were bombed [33]), would absorb sunlight and drastically lower ambient temperatures for months. A major effect of this would be the effective loss of a growing season and rapid depletion of world food reserves. When one considers the destruction of the complex food production, storage, and distribution network on which modern civilization depends, it becomes clear that a rapid return to labor-intensive husbandry would occur, along with widespread starvation. The resistance of insects to radiation would be another unpleasant factor depleting food supplies and would synergize in a negative fashion with the widespread disease and radiation-depleted immune systems of the survivors. Dependence of developing countries on the major grain-exporting regions would leave the developing nations intertwined in the winding spiral of starvation and disease. Thus it has been predicted by the World Health Organization that the resulting global starvation would cause more deaths in the long run than all the direct effects of nuclear war combined [40].

RESPONSE OF DISASTER PHYSICIANS

All projections of numbers of casualties and viability of medical assistance in the event of nuclear war are just that—projections. They are untestable in a mass setting. Speculations that the extinction of our species might occur from the above effects are just that: speculations. Unfortunately, such questions have been raised and will never be answerable. We just do not know. We do know that the energy released by the combination of two hydrogen atoms to form helium, or by the splitting of uranium atoms to form cesium, strontium, and other "hot" byproducts is incredible (Fig. 15-5). We do know that "megaton" explosions are fearsome events beyond our comprehension and that we have assembled, in the world's arsenals, many thousands of devices capable of producing such explosions. The "doomsday machine" of popular science fiction is, unfortunately, not fiction but cold reality. What should we do, as responsible disaster management physicians, in such an unpleasant situation?

First, we might do what the majority of persons in the world do to deal with such an uncomfortable reality: pretend it doesn't exist. "If it comes, it

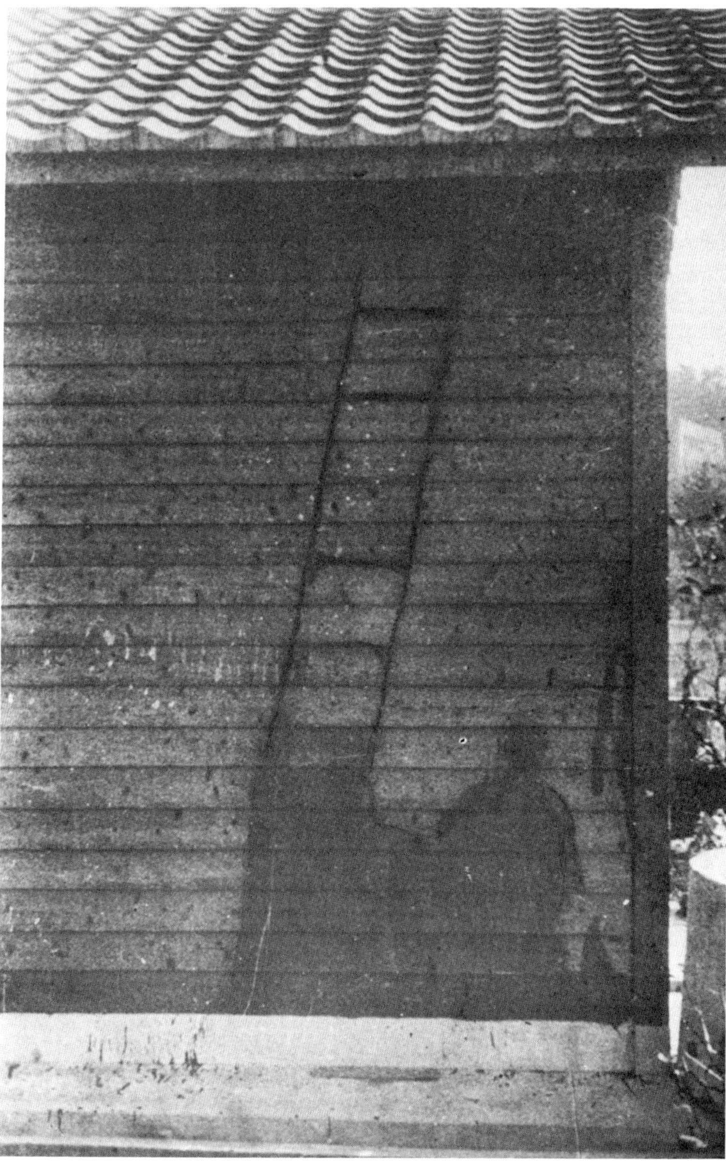

Fig. 15-5. Flash shadows at Nagasaki. A soldier descended from an observation post as the "all clear" sounded. He unfastened his sword, hooked it onto a clapboard, and unbuttoned his jacket when he saw the flash. His shadow is burned into the plank wall (3.5 km from the hypocenter.) (From Hiroshima-Nagasaki Publishing Committee, Shiba, Japan. Photo by Eiichi Matsumoto. Courtesy of the Japan Peace Museum.)

comes. We all die, and that's that. Now, what else shall we talk about?" This "head-in-the-sand" or "ostrich" attitude has been labeled "psychic numbing" by Lifton [41]. It is his thesis that, unfortunately, fear of the reality of the nuclear dilemma, instilled in all of us at one time or another, is repressed but only to reappear in other deleterious ways. "Live for the moment," the mad pursuit of pleasure, power, or money, the use of drugs, hopelessness, and so on can all be ascribed to a suppressed consciousness that all of civilization is threatened at all times.

Second, we might decide to side with the Doctors for Disaster Preparedness [26], who have stated that it is our moral duty as physicians to face reality, however unpleasant, and do our best to prepare for all those millions (billions?) of casualties. This author sympathizes with this group that an all-out international health effort could aid the victims of an isolated thermonuclear explosion and that such preparations should perhaps be made. However, in examining as objectively as possible the hypothetical world that would exist following a nuclear war, it becomes clear that no medical response would be meaningful and that the more realistic question would be whether mankind is reduced to the Bronze Age, the Stone Age, or extinction.

The third option is to recognize the problem and deal with it by efforts at prevention. Initially, to read such documents as the previously mentioned report by the NAS (*The Medical Implications of Nuclear War*) [29] releases depression, an emotion that "psychic numbing" has kept in check. Only by actions that attempt to prevent nuclear war, whether education, cultural exchange, political interaction, or other activities, can the knowledge of the grim reality and the depression it produces be surmounted.

In considering disaster planning for nuclear attack and explosion, or civil defense, one must recognize that there may be fundamental differences in the ethics of disaster preparation in different countries. Between a country such as Switzerland, which does not possess offensive nuclear weapons and does exert considerable energy in preparations, however futile, for defense against nuclear attack, and countries such as ours or the U.S.S.R., there exists a great moral chasm. The United States has a fundamentally offensively oriented military (i.e., tanks are favored over antitank devices, missiles over antimissiles). If we tried to initiate a massive civil defense effort such as Switzerland's or to manufacture such a dubiously effective and complicated system as the Strategic Defense Initiative (SDI), the presence of our offensive weaponry can only lead our rivals to view such efforts as support for an aggressive posture. Any defensive measures we take become offensive gestures in this perspective, as do defensive measures undertaken by the Soviet Union. Only when all parties have defused their offensive capabilities can defensive measures and effective civil defense decrease tension. Thus, in the absence of active reduction in offense, physicians become soldiers in assisting civil defense preparations.

The historic Intermediate Nuclear Forces (INF) treaty is a major first step in such reductions. For the first time, not only will the two superpowers dismantle weapons (admittedly, only 4 percent of the total), but bilateral on-site inspection procedures will be initiated. But as the initial wave of euphoria over the treaty wanes, the realization that new weapons and technologies will continue to be developed must be tempered by the fundamental philosophic change represented by this treaty—i.e., that nuclear weapons do not add to any nation's security. To break the vicious cycle of the arms race, new technologies must be evaluated, not on the basis of "kill-power" or "first strike accuracy" but on the basis of their providing both safety from accidental use and deterrence to war [42].

In summarizing this topic, let us consider three often asked questions regarding physicians and nuclear war.

Question 1. *Why should physicians concern themselves with war and peace?*

In 1945, with the onset of the nuclear age, all previous historical definitions of war became obsolete. Clausewitz, for example, classically defined war as "the advancing of objectives through other than political means." In the nuclear age, as evidenced by the lack of use of nuclear weapons in such conflicts as Vietnam and Afghanistan, the destructive capabilities of the weapons make their use irrational. The above-mentioned works of Turco et al. and Ehrlich et al. predict climatic aberrations following a large nuclear war of such magnitude that secondary effects, such as disease and famine, could endanger the continued existence of the human species [38, 39]. Thus, the issues are not so much war and peace but survival and health.

Physicians have increasingly concerned themselves with group health as opposed to individual health. Observe the interest of physicians in combating cigarette smoking, drug (including alcohol) abuse, the consumption of fatty foods, and the failure to use seat belts and motorcycle helmets. Often this attitude involves politics, and the pitting of the health profession head on against groups that have a vested economic interest, such as the tobacco industry, the liquor industry, or the fast food industry. In the examples above, we see the results of the problems everyday in our patients (lung disease, liver disease, atherosclerosis). But in the question of nuclear weapons and the arms race, we often see only a positive economic spin-off, especially in states with large arms industries such as California and Massachusetts. The negative aspects of the arms race are less obvious but can still be seen in our national debt and trade deficit, in the booming and essentially military-free West German and Japanese economies, and in the misery of the developing countries. Health problems from radioactive mine tailings and other waste products of nuclear weapons manufacture [43] show up only years later as cancers and thyroid disease that are difficult to link to their source. By the time we experience the immediate negative health effects of nuclear weapons, it will be too late to offer effective treatment. Hence the preoccupation with prevention.

Traumatologists, whether surgeons, anesthesiologists, or emergency physicians, are natural candidates to help this conflict owing to the nature of their work and especially their involvement in disaster planning. Other specialists who have become interested in nuclear weapons include psychiatrists, who report widespread (and rational) subconscious fears of nuclear war, radiologists, geneticists, public health physicians, oncologists, and so on.

Because civilians are targeted by present nuclear weapons, it is our duty as physicians, of whatever country, to act as defenders of the citizenry from the ultimate disaster. The fact that we are physicians opens doors to military and political leadership, and international travel and bridge-building become easier through the common language of medicine. Our scientific background enables us to understand better than our political leaders the physics of nuclear fission and fusion and the effect of explosions on the populace and, by nature of our work, we often possess the social skills needed to assist in the education of the populace, leadership, and military in the medical meaning of what kind of disaster each megaton contains.

Question 2. *After the downing of that Korean jetliner and the invasion of Afghanistan, not to mention the situation in Eastern Europe since World War II, how can we trust the Russians?*

The people of the Soviet Union, a diverse ethnic lot, seem to be the same as people anywhere. Mostly they want to be left alone to the pursuit of happiness. The Soviet military regime, on the other hand, is also like a military organization anywhere. They can be trusted, but trusted to act in their own, or their leader's own, interest. That interest may involve invading, shooting, and killing because that is what military establishments, our own included, are trained to do. Luckily, it is not in the interest of the Soviet military, or any military, to start a nuclear war, for reasons discussed above. In fact, largely through the efforts of physician-mediated international groups, national media attention in the U.S.S.R. has left the Soviet public and the military with few factual delusions about the chances for survival after a nuclear war.

Certainly any arms agreement must include verification and inspection agreements. In great part due to the on-site inspection requirements of the INF treaty, military forces on both sides are developing new, positive attitudes to replace the enemy stereotypes that have fueled the Cold War for so long [44, 45].

This leaves the greater question of how to trust and control the military in any country, again, our own included. As long as sociopaths such as Hitler, Pol Pot, or Stalin appear through history and commit mass militaristic murder, there will be need for a military, even in peaceloving nations. Yet how can we trust the military of India, Pakistan, Israel, Syria, Iran, China, Argentina, France, or any other of the growing number of countries who have, or plan to have, nuclear weapons? An educated, informed, involved, and well-traveled civilian and military population, qualities lacking in many countries with military junta governments or dictatorships, may be the key. If the best way to engender trust is by education, communication, and mutual economic propserity, then somehow the enormous arms export industry of the United States, U.S.S.R., and other countries must be converted to more beneficial commerce that is not so dangerous, ultimately, to the well being of all. A final determinant of whether human civilization really makes us something special in the course of evolution will depend on mankind's ability to restrain its military and their destructive weapons.

Question 3. *With the Russians' superior conventional strength, aren't you physicians just dupes for Soviet desires to negotiate Western nuclear strength and give them the advantage?*

The entrenched notion of the conventional superiority of the U.S.S.R. in Europe, which serves NATO defense ministries very well during budget season, has been questioned [46, 47, 48]. For example, the superiority of the Warsaw Pact's 18,000 tanks over NATO's 12,700 tanks (International Institute for Strategic Studies, [47]) is diminished by the fact that 45 percent of these 18,000 tanks entered service before 1965, whereas only 5 percent of the NATO tanks are of the same vintage. If "bean-counting," or the consideration of numbers only, was a predictor of war outcome, then Israel would be destroyed today, and the Spanish Armada would have ruled the seas [47].

But let us assume that this conventional superiority truly exists. Because there has been no global war since 1945, any change in the balance of forces is risky and places the responsibility for failure with the initiators. Yet, as we have mentioned, there have been major changes that place us at increasingly greater risk of accidental nuclear war, principally advances in technology such as MIRVed missiles and offshore submarines, which have forced the deployment of the computer-operated launch-on-warning systems mentioned earlier. A number of computer malfunctions have already nearly started a nuclear war, the most famous being the inadvertent placement of the simulated attack computer tape into the NORAD defense systems [22, 49, 50]. Technology can fail, as the events of Chernobyl and Challenger attest. To leave the fate of the earth up to our computers, however sophisticated, seems unreasonable.

Although physicians groups such as IPPNW have focused on nuclear weapons as an immediate emergency and a common meeting ground for all countries (and more than 50 are represented), most embrace the notion that conventional weapons must be controlled as well, especially as they become more deadly and include biologic weapons. Global problems, like any other problems, must be broken down into components, and efforts must be focused to achieve a result. Hence the centering on nuclear weapons. The negotiating skills and communicative apparatus formed to solve this problem can carry over to solve other pressing, related problems such as conventional weapons, human rights, and global ecologic problems.

CONCLUSION

Responsible physicians, and certainly every physician involved in trauma management, should become involved in disaster preparation and prevention. Active preparation for such events as large earthquakes will require national and international activity. Nuclear war is another story. Active participation in the pursuit of peace by physicians and public alike of all countries will be the only salvation from this entity. A landmark document presented by the American College of Emergency Physicians (ACEP) in 1983 concluded that:

> . . . no organized medical treatment exists or can currently be developed to meet the public health threat of a thermonuclear war. As with other nontreatable disease threats, prevention is society's only recourse [24].

But it was Dwight Eisenhower, thirty-fourth President and Supreme Commander, Integrated European Defense Forces, who said it best:

> Every gun that is made, every warship launched, every rocket fired signifies, in the final sense, a theft from those who hunger and are not fed, those who are cold and are not clothed. This world in arms is not spending money alone. It is spending the sweat of its laborers, the genius of its scientists, the hopes of its children. . . . This is not a way of life at all in any true sense. Under the cloud of threatening war, it is humanity hanging from a cross of iron [51].

And, in a more optimistic light:

> I like to believe that people in the long run are going to do more to promote peace than are governments. Indeed, I think that people want peace so much that one of these days governments had better get out of the way and let them have it [52].

REFERENCES

1. Mahoney, L. E., and Reutershan, T. P. Catastrophic disasters and the design of disaster medical care systems. *Ann. Emerg. Med.* 16:1085–1091, 1987.
2. Brandt, E. N., Mayer, W. N., Mason, J. O., et al. Designing a national disaster medical system. *Public Health Reports* 100:455–461, 1985.
3. Kornfeld, H. Nuclear weapons and civil defense. *West. J. Med.* 138:207–212, 1983.
4. Leaning, J., and Keyes, L. (eds.), *The Counterfeit Ark: Crisis Relocation for Nuclear War.* Cambridge, Mass.: Ballinger, 1984, 337 pp.
5. Moritsugu, K. P., and Reutershan, T. P. The National Disaster Medical System: A concept in large-scale emergency medical care. *Ann. Emerg. Med.* 15:1496–1498, 1986.
6. Chipman, M., Hackley, B. E., and Spencer, T. S. Triage of mass casualties: Concepts for coping with mixed battlefield injuries. *Military Medicine* Feb., 1980, pp. 99–100.
7. Baker, F. J. The Management of Mass Casualties. In H. W. Meislin (ed.), *Priorities in Multiple Trauma.* Germantown, MD: Aspen Systems, 1980.
8. Wiener, S. L., and Barrett, J. Mass Casualties and Triage. In *Trauma Management for Civilian and Military Physicians.* Philadelphia: Saunders, 1986. Pp. 536–549.
9. Savage, P. E. A. Area disaster planning in the UK: A preliminary report. *Disaster Medicine* 1:330–331, 1983.
10. De Bruycker, M., Greco, D., and Lechat, M. F. The 1980 earthquake in southern Italy—morbidity and mortality. *Int. J. Epidemiol.* 25:113–117, 1985.
11. Walt, A. J. (ed.), Disaster Planning for Mass Casualties. In *Early Care of the Trauma Patient.* Philadelphia: Saunders, 1982.
12. Whiffler, K., and Leiman, B. C. The application of regional anesthesia in a disaster situation. *South Afr. Med. J.* 63:409, 1983.
13. Boulton, T. B. Anaesthesia and resuscitation in difficult environments. *Int. Anesth. Clin.* 11:143–238, 1973.
14. Madjidi, A., and Frey, R. Anesthesia for victims of the earthquake in Iran, 1978. *Disaster Medicine* 1:431–432, 1983.
15. Shulman, D., Bar-Yishay, E., Beardsmore, C., et al. Determinants of end-expiratory volume in young children during ketamine or halothane anesthesia. *Anesthesiology* 66:636–640, 1987.
16. Bourke, D. L., Malit, L. A., and Smith, T. C. Respiratory interactions of ketamine and morphine. *Anesthesiology* 66:153–156, 1987.
17. Fineberg, H. V., Pearlman, L. A., and Gabel, R. A. The case for abandonment of explosive anesthetic agents. *N. Engl. J. Med.* 303:613–617, 1980.
18. Konarzewski, W. H., Richards, G., Thomson, S., et al. Explosive anaesthetic agents: A regional survey on the use of ether and cyclopropane. *Anaesthesia* 42:186–189, 1987.
19. Kurzman, D. *Day of the Bomb: Countdown to Hiroshima.* New York: McGraw-Hill, 1986.
20. Hersey, J. *Hiroshima.* New York: Knopf, 1946.
21. Abrams, H. L. The problem of accidental or inadvertent nuclear war. *Preventive Med.* 16:319–333, 1987.
22. Goldwater, B., and Hart, G. Committee on Armed Services Report, U.S. Senate. Recent false alerts from the nation's missile attack warning system. Washington, D.C.: U.S. Government Printing Office, Oct. 8, 1980.
23. Chivian, E., Chivian, S., Lifton, R. J., et al. (eds.), *Last Aid: The Medical Dimensions of Nuclear War.* New York: W.H. Freeman, 1982.

24. American College of Emergency Physicians. Nuclear war and emergency health care (position paper). *Ann. Emerg. Med.* 12:635, 1983.
25. Vanstrum, G. S. A unified voice to denounce the nuclear arms race (Letter). *Ann. Emerg. Med.* 13:641, 1984.
26. Maccabee, H. D., Looney, G., Williams, S. D., et al. (Letter). On nuclear war and emergency health care. *Ann. Emerg. Med.* 13:212–213, 1984.
27. Linnemann, R. E. Soviet medical response to the Chernobyl nuclear accident. *J.A.M.A.* 258:637–643, 1987.
28. Gale, R. P. Immediate medical consequences of nuclear accidents: Lessons from Chernobyl. *J.A.M.A.* 258:625–628, 1987.
29. Solomon, F., Marston, R. O. (eds.), *The Medical Implications of Nuclear War.* Institute of Medicine, National Academy of Sciences, Washington, D.C.: National Academy Press, 1986.
30. Relman, A. S. The physician's role in preventing nuclear war. *N. Engl. J. Med.* 315:889–890, 1986.
31. Leaf, A. New perspectives on the medical consequences of nuclear war. *N. Engl. J. Med.* 315:905–912, 1986.
32. Geiger, H. J. The Medical Effects on a City in the United States [of a Nuclear Explosion]. In E. Chivian, S. Chivian, R. J. Lifton, et al. (eds.), *Last Aid: The Medical Dimensions of Nuclear War.* New York: W.H. Freeman, 1982.
33. Postol, T. A. Possible Fatalities from Superfires Following Nuclear Attacks in or Near Urban Areas. In F. Solomon and R. Q. Marston (eds.), *The Medical Implications of Nuclear War.* Washington, D.C.: National Academy Press, 1986.
34. Leonard, R. B., and Ricks, R. C. Emergency department radiation accident protocol. *Ann. Emerg. Med.* 9:462–470, 1980.
35. Curreri, P. W., Luterman, A., Braun, D. W., et al. Burn injury: Analysis of survival and hospitalization time for 937 patients. *Ann. Surg.* 192:472–478, 1980.
36. Mark, J. C. Nuclear Weapons: Characteristics and Capabilities. In R. Adams, and S. Cullen (eds.), *The Final Epidemic.* Chicago: University of Chicago Press, 1981. Pp. 93–109.
37. Caldicott, H. *Missile Envy.* Toronto: Bantam Books, 1986.
38. Ehrlich, P. R., et al. Long-term biological consequences of nuclear war. *Science* 222:1293–1300, 1983.
39. Turco, R. P., et al. Nuclear winter: Global consequences of multiple nuclear explosions. *Science* 222:1283–1292, 1983.
40. World Health Organization. Effects of nuclear war on health and health services. Report of the International Committee of Experts in Medical Sciences and Public Health to implement resolution WHA34.38. Geneva: World Health Organization, 1984.
41. Lifton, R. J. In a Dark Time. In R. Adams, and S. Cullen (eds.), *The Final Epidemic.* Chicago: University of Chicago Press, 1981. Pp. 7–20.
42. Evangelista, M. How technology fuels the arms race. *Technol. Rev.* (Mass. Institute of Technol) 91(5):42–49, 1988.
43. Alvarez, R., and Makhijani, A. Radioactive waste: Hidden legacy of the arms race. *Technol. Rev.* (Mass. Institute of Technol) 91(6):42–51, 1988.
44. King, P. H. Soviets set up shop near Nevada nuclear test site. *Los Angeles Times* July 14, 1988. P. 1.
45. Parks, M. U.S., Soviets build trust as missiles are destroyed. *Los Angeles Times* October 25, 1988. P. 1.
46. Mako, W. P. *U.S. Ground Forces and the Defense of Central Europe.* Washington: Brookings Institute, 1983. 134 pp.
47. Sigal, L. V., and Mendelsohn, J. The stage shifts in arms control. *Technol. Rev.* (Mass. Institute of Technol) 91(6):52–61, 1988.

48. Mearsheimer, J. J. *Conventional Deterrence.* Ithaca, NY: Cornell University Press, 1983. 296 pp.
49. Sulzberger, A. O. Error alerts U.S. forces to a false missile attack. *New York Times* November 11, 1979. P. 30.
50. Halloran, R. Computer error falsely indicates a Soviet attack. *New York Times* June 6, 1980. P. 14.
51. Eisenhower, D. D., quoted in H. Caldicott. *Missile Envy.* New York: Bantam Books, 1986, 346 pp.
52. Eisenhower, D. D., from television talk with British Prime Minister Harold Macmillan, September 6, 1959, quoted in G. R. La Rocque (ed.), *Nuclear War Quotations.* Washington, D.C.: Center for Defense Information, 1986.

Index

A fiber, 204
Abdominal distention
    airway management in, 24–25
    ventilatory capability and, 80
ABO blood groups, 323–324
Abortion
    missed, 263
    spontaneous, 199–200
    threatened, 262
Abruptio placentae, 263
Acetylcholinesterase inhibitor, in
        neuromuscular relaxant reversal,
        164
Acid-base balance, in cardiac arrest, 112
Acidosis
    cardiac arrest and, 112
    in chronic renal failure, 284
Acquired immunodeficiency syndrome
        (AIDS), 297–299
Acromegaly, airway management in, 65–66
Acupuncture, 218
Adam's apple, 39
Addison's disease, steroid supplementation
        in, 20
Adolescent, 224
Adult respiratory distress syndrome, 94
    transfusion and, 322, 324
Aerobic metabolism, 18
Afterload, 105
Agitation, during mechanical ventilation,
        95
Agonist drug, receptor pharmacology for,
        150
Agonist-antagonist drug, receptor
        pharmacology for, 150
AIDS, 297–299
Airway management, 13–67
    abdominal distention and, 24–25
    accessory musculature and, 21
    in acromegalic patient in arrest, 65–66
    anatomic problems in, 65–67
    anatomy and, 20
    aspiration prevention in, 15
    assessment, 19–29
    in asthmatic, 64
    auscultation in, 25–26
    blood gas tensions and, 26–27
    in blunt multiple trauma, 60–61
    in cardiogenic shock, 13, 63
    case studies of, 59–67
        of anatomic problems, 20, 65–67
        of medical problems, 63–65
        of trauma airway problems, 60–63

cervical spine and, 15, 24
in cervical spine fracture, 62
in children, 230–234
color of skin and mucous membranes
        and, 20
in combative trauma patient, 13–14
in congenital lobar emphysema, 250
in coronary catheterization, 13
coronary supply and demand and, 101–
        103
"crash" induction in, 276
crepitus and, 24
cricothyroidotomy in, 34–35
dental damage in, 15
depolarizing agents in, 17
endotracheal intubation in. *See*
        Endotracheal intubation
endotracheal tube in, 23
end-tidal carbon dioxide monitors for,
        28–29
in esophageal atresia with
        tracheoesophageal fistula, 251
esophageal obturator airway for, 34
goals in, 14–19
in Goldenhar's syndrome, 233
in hanging victim, 63
in head injury, 23, 60, 366–369
history taking for, 19–20
initial, 30–38
inspection for, 20–24
intracranial pressure and, 16
jugular venous pressure and, 23
in laryngeal tumor, 64
location and personnel for, 58–59
in maxillofacial trauma, 62–63
mechanics of breathing and, 19
medical problems in, 63–65
muscle relaxants in, 16–17
nasal trumpets in, 33
noninvasive monitoring in, 27–29
oral, 33
in overdose patient, 65
oxygen delivery systems for, 35–38
    for patients with doubtful or absent
        respiratory effort, 36–38
    for patients with good respiratory
        effort, 35
        with dyspnea, hypotension, and
        elevated CVP, 38
oxygen saturation and, 27–28
oxygenation in, 18
palpitation in, 24–25
paradoxical chest motion and, 21–23